Glucocorticoids: Advanced Concepts

Glucocorticoids: Advanced Concepts

Edited by **Reginald Thornburg**

hayle
medical

New York

Published by Hayle Medical,
30 West, 37th Street, Suite 612,
New York, NY 10018, USA
www.haylemedical.com

Glucocorticoids: Advanced Concepts
Edited by Reginald Thornburg

International Standard Book Number: 978-1-63241-234-8 (Hardback)

Printed in the United States of America.

Contents

Preface   VII

Section 1   Prenatal Glucocorticoids and Placental Development   1

Chapter 1   **Prenatal Glucocorticoids:**
Short-Term Benefits and Long-Term Risks   3
Milica Manojlović-Stojanoski, Nataša Nestorović
and Verica Milošević

Chapter 2   **The Effects of Glucocorticoids on**
Fetal and Placental Development   57
Emin Turkay Korgun, Aslı Ozmen,
Gozde Unek and Inanc Mendilcioglu

Chapter 3   **Sex-Specific Effects of Prenatal**
Glucocorticoids on Placental Development   89
Hayley Dickinson, Bree A. O'Connell,
David W. Walker and Karen M. Moritz

Chapter 4   **Glucocorticoids: Biochemical Group**
That Play Key Role in Fetal Programming
of Adult Disease   105
Aml Mohammed Erhuma

Chapter 5   **The Role of Glucocorticoids in Pregnancy:**
Four Decades Experience with Use of Betamethasone
in the Prevention of Pregnancy Loss   135
Fortunato Vesce, Emilio Giugliano, Elisa Cagnazzo,
Stefania Bignardi, Elena Mossuto,
Tarcisio Servello and Roberto Marci

Section 2   Glucocorticoids in Modern Clinical Therapy   177

Chapter 6   **The Use of Glucocorticoids in the Treatment
of Acute Asthma Exacerbations**   179
Abdullah A. Alangari

Chapter 7   **Glucocorticoid Therapy in Systemic Lupus Erythematosus –
Clinical Analysis of 1,125 Patients with SLE**   201
Hiroshi Hashimoto

Chapter 8   **Glucocorticoid Resistance in
the Upper Respiratory Airways**   221
Fabiana C.P. Valera, Edwin Tamashiro and Wilma T. Anselmo-Lima

Chapter 9   **Assessment of Glucocorticoids -
Induced Preclinical Atherosclerosis**   237
Amr Amin and Zeinab Nawito

Chapter 10   **The Role of Corticosteroids in Today's
Oral and Maxillofacial Surgery**   249
Mohammad Zandi

Chapter 11   **Steroids in Asthma: Friend or Foe**   267
Mahboub Bassam and Vats Mayank

Section 3   New Formula of Glucocorticoids in Clinical Treatment   291

Chapter 12   **Soft Glucocorticoids: Eye-Targeted Chemical
Delivery Systems (CDSs) and Retrometabolic Drug Design:
A Review**   293
Pritish Chowdhury and Juri Moni Borah

Chapter 13   **Corticosteroids for Skin Delivery:
Challenges and New Formulation Opportunities**   327
Taner Senyigit and Ozgen Ozer

Permissions

List of Contributors

Preface

This book has been a concerted effort by a group of academicians, researchers and scientists, who have contributed their research works for the realization of the book. This book has materialized in the wake of emerging advancements and innovations in this field. Therefore, the need of the hour was to compile all the required researches and disseminate the knowledge to a broad spectrum of people comprising of students, researchers and specialists of the field.

As one category of the most essential steroid hormones, glucocorticoids have been acknowledged for long, and their therapeutic benefits have been broadly used in clinical treatment, particularly in anti-inflammation cases. Glucocorticoids controls several processes in the body also with the mobilization of energy stores, immune system, gene expression, and upholding of the homeostasis as well as the stress response, this is not unexpected that the theory of "glucocorticoids" is talked about in almost all medical books that aims on definite organs or systems such as the cardiovascular system, the immune system, and the neuroendocrine system. This book aims to reveal the newest researches linked to glucocorticoids, also examines prenatal glucocorticoids affecting the placental development and its consequences on adulthood and the clinical use of glucocorticoids in the treatment of various diseases.

At the end of the preface, I would like to thank the authors for their brilliant chapters and the publisher for guiding us all-through the making of the book till its final stage. Also, I would like to thank my family for providing the support and encouragement throughout my academic career and research projects.

Editor

Prenatal Glucocorticoids
and Placental Development

Prenatal Glucocorticoids:
Short-Term Benefits and Long-Term Risks

Milica Manojlović-Stojanoski, Nataša Nestorović and Verica Milošević

Additional information is available at the end of the chapter

1. Introduction

Glucocorticoids are steroid hormones synthesized in the adrenal gland cortex, and most of their physiological effects are mediated by the glucocorticoid receptor (GR), that acts as a ligand-dependent transcription factor. Coordinate changes in metabolism under glucocorticoid influence provide energy that is instantly and selectively available to vital organs, an enables them to deal with immediate environmental demands, at the expense of anabolic pathways, such as bone formation, reproduction, immunological responses and other, that are being blunted or delayed, under glucocorticoid influence [1-3].

During fetal development the synthesis of adrenal glucocorticoids precedes the establishment of a definitive structure of the gland. In rats, secretion of the main glucocorticoid – corticosterone starts as early as on day 13 of development [4] (term=22 days, short gestation period), while in humans secretion of the main glucocorticoid – cortisol starts in the 8th week of pregnancy (term=40 weeks, long gestation period) [5]. Glucocorticoid receptor mRNA is present in the tissue derivatives of all three germ layers from fetal day 13 onwards, and increases gradually during rat fetal development [6]. Human fetal tissues express GR at the gestational age of 6 weeks, meaning that the machinery for hormone action is prepared at the early stages of development [5]. These facts suggest that endogenous glucocorticoids produced by the fetal adrenal glands have a crucial role in fetal growth and the development of individual fetal tissues [7]. In response to the prepartum rise in glucocorticoids a wide variety of changes known as "preparation for birth" occurs, meaning that the maturational changes in many fetal tissues, essential for neonatal survival, are intensified during the last third of gestation. Namely, circulating glucocorticoids induce fetal lung maturation and surfactant production, trigger a variety of physiological effects on brain cell differentiation and synaptogenesis, stimulate the production of hepatic gluconeogenic enzymes, affect pancreatic β-cell development and insulin content, influence renal development and affect the maturation of the immune system [8-10]. Metabolic, cardiovascular and immune adaptations under glucocorticoid influence are fundamental to successfully overcoming birth-related stress and postnatal adaptation of the newborn to environmental challenges [11, 12].

Environmental conditions influence the prevailing nutritional and endocrine status in mothers and fetuses. Numerous animal and human studies have shown that adverse environmental conditions during pregnancy, such as maternal undernutrition [13, 14], stress [15, 16], illness, placental insufficiency [17, 18], as well as prenatal glucocorticoid exposure [19, 20] affect fetal development and postnatal outcome. Changes in the maternal hypothalamic-pituitary-adrenal (HPA) activity, transplacental diffusion of nutrients, hormones and growth factor supply, potently affect the fetal HPA axis influencing glucocorticoid output as well as other developing systems [21, 22]. Gestational age, at which an insult occurs, its nature and intensity, determines the specific tissue or organ which will be affected by the insult. Glucocorticoids are the key mediators between maternal environment and the fetus, and as such are involved in adaptations of the fetus to predicted postnatal environment. Even transient changes in glucocorticoid levels could have long-lasting consequences. The outcome might be growth retardation and change in the developmental trajectory, in the direction that best suited to the expected environment [23, 24]. This phenomenon is known as programming. The adaptations caused by suboptimal intrauterine conditions are appropriate if the predicted and actual postnatal environments match, and lead to survival to reproduce in a deprived environment [25, 26]. If there is a mismatch between the environment predicted and the actual environment experienced postnatally, adaptations are inappropriate and result in the development of disease like hypertension, ischemic heart disease, glucose intolerance, insulin resistance and type 2 diabetes [27-29].

In this chapter the latest findings, with clear statements from the literature, as well as own results regarding the endocrine mechanisms of intrauterine programming mediated by glucocorticoids will be analyzed. The causal relationship between a prenatally programmed endocrine axes and their postnatal functioning that affect growth, stress response, metabolism and reproduction will be discussed. In order to better understand mechanisms of fetal glucocorticoid programming of endocrine axes, special attention will be paid to key points of their development.

2. Development of endocrine axses

2.1. Development of hipothalamic-pituitary-adrenal axis

Functional differentiation of anterior pituitary cells is under the control of transcription factors and their cofactors. The transcription factors expressed in early pituitary development such as Rpx/Hesx1, Ptx1, Ptx2, Lhx3 regulate the formation of Rathke's pouch and maintain the formation of the baseline cellular structure. Signaling between the developing hypothalamus and the Rathe's pouch is also involved in the initial formation of pituitary primordia and further differentiation of the pituitary gland. Hypothalamic BMP 4 and FGF 8 are required for the activation of expression and maintenance of expression of the early transcriptional factors in the pouch. The lineage of adrenocorticotropin (ACTH) producing cells arises first during organogenesis, and thus represents a separate lineage. Pituitary homeobox 1 (Ptx1/Pitx1) was reported as factor for differentiation towards proopiomelanocortin (POMC) cells [30]. In the fetal pituitary the first cells that are immunopositive for ACTH can be found on fetal day 13 in the pars tuberalis anlage, whereas ACTH immunostaining is found 1 day later in the pars distalis [31]. The pars intermedia of the fetal rat pituitary is the last part to display ACTH staining [32]. Although pituitary precursor cells are influenced by spatial cues and extrinsic signals, for the initiation of ACTH synthesis in the fetal pituitary, a certain degree of autonomy exists. Moreover, ACTH immunostaining was found in 11-day-old fetal rat pituitary primordia cultured for 4 days in a serum-free medium, thus without endocrine or neuroendocrine signals [33]. Furthermore, ACTH-containing cells were detected in anencephalic human fetuses [34].

In the next stage of differentiation of ACTH-producing cells, the hypothalamic (corticotropin-releasing hormone) CRH control over ACTH cells has an indispensable role. In rats, the appearance of hypothalamic CRH-containing neurons occurs in lateral hypothalamic areas and in the paraventricular nucleus (PVN) on days 15.5 and 16.5 of gestation, respectively, whereas beaded fibers are visible in the external layer of the median eminence on day 17.5 of gestation [35]. Expression of CRH is correlated with a progressive rise in ACTH in the fetal circulation. A progressive 10-fold increase in ACTH concentration occurs in the pars distalis on days 17–20 of gestation [36], which suggests a crucial role of the developing hypothalamus. From the 20th day of gestation until term, the ACTH concentration remains unchanged. The existence of a mechanism that overcomes the negative feedback effect of elevated glucocorticoid levels on POMC gene expression during late pregnancy was demonstrated [37]. From that period onwards, ACTH is stored in the fetal pituitary gland as a readily releasable pool. Its location near the fenestrated capillary network enables momentary depletion of significant amounts of ACTH, and a subsequent considerable increase in ACTH concentration in the circulation, if physiologically demanded [38].

The cells of the adrenal cortex arise early in development due to the local proliferation of cells from the splanchnic mesoderm. The genes coding the orphan nuclear receptors SF-1 and DAX-1 control the early fetal adrenal cortex development. Knockout mice for these genes manifest adrenal and gonadal agenesis, gonadotropin deficiency and the absence of the hypothalamic ventromedial nucleus [39]. The potential for steroid synthesis occurs early, in 12-day-old rat fetuses [40]. In the later stages of fetal life, ACTH controls growth and development, as well as steroidogenic maturation of the adrenal glands [41]. Histological analysis of a near term rat fetal adrenal glands showed that the main part of the gland is steroidogenic tissue composed of a zona glomerulosa (ZG) and an inner zone (IZ), while the number of migrating chromoblasts is still modest [42]. Both cortical zones are functionally competent and able to produce aldosterone and corticosterone in 19-day-old fetuses [43]. The proliferative activity of adrenocortical cells is most intensive in the outer portion of the glands, in the subcapsular ZG region and outer portion of IZ from where the cells migrated centripetally [44]. A balance between proliferation and cell death enables proper functioning and integrity of the developing adrenal glands. Programmed cell death appears to occur in the inner cortical layers, where many resident macrophages are present [4], as well as in the resorption zones and giant cells [45, 46].

The development of the human adrenal glands exhibits a number of important differences in histological organization and steroidogenic activity in relation to species with a short-term gestation period. The primordium of the human fetal adrenal glands can be recognized by 3–4 weeks of gestation, but by the 8th week of embryonic development the adrenal cortex is clearly identifiable with its characteristic zonal partitioning [47]. The principal steroids of primate fetal adrenal gland, i.e. fetal zone situated in the inner part of the gland, are dehydroepiandrosterone (DHEA) and DHEA sulfate (DHEAS). DHEA serves as a substrate for placental estrone and estradiol production. Rapid growth of the fetal adrenal cortex, especially the fetal zone, with a significant increase in steroidogenic activity begins after week 10 of gestation and continues until term [47]. The definitive zone, positioned at the peripheral part of the gland, is steroidogenically inert, at last until the second trimester of pregnancy. After this period mineralocorticoid production were found, although aldosterone synthesis in the fetal adrenals is in poor correlation with plasma renin activity. The transitional zone that becomes distinguishable between fetal and definitive zone at the end of the second trimester of pregnancy represents a precursor of the adult zona fasciculata (ZF). The expression of enzymes 3β hydroxysteroid dehydrogenase (3βHSD) and cytochrome P450 17α-hydroxylase/lyase (CYP17) in the transitional zone enables the capacity for cortisol production [48]. In the initial phase, the fetal adrenals begin to produce cortisol between weeks 10 and 20 of gestation, possibly utilizing progesterone as a precursor. However, *de novo* synthesis of cortisol from cholesterol is established fairly late in gestation, leading to a remarkable increase in cortisol concentrations in the third trimester. Immediately after birth, the fetal zone of the adrenal cortex degenerates extensively, whereas the ZF matures in the subsequent period. [48]. Although the presence of ACTH is established in circulation from week 15 of gestation, cortisol and androgen production by the definitive and fetal zone are maximally stimulated by circulating ACTH from midgestation [49].

The functional state of the fetal HPA axis is important for several reasons. Firstly, glucocorticoids play a role in the maturation of numerous organs necessary for intrauterine development and extrauterine existence. Organ systems involved in reaching metabolic homeostasis, stress response and electrolyte balance in outer space are strongly controlled by glucocorticoids [50]. Secondly, the fetal HPA negative feedback mechanism begins to operate between days 15 and 17 of rat gestation [51]. Thus, near term fetuses are able to regulate their own homeostasis and glucocorticoid production in response to different maternal stressors [52] and adverse conditions [37]. Finally, the fetal HPA axis activity strongly affects the timing of parturition [48]. In a number of species at the end of gestation there is an increase in HPA activity, with increased plasma glucocorticoid levels that reflects on the placental trophoblast cells, causing enhanced output of prostaglandins [37]. The effects of prostaglandins on the myometrium associated with increased oxytocin activity represent an important step in the initiation of birth [50].

2.1.1. Effects of glucocorticoids during fetal development

Strictly defined spatial and temporal effects of glucocorticoids are actually determined by the previous appearance of the GR. *In situ* hybridization histochemistry revealed GR gene expression in the tissue derivatives of all three germ layers. The facts that intense GR mRNA labeling happened just before the final differential step for each glucocorticoid target tissue, and that upon differentiation reduced amounts of GR mRNA were found further support the crucial morphogenic role of glucocorticoids during fetal development [6].

Sufficient glucocorticoid levels are essential for the normal maturation of many parts of CNS during the prenatal period. In general, glucocorticoids act on neuronal maturation, replication, differentiation, and programmed cell death [8, 12]. In parallel with reducing the rate of neuronal replication, glucocorticoids promote the differentiation of central noradrenergic, serotonergic and dopaminergic neurons, enhance axonal growth, dendritic arborisation and synaptogenesis in a regionally selective manner, and control programmed cell death [53, 54].

Glucocorticoids promote the differentiation of sympathoadrenal precursors, initially expressed multiple neuronal markers, into endocrine chromaffin cells in the adrenal gland medulla. As sympathoadrenal precursors invade the primordium of the fetal adrenal gland and migrate centripetally, they are exposed to adrenal steroids. The initial adrenaline synthesis occurs in parallel with a sharp rise in the adrenal tissue and plasma glucocorticoid concentrations, and the appearance of GR in the sympathoadrenal precursor cells in 17-day-old rat fetuses [55]. Thus, glucocorticoids represent an important signal for the induction and maintenance of adrenaline synthesis in the adrenal medulla, but initial induction of the adrenaline-synthesizing enzyme, phenylethanolamine-N-methyltransferase is rather determined by a cell-intrinsic timed process in the chromaffin precursors [56].

Glucocorticoids accelerate lung maturation as they speed up the thinning of the double capillary loop to form the thin gas exchanging walls of the alveoli. By enhancing the production of surfactant by type II pneumocytes, glucocorticoids allow the newborn to draw its first breath and enable the start of the breathing process [57].

In the fetal liver, glucocorticoids promote the activity of the key gluconeogenic enzyme systems and hepatic glycogen deposition in preparation for the nutritional transition at birth. Inability of the adrenalectomised sheep fetuses to induce glucogenesis during extreme circumstances such as maternal undernutrition with reductions in hepatic glycogen content was associated with lower circulating concentrations of cortisol [10]. It might be concluded that birth-related stress and subsequent environmental challenges trigger glucocorticoid actions essentially involved in the activation of fetal glucogenesis and glucose availability necessary for maintaining homeostasis after birth.

By combining *in vitro* studies with *in vivo* investigations in mice lacking the GR in the whole organism or in specific pancreatic cell populations, it has been shown that glucocorticoids are important hormones in pancreatic development. Acting before insulin expression onset, glucocorticoids decreased the differentiation of the embryonic pancreas into β-cells favoring acinar cells differentiation. Deletion of the GR in pancreatic precursor cells led to increased β-cell mass. Thus, glucocorticoids unable β-cells mass expansion in later stages, by modifying the balance of specific transcription factors, mostly Pdx-1 [9]. At birth, as the placental source of glucose is lost, tight glycemic control must be established. A prepartum rise in glucocorticoid levels in fetal horse and sheep increases pancreatic β cells sensitivity to glucose and influences the fetal insulin level, enabling active regulation of the glucose level after birth, and thus the transition to enteral supply [10, 22].

The highest expression of the GR mRNA was identified during early kidney development in the developing glomeruli, epithelial cells of the proximal and distal renal tubule, and the central collecting duct. Reduction of GR levels in the fully differentiated glomeruli pointed out the importance of glucocorticoids during a defined period of establishment of the definitive renal structure and function [5].

Effective thermoregulation in response to cold exposure in the extrauterine environment post birth is crucial to prevent hypothermia in newborns. The expression of mitochondrial uncoupling protein (UCP), that catalyzes adaptive thermogenesis in mammalian brown adipose tissue increases dramatically during the final week of gestation in fetal adipose tissue [58]. The late-gestation augment in fetal plasma glucocorticoid levels as well as application of synthetic glucocorticoids enhance mitochondrial UCP expression, suggesting that glucocorticoids are crucially involved in increasing the thermogenic potential of fetal adipose tissue near term [59, 60].

2.2. Development of the somatotropic axis

Growth hormone (GH) is secreted from the anterior pituitary gland under the control of two hypothalamic hormones: the releasing hormone is growth hormone-releasing hormone (GHRH), and the release-inhibiting hormone is somatostatin (SRIH). In addition to these two neurohormones, a number of factors such as free fatty acids, acetylcholine, amino acids, opiates, glucocorticoids and some neuropeptides also have direct or indirect effects on GH release. Most of the metabolic actions of GH are mediated by insulin-like growth factor I (IGF-I), which is produced in many different tissues, with most of the circulating IGF-I being derived from the liver. IGF-I has anabolic as well as metabolic effects in many cell types, acting through autocrine, paracrine and classical endocrine mechanisms. IGF signaling has been recognized as one of the major molecular regulators of cell growth and proliferation [61]. Moreover, it is generally accepted that GH, by controlling important aspects of IGF activity in many tissues and cell types of mammals, is able to coordinate somatic growth in a defined spatio-temporal manner at the whole body level [62]. IGF signaling, however, not only regulates growth but also affects differentiation and may, through epigenetic processes, steer adult cell function as a result of particular conditions during postnatal development [63].

In rat, GHRH neurons are detected at the 16th day of fetal development [64], while SRIH mRNA in the periventricular nucleus of the hypothalamus is expressed on the 14th fetal day [65]. Initial pituitary GH expression is detected on day 15 of gestation using sensitive methods such as the reverse transcriptase-polymerase chain reaction (RT-PCR) [66]. In the following phase of GH cell development the expression of Pit-1 occurs. Pit-1 is a pituitary-specific transcriptional factor that mediates cell proliferation and differentiation into specific hormone-producing cell types – thyrotropes, somatotropes or lactotropes [67]. During this period, the quantity of GH transcripts remains at an extremely low level. A marked increase in cell number and GH production occurs between days 18 and 19 of fetal development [68]. The expression of the GHRH receptor also occurs on fetal day 19 in rats [69, 70].

It has been considered that pituitary GH promotes and controls fetal development and body weight by stimulating the family of hepatic growth factors. Recent investigations showed that extrapituitary GH as well as local production of growth factors had great paracrine/autocrine influence on fetal developmental processes and differentiation. The expression of GH and GH receptor in a wide variety of tissues is established before the pituitary gland and circulatory system become functional [71]. In rats and mice a contribution of the pituitary GH to growth, development and body weight has been demonstrated postnatally, during the second week of life [72]. The influence of pituitary GH on normal growth and body weight in near-term fetuses, immediately after the GH cells become functional, is still difficult to understand and not well defined.

In humans, GH cells are evident at 8 weeks of gestation, with abundant immunoreactive cytoplasmic GH expression. Plasma GH concentrations are highest at midgestation and thereafter fall until term. The pattern of ontogenesis of plasma GH reflects the progressive maturation of hypothalamic–pituitary and forebrain function. The responses of GH to SRIH and GHRH are mature at term in human infants [73].

IGF-1 and IGF-2 mRNA transcripts are present in virtually all fetal tissues [74]. Both IGFs are also detected in the fetal circulation from early gestation, but the plasma concentrations of IGF-II are 3–10 fold higher than those of IGF-I during late gestation [75]. They are present in serum and other extracellular fluids associated with highly specific binding proteins (IGF binding proteins (IGFBPs)). In the fetus, IGFs are predominantly complexed with IGFBP-1 and -2, and the liver is the predominant production site for these IGFBPs [76]. Tissue and plasma IGF-II are higher in the fetus than in newborn or adult animals in most species [77]. In rodents, IGF-II expression disappears from most tissues except the brain by weaning, with the consequence that IGF-II is virtually undetectable in adult plasma [78]. In contrast, plasma IGF-I levels increase rapidly after birth, primarily as a result of the onset of GH stimulated IGF-I production by the liver [79], since IGF regulation is GH-independent during the fetal period [74]. There is, therefore, a shift in IGF predominance from IGF-II before birth to IGF-I after birth, which has led to the concept that IGF-II is the IGF primarily responsible for fetal growth [80].

2.3. Development of hypothalamic-pituitary-thyroid axis

The development of thyroid-stimulating hormone (TSH) cells in the fetal rat pituitary pars distalis is determined by the expression of Pit-1 and TEF transcription factors [67]. Differentiation from precursor cells enables detection of TSH cells mRNA on day 15 of gestation [81], while immunocytochemically recognized TSH cells can be observed in 16.5- to 17.5-day-old fetuses. TSH cells were few in 17.5-day-old rat fetuses, but their number increased thereafter, particularly during the 2nd week after birth [68].

In the rat fetal hypothalamus, thyrotropin-releasing hormone (TRH), which promotes prompt synthesis and secretion of anterior pituitary TSH, is first detected on the 16th day of gestation [82]. The destruction of paraventricular nuclei (PVN), which contain TRH neuronal cell bodies, results in a significant decrease in anterior pituitary TSHβ- and α-subunit mRNA levels, as well as in serum TSH concentrations [83]. During the fetal period a major influence of TSH is to control the morphological and functional maturation of the fetal thyroid gland.

The thyroid gland is derived from the fusion of a medial outpouching from the floor of the primitive pharynx and bilateral evaginations of the fourth pharyngeal pouch, giving rise to the precursors of follicular (thyroxine-producing cells) and parafollicular (calcitonin-producing C cells) cells. Coordinate action of numerous transcription factors is involved in thyroid morphogenesis. Titf1, Hhex, Pax8 and Foxe1 are expressed in the rat just prior to the first appearance of the thyroid diverticulum on fetal day 9.5–10, controlling the proliferation, survival and migration of precursor cells [84]. Targeted disruption of Titf1 in mice results in total absence of the thyroid tissue, while the lack of Pax8 results in follicle agenesis, with the remaining tissue being composed almost exclusively of C-cells [85, 86].

In rats on fetal day 17 significant growth and rapid functional and structural development of the thyroid gland are established. The first appearance of follicles, iodine organification and thyroid hormonogenesis occur in parallel with a marked increase of TSH in fetal circulation and the expression of TSH receptors (TSHR) in thyroid tissue. Thus, upregulation of TSHR gene expression by TSH in fetuses is crucial for further maturation of the thyroid [81].

Deiodinase enzymes provide biologically active triiodothyronine (T3) to developing tissues by activating and/or deactivating systemic serum thyroid hormones (TH). Three types of iodothyronine deiodinases (D1, D2, D3) have been identified, which differ in tissue distribution, substrate specificity and sensitivity to inhibiting compounds [87]. Expression of D1 is low through gestation, while D2 and D3 are the major isoforms in the fetus [88]. D2 is the activating enzyme that catalyzes the removal of one iodide from the outer tyrosine ring of thyroxine (T4) and production of active T3. D3 is the inactivating enzyme that catalyzes the cleaving of one iodide from the inner tyrosine rings of T4 or T3, thus generating reverse T3 (rT3) or T2. Action of D2 and D3 preserves the safe level of T3 in the developing brain and the pituitary [87], while the activity of D3 in the utero-placental unit protects fetal tissues against high maternal T4 concentrations. Local tissue deiodinase activity is essential for compensation and adaption to potential malfunctions in the fetal hypothalamic-pituitary-thyroid (HPT) axis, i.e. in the case of congenital hypothyroidism and normal maternal T4, the transfer of the latter, together with increased brain D2 activity, protects the fetal brain from T3 deficiency [89].

In humans, thyroid gland reaches maturity by the 11th–12th week of gestation, when tiny follicle precursors with thyroglobulin in follicular space can be seen and iodine binding is detected. In this period both T4 and T3 are measurable in fetal serum [90]. At this stage of early development maternal T4 transplacental passage contributes to the fetal hormonal status, which is essential for normal early fetal neurogenesis. In the later stages of development, if fetal thyroid function is normal, placental TH passage is relatively limited due to the presence of D3 [91]. The increase in total T4 and free T4 levels between weeks 18 and 36 of gestation indicates maturation of the HPT axis function, with the establishment of feedback control about midgestation.

2.4. Development of the endocrine pancreas

The embryogenesis of pancreas is mediated by a series of transcription factors involved in morphogenesis. The expression of Pdx1 has been found early in organ formation, in cells that give rise to endocrine and exocrine cells of the mouse neonatal pancreas. In Pdx1 null mice pancreas agenesis occurs. The appearance of insulin and glucose transporter GLUT2 is also regulated by this transcription factor [92]. Transcription factors Hlxb9 and Isl1 are necessary for the initial induction of Pdx1. Hlxb9 is observed during the formation of pancreatic anlage and later during the differentiation of β cells. Neurogenin 3 has been identified as the key regulator of endocrine development, giving rise to all pancreatic endocrine lineages [93].

The pancreas arises from a multipotent endodermal cell population that will produce ductal, exocrine and endocrine cells [94]. The human fetal pancreas develops during the 5th week of gestation, while endocrine cells are identifiable by the 8th or 9th week of gestation. Scattered single endocrine cells are recognized to produce insulin (β-cell), glucagon (α-cells), somatostatin (δ-cells) and pancreatic polypeptide (PP cells). Clusters of epithelial endocrine cells form primitive islets of Langerhans a few weeks later, in parallel with the expression of neural adhesion molecule (N-CAM) [95]. The largest expansion of the β-cell mass has been shown to take place in the second half of prenatal development, from approximately 20 weeks in humans. This developmental period is critical to achieve a β-cell mass required to ensure proper insulin secretion throughout life. It is thought to result from β-cell neogenesis from rapidly dividing undifferentiated progenitor cells [96]. Thereafter, some degree of β-cell expansion persists at least until adolescence due to β-cell neogenesis, mitosis and perhaps to transdifferentiation of α-cells, acinar or ductal cells [97].

During the development of insulin-expressing cells there is a changing phenotype, from progenitor cells to immature β-cells, and finally, to mature adult β-cells. Using gene expression and immunohistochemistry, differences among late-embryonic, neonatal, and adult β-cells were found in a series of markers with transient expression patterns during the perinatal period. Of these, cytokeratin-19, matrix metalloproteinase-2 and surfactant protein-D can be considered as true markers of new and immature β-cells, as their expression is transient and not entirely synchronous, but absent in adults [98]. Sympathetic innervation and vascularization of islets play important roles in normal islet morphogenesis during prenatal life, and have trophic effects on β-cells survival, maturation and insulin secretion [99].

Human and rodent fetal islets are insensitive to glucose, as fetal β-cells do not discriminate between different glucose levels, despite adequate insulin reserves. Relative functional immaturity *in utero* was also recorded in response to circulating amino acids, particularly leucine, catecholamines and neural stimulation, with regard to the capacity to secrete both insulin and glucagon [100]. For blunted capacity for insulin and glucagon secretion several causes are proposed. Firstly, during fetal development in mammals glucose homeostasis is mainly achieved by the mother because of a constant supply of glucose by placental transfer through facilitated diffusion. Secondly, the mechanisms that mediate insulin secretion in adults are immature in fetuses, meaning that the production of cAMP is decreased, expression of glucose transporter GLUT2 is lower and expression of voltage-gated L-type Ca^{2+} channels is diminished in β-cells [100, 101]. Furthermore, generalized immaturity of the metabolic enzyme expression in pancreatic β-cells during the fetal and neonatal period in the rat has been recorded. Lower expression levels of the metabolic enzyme genes such as malate dehydrogenase, glycerol-3-phosphate dehydrogenase, glutamate oxaloacetate transaminase and pyruvate carboxylase were established and confirmed by quantitative PCR during fetal development and several weeks after birth than in adults [102]. During fetal life GH might be involved in the process of β-cell mass expansion and maturation that finally leads to an effective response to hyperglycaemia [103].

2.5. Development of the hypothalamic-pituitary-gonadal axis

Reproductive physiology in mammals is centrally regulated through the hypothalamic–pituitary–gonadal (HPG) axis and depends on gonadotropin-releasing hormone (GnRH). GnRH, a decapeptide, is released into the hypophyseal portal vasculature from axon terminals at the median eminence and binds to the GnRH receptor (GnRHR), which is specifically expressed in gonadotrope cells in the anterior pituitary gland. GnRH signaling controls the biosynthesis and release of luteinizing hormone (LH) and follicle-stimulating hormone (FSH), which in turn regulate the development and activity of the ovaries and testes. LH and FSH, together with TSH, are heterodimeric glycoproteins composed of a common α-subunit (αGSU) and a hormone-specific β-subunit (LHβ, FSHβ).

The crucial maturation events at the hypothalamic–pituitary level are the onset of GnRH synthesis, access of GnRH to the hypothalamic–hypophysial circulation, appearance of GnRH receptors in the pituitary gonadotropes, and the onset of gonadotropin synthesis and secretion. Traces of GnRH in whole rat brain extracts were detected as early as on day 12 of gestation, and by the 17th day of gestation immunoreactive GnRH cells within the brain were distributed in a pattern similar to that of the adult, projecting neurosecretory axons to the median eminence [104].

Although gonadotrope is the last cell type in the anterior pituitary to reach maturation with the expression of terminal differentiation markers LHβ, FSHβ, and GnRHR, αGSU is the first pituitary hormone transcript expressed during development. In mice, it is first detected at fetal day 10.5 in the most ventral region of Rathke's pouch [105]. Gonadotrope specific expression of αGSU is regulated by SF1, which plays essential roles at multiple levels of the reproductive axis, reviewed in [106]. However, no single transcription factor has been demonstrated to be necessary and sufficient for gonadotrope lineage commitment [107]. In the rat pituitary, on fetal day 16 rare LHβ were detected by *in situ* hybridization. Many more cells hybridizing LHβ and FSHβ were observed on day 17. At this stage, the fetal pituitary gland becomes GnRH responsive [104]. Recently, it has been shown that two types of gonadotropes may become responsive to GnRH at different time points during development [108].

In humans, fetal pituitary gonadotropins are secreted as early as at 12 weeks of gestation. Marked rises in the pituitary and plasma concentrations of FSH and LH are observed during the second trimester of gestation, and significantly higher levels of circulating gonadotropins are detected in female than in male fetuses [109].

Gonad development is a unique system in which a single rudimentary tissue can be induced to form one of two different organs, the ovary or the testis. The gonads originate from the thickening of the ventrolateral epithelium along the embryonic mesonephros surface, called the genital ridge, and in mice are visible at fetal day 10. Proliferation of these epithelial cells gives rise to somatic cells of the gonad. By contrast, the germ cell lineage arises outside the urogenital ridge before the formation of gonads. Mouse primordial germ cells (PGCs) are specified in the epiblast, and are first detected at about fetal day 7.25 using alkaline phosphatase as a marker [110]. PGCs proliferate and migrate through the gut mesentery into the urogenital ridge, populating the gonads between the 10th and 11th day of fetal development. The exact trigger that initiates PGCs migration to the genital ridge and the chemoattractants that are required for the directional movement toward the genital ridge are slowly beginning to be understood [111].

In mammals, the choice between the male or the female gonad, is initiated by a single gene on the Y chromosome, Sry (sex-determining region of the Y chromosome). Sry is expressed in the somatic cells of the XY gonad between 10.5 and 12.0 of gestation [112] and encodes a putative transcription factor that acts as a genetic switch for male development. The Sry protein is expressed in each pre-Sertoli cell during a narrow window of several hours in the period of gonadal differentiation, between fetal days 10.5 and 12.5, resulting in up-regulation of Sox9, the major gene transcriptionally downstream of Sry [113]. If Sry is expressed in the rudimentary gonad, either from the Y chromosome or from an ectopic transgene, a testis forms [114]. If Sry is not expressed, as in XX individuals or in cases where Sry is mutated or deleted, an ovary forms [115]. Based on this, it was believed that the presence of Sry actively caused testis development to occur, and that in the absence of Sry the ovary developed passively (i.e. the so-called "default" pathway). Recent discoveries have now made it clear that early ovarian development is an active process that involves the interaction and competition of multiple signaling pathways that specify male or female development. The two alternative sex fates are thought to emerge through the antagonistic activities of sex-specific transcription factors in a restricted number of gonadal cells. This initial cell fate decision is further expanded by extracellular non-cell-autonomous signals that promote one developmental program, while at the same time suppressing the other [116]. Studies have identified two secreted factors, Wnt4 and follistatin, which are required during early gonad development to repress the aspects of testis differentiation in XX gonads, reviewed in [111].

By fetal day 13.5, germ cells in XX and XY gonads have taken different developmental paths. In XY gonads germ cells undergo mitotic arrest as prospermatogonia, whereas in XX gonads the germ cells enter the prophase of the first meiotic division. The fate of germ cells is dependent on the somatic environment, and not on the chromosomal sex of the germ cells [117]. Thus, signals from adjacent somatic cells must direct the differentiation of germ cells in the embryonic gonads, although these signals have not been identified.

The onset of gonadal endocrine activity is very clearly sexually dimorphic. During embryogenesis, male differentiation requires the secretion of three testicular hormones. Anti-Müllerian hormone (AMH), produced by fetal Sertoli cells, induces regression of the Müllerian ducts. Testosterone, produced by Leydig cells, promotes the development of Wolffian duct derivatives and masculinization of the external male genitalia. Finally, insulin-like 3 (Insl3) mediates transabdominal testicular descent into the scrotum [118]. The action of LH and production of testosterone start simultaneously in the rat testis on fetal day 15.5 [119]. In females, differentiation occurs when the absence of AMH allows development of Müllerian structures. The lack of androgens permits degeneration of Wolffian ducts, and the absence of Insl3 maintains the gonads in the abdomen. In the ovary, the responsiveness to LH appears postnatally at the end of the first week of life [120] concomitantly with the onset of steroidogenesis [121]. Functional FSH receptors can be detected some days earlier in the perinatal rat ovary, at the age of 4–5 days [122].

Steroid hormones play a crucial role in fetal gonadal development and ovarian cell wellbeing. Estrogen action is needed for normal ovarian development, follicle survival and the regulation of female reproduction. The role of estrogens in female sexual development has been demonstrated in many studies utilizing mice lacking functional estrogen receptors or estrogen-converting enzymes [123, 124]. However, the developmental role of estrogens in human fetal ovaries is not well known. In contrast, testicular hormones are crucial for testicular formation and function, i.e. induction and maintenance of the male phenotype at all stages of development.

In humans ovarian development starts at around the 5th week of gestation, when primordial germ cells migrate into the undifferentiated gonad. Thereafter, the germ cells undergo multiple mitotic divisions, and the number of oogonia reaches its peak by the 20th week of development. At this time about 7–8 million germ cells are present in the ovary [125]. Simultaneously with mitotic divisions, starting around the fetal age of 11–12 weeks, primordial germ cells begin to enter meiosis [126]. After the 10th week of gestation granulosa cell precursors start to form, and at 24 weeks of development almost all oocytes are enveloped in a primordial follicle structure [127]. The human fetus is exposed to high concentrations of maternal and placental estrogens, and estrogens are produced in several fetal tissues [128, 129]. However, minimal amounts of fetal circulating estrogens are produced in the fetal ovarian follicles [109].

In the human male at 7 weeks of gestation, the presence of germ cells in the embryonic gonadal ridge and of coelomic epithelial cells that give rise to Sertoli cells was observed. This was followed by the appearance of Sertoli cells in the testicular tubules and of Leydig cells at 9 weeks, and also by the appearance of vascular endothelial cells and peritubular myoid cells at 12 weeks [130]. The production of testosterone peaks at around 11 or 12 to 14 weeks of gestation, as determined by measurements in the testis and fetal blood [131]. Between weeks 12 and 20, serum testosterone levels in the male fetus are from 3- to 8-fold higher than in the female [132].

3. Programming

During development, there are critical periods in the course of which a system or an organ has to mature. The critical periods are defined by the epochs of rapid cell division within an organ, and different organs develop at different rates and different times. At these critical periods organs are especially vulnerable to challenges such as decreased oxygenation, nutrient supply, and altered hormone exposure. If adverse conditions are experienced in the window of vulnerability, then the trajectory of development of the responding organ may be changed in ways that result in persistent malfunction. The concepts of "nutritional programming", "fetal programming", "fetal origins of adult disease", "developmental origins of health and disease", "developmental induction", and "developmental programming" [26, 133-135] imply that some stimulus or an insult at these critical, restricted periods in development has long-lasting consequences, setting in train a series of events that culminate in the adult onset of disordered function, while the same environmental stimulus outside that critical period induces only reversible changes. The concept evolved from human epidemiological studies that have shown that impaired intrauterine growth is associated with an increased incidence of metabolic, cardiovascular and other diseases in later life. Low birth weight, in particular, has been linked to hypertension, glucose intolerance, insulin resistance, type 2 diabetes, dyslipidaemia, obesity and reproductive disorders in the adult (Figure 1) [133]. The Dutch famine, a unique "natural experiment" with a well-defined period of food shortage in an otherwise well-nourished population, has shown that maternal undernutrition during gestation compromises health in later life, and that these long-term effects depend on its timing during gestation [136]. Intrauterine growth retardation (IUGR) and/or delays in attaining motor, verbal and social skills were recorded in the offspring of mothers exposed to the influence of a large variety of "stresses" such as loud, unanticipated noise (as experienced by people living under the flight paths of busy airports) and living in a country preparing for and ultimately going to war (e.g. the six-day Israeli war) [137].

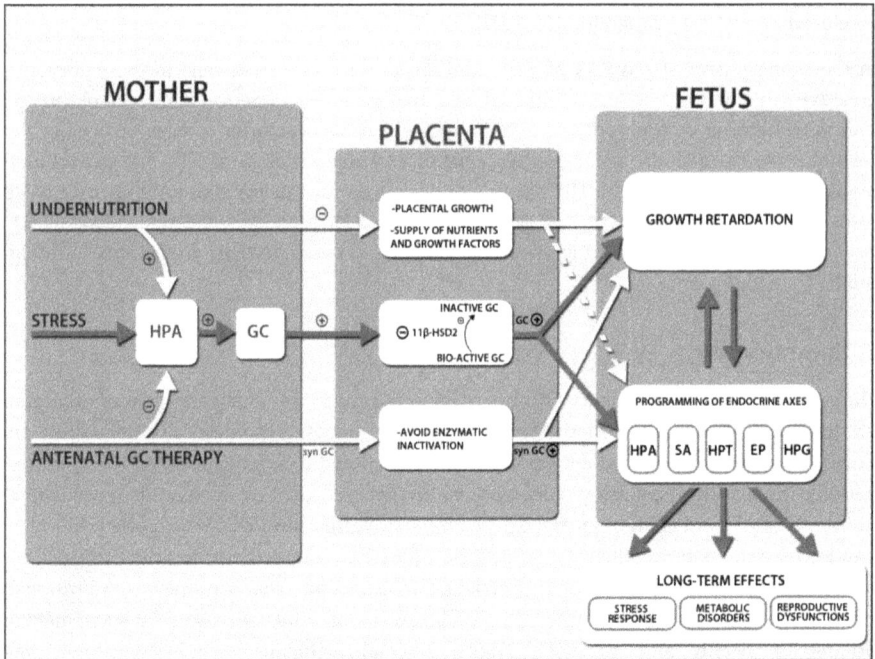

Figure 1. Maternal undernutrition or stress increase maternal glucocoticoid levels and decrease the rate of their inactivation by 11ß-HSD2 in the placenta that results in fetal glucocorticoid overexposure. The synthetic glucocorticoids pass through the enzymatic placental barrier and reach the fetal circulation. Consequences of fetal glucocorticoid overexposure are growth retardation and programming of endocrine axes with long-term effects. HPA-hypothalamic-pituitary-adrenal axis; GC-glucocorticoids; synGC-synthetic glucocorticoids; 11ß-HSD2-11ß-hydroxysteroid dehydrogenase type 2; SA-somatotropic axis; HPT-hypothalamic-pituitary-thyroid axis; EP-endocrine pancreas; HPG-hypothalamic-pituitary-gonadal axis.

The concept of programming has been tested experimentally in numerous species using a wide range of experimental approaches to impair fetal growth. Some of the most commonly used experimental models are maternal undernutrition (calorie restriction, protein deprivation, iron deficiency), placental insufficiency and exposure to glucocorticoids that includes maternal stress, maternal treatment with synthetic glucocorticoids and inhibition of placental 11ß-hydroxysteroid dehydrogenase (11β-HSD2) (Figure 1) [138].

Majority of these experimental models ultimately result in fetal glucocorticoid overexposure, since they mediate the programming effects of nutritional and other environmental challenges during pregnancy [139]. Maternal low-protein diet and placental 11β-HSD2 deficiency cause fetal growth restriction via distinct pathways but with a common component: overexposure of fetoplacental tissues to glucocorticoids. Whatever the source, glucocorticoids play an important role in the regulation of fetal growth, and through this in developmental programming [140]. Glucocorticoids are growth inhibitory and affect development of all the tissues and organ systems that are at increased risk of adult pathophysiology when fetal growth is impaired [11]. Glucocorticoids signal adverse intrauterine conditions and adapt fetal development to ensure the maximum chances of survival both *in utero* and at birth. They act at cellular and molecular levels to induce changes in tissue growth and differentiation by direct and indirect mechanisms. At the cellular level, glucocorticoid exposure *in utero* alters receptors, enzymes, ion channels and transporters in a wide range of different cell types during late gestation. They also change the expression of various growth factors, cytoarchitectural proteins, binding proteins and components of the intracellular signaling pathways [139]. These changes will influence the basal functioning of the cell and its responses to endocrine, metabolic and other stimuli, with consequences for its size, proliferation rate and terminal differentiation. In addition to these direct effects, glucocorticoids can act indirectly on tissue proliferation and differentiation through changes in the cellular secretion of proteins, hormones, growth factors and metabolites [139].

Another major mechanism by which glucocorticoids act on physiological systems is through changes in hormone bioavailability. They alter the production and secretion by the placenta and fetal endocrine glands of a number of hormones, such as estrogen, insulin, gastrin, neuropeptide Y, angiotensin II, T3, noradrenaline and adrenaline. They also regulate hormone receptor densities and the activities of several enzymes involved in activating and inactivating hormones in the fetal tissues. One of the recently proposed mechanisms of programming, with particular emphasis on glucocorticoids, is epigenetic programming. Glucocorticoids act as epigenetic signals that allow transgenerational transmission of non-genomic factors important in developing the optimal phenotype for survival to reproductive age [141]. The consequences of fetal overexposure to either endogenous or exogenous glucocorticoids lead to hypertension, glucose intolerance, insulin resistance, and abnormalities in the HPA function after birth [142].

3.1. Placental 11ß-hydroxysteroid dehydrogenase 2 (11ß-HSD2)

Transcriptional activation of GR is known to be determined by intracellular glucocorticoid availability that is regulated by two distinct isoforms of the enzyme 11ß-HSD. These enzymes control the first critical step for GR activation and target gene expression, while the process has been termed pre-receptor ligand control [2]. 11ß-HSD1 is NADPH-dependent with reductase activity, converting cortisone to the bioactive cortisol in the human, and 11-dehydrocorticosterone to corticosterone in the rat. 11ß-HSD2 is NAD-dependent and catalyzes the rapid metabolism of cortisol and corticosterone to inactive 11-keto forms, cortisone and 11-dehydrocorticosterone, respectively [143]. These enzyme systems function in most fetal gucocorticoid sensitive tissues modulating ligand access to GR. This is especially important for mineralocorticoid sensitive tissues. In the developing kidney, for example, in the presence of 11ß-HSD2, cortisol was efficiently metabolised to inert cortisone, which does not bind to receptors allowing aldosterone action. As a consequence, sodium retention, potassium loss and hypertension are prevented [5].

11ß-HSD2 is highly expressed in the placenta, in the syncytiotrophoblast in humans, and in the labyrinthine zone in rodents, i.e. at the interface between maternal and fetal circulations. Besides the mentioned function, it has an additional role in the placenta: it selectively regulates passage of glucocorticoids from the mother to the fetus, since highly lipophilic glucocorticoid molecules are able to pass freely across the placenta [144, 145]. As glucocorticoid levels are significantly lower in the fetus than in the mother, the 11ß-HSD2 placental enzymatic barrier prevents most of the maternal glucocorticoids from reaching the fetus, protecting the very sensitive fetal tissues from high glucocortivoid levels during development. Although 11ß-HSD2 limits fetal exposure to maternal glucocorticoids, a certain amount avoids enzymatic inactivation and reaches the fetus [146]. 11ß-HSD2 maintains a gradient of glucocorticoids from the maternal to the fetal circulation, although its magnitude varies between species. There is a positive correlation between the materno-fetal gradient and the activity of placental 11ß-HSD2 [139].

Reduced 11ß-HSD2 placental activity results in higher levels of glucocorticoids reaching the fetus, which induces growth retardation and program later disease susceptibility (Figure 1). In rats the lowest placental 11ß-HSD2 activity caused the highest fetal exposure to maternal glucocorticoids is seen in the smallest fetuses with the largest placenta [146]. In addition, low levels of 11ß-HSD2 placental activity decrease birth weight in humans, and can lead to adult hypertension [143]. Furthermore, in 11ß-HSD2 knockout mice fetal weight is significantly reduced in relation to wild type controls, as a consequence, not only of the increased fetal exposure to maternal glucocorticoids, but also altered placental function, i.e. decreased transport of nutrients. Thus, absence of 11β-HSD2 compromises not only fetal but also placental growth, function and morphology, representing an additional mechanism of fetal programming [147]. Since maternal glucocorticoid levels are significantly higher then those in the fetus, even modest perturbations of the placental 11β-HSD2 levels or activity can have a profound impact on fetal glucocorticoid exposure [148]. Inhibition of 11β-HSD2 activity by the application of carbenoxolone to gravid females, a potent inhibitor of 11β-HSD2, reduces birth weight in rats and elevates blood pressure in the adult rat offspring. These effects require the presence of maternal adrenal products, since carbenoxolone given to adrenalectomized pregnant rats had no effect on birth weight or blood pressure [149].

Placental 11ß-HSD2 can be avoided by the application of synthetic glucocorticoids. It has been demonstrated that treatment of pregnant rats with dexamethasone and betamethasone, synthetic glucocorticoids that are poorly metabolized by the enzyme, results in reduced birth weight, higher activity of the HPA axis and elevated blood pressure in the adult offspring (Figure 1) [143]. Synthetic glucocorticoids have been shown to up-regulate the activity of 11ß-HSD2, and, hence, amplify the placental barrier for physiological glucocorticoids [150].

It can be concluded that fetuses are protected from environmental perturbations by an enzymatic placental barrier that, by regulating fetal exposure to maternal glucocorticoids, crucially determines foeto-placental growth. Its deficiency causes programming effects in the offspring.

3.2. Stress during pregnancy and maternal undernutrition

Exposure to stress during pregnancy has been associated with offspring behavior, morphology, physiology, and immunology [151]. Although the mechanisms by which stress during pregnancy can influence the development of the offspring are not entirely known, elevation of the maternal glucocorticoid levels after stress exposure could be the first step in early life programming that predisposes individuals to several illnesses and psychiatric disorders. Maternal exposure to alcohol, repeated restraint stress, electric tail shocks, and undernutrition during pregnancy induced a corticosterone increase [152, 153]. In the offspring of these mothers growth retardation with altered function of the HPA axis and glucocorticoid responses under stress challenge, hyperglycemia and other dysfunctions related to type 2 diabetes, as well as hypertension were established (Figure 1) [14, 15, 153].

Adrenalectomy, as a blockade of the maternal stress-induced corticosterone secretion, suppresses the changes established in the offspring of prenatally stressed dams. The effects of repeated restraint stress during pregnancy on the offspring HPA axis activity and hippocampal mineralocorticoid receptor (MR) level are suppressed by adrenalectomy, while the administration of corticosterone to adrenalectomised mothers reinstates the effects induced by prenatal stress [153]. Furthermore, a pharmacological blockade of the maternal glucocorticoid synthesis with metyrapone also prevented hypertension, which is induced by fetal exposure to maternal low-protein diet [154]. Adrenalectomy carried out during pregnancy (without stress exposure), although it causes the opposite result in relation to stress exposure due to circulating corticosterone levels, also affects offspring development. Maternal adrenalectomy performed during gestation results in a compensatory increase in fetal corticosterone levels [152], decreases body weight in both male and female offspring, while the HPA axis shows a sex-specific pattern of vulnerability. In females, a dramatic increase in hypothalamic CRH and GR mRNA levels was established on day 14 [155]. All this together points out that highly regulated maternal glucocorticoids are indispensable during normal fetal development.

Various types of stress applied during gestation cause a broad spectrum of effects in the offspring at any age. Effects of prenatal stress caused by the restraining of pregnant rats influence the development of fetal hypothalamic PVN neurons in a duration-dependent manner. Long-lasting stress causes neurotoxic changes of the fetal PVN neurons, including CRH neurons that showed significantly shorter total length of the neuronal processes and an increased number of apoptotic cells. On the contrary, short-lasting stress facilitates the development of these fetal PVN neurons that showed enhanced CRH messenger RNA expression, while the varicosities of CRH-containing axons at the median eminence revealed more mature morphology. A greater degree of neuronal differentiation, as manifested by an increase in both the number of branch points and the total length of the processes from the cell body, was also demonstrated [156].

Chronic maternal restraint stress during late gestation decreases placental 11β-HSD2 expression and activity, and reduces body weight in rat fetuses at term. These alterations were associated with reduced pancreatic β-cell mass, growth hormone level, and decreased glucose concentration in fetal plasma [18]. Other results established hyperglycaemia, glucose intolerance and decreased basal leptin levels in prenatally stressed aged male rats as dysfunctions related to type 2 diabetes mellitus [15]. These data suggest that maternal stress and later dysfunctions such as type 2 diabetes could be linked to the restricted fetal growth and the adverse glucocorticoid environment *in utero* as the consequences of decreased placental 11β-HSD2 expression.

Observations from animal and human studies have linked maternal nutritional status and fetal growth retardation with the programming of hypertension and coronary heart disease in later life [27]. In the ewe, undernutrition in early pregnancy leads to placental enlargements, as adaptation to extract more nutrients. There is a correlation between placental weight and systolic blood pressure in adults that tends to rise as placental weight increases [157]. Mild protein restriction during pregnancy attenuates placental 11β-HSD2 expression which leads to overexposure of the fetus to maternal glucocorticoids (Figure 1) [14, 143]. Intrauterine growth retardation and disturbed development of the HPA axis appear as an outcome [15]. In addition, in the adult offspring subjected to maternal undernutrition during pregnancy persistently elevated expression of GR and decreased expression of 11β-HSD2 in the kidney, liver and brain mediated tissue-specific increases in glucocorticoid action. These changes represent potentially important mechanisms contributing to the programming of hypertension *in utero* [158].

As presented, it has so far been established that certain types of stress affect the reduction of placental 11β-HSD2 expression in rats, suggesting that the fetus and placenta are exposed to excessive amounts of glucocorticoids. Thus, deficiency of the placental barrier to maternal glucocorticoids may represent a common pathway between the maternal environment and feto-placental programming of later disease [12, 18]. Secondly, disturbances in placental growth and function, as a consequence of maternal stress exposure, decrease fetal nutrient supply and may further contribute to suboptimal fetal growth [14, 145]. Both changes, i.e. the reduced maternal glucocorticoid inactivation and decreased nutritional supply reflect on the HPA axis activity in fetuses and offspring, although the HPA axis response is differentially affected by the gestational stress procedure (Figure 1) [151]. Thus, the fetal HPA axis is a possible primary target and is intricately involved in early life disturbance caused by maternal stress exposure with far-reaching physiological consequences.

3.3. Antenatal glucocorticoid therapy

Because glucocorticoids have potent influence on maturation of fetal lung and other tissues they have been used for more than 40 years in human pregnancies at risk of preterm delivery. Use of antenatal corticosteroid therapy reduced the complications associated with preterm delivery such as neonatal respiratory distress syndrome (RSD), periventricular hemorrhage, necrotizing enterocolitis and, most importantly, neonatal mortality [159]. According to the National Institute of Health [160] all fetuses between the 24th and 34th week of gestation at risk of preterm delivery should be considered as candidates for the beneficial effects of antenatal glucocorticoid treatment. The recommended treatment consists of two doses of 12 mg betamethasone given 24 h apart, or alternative regimen of four doses of 6 mg dexamethasone given 12 h apart [161]. However, antenatal glucocorticoid therapy may produce growth retardation, affective and cognitive disturbances as well as other disorders in children and adults [162], thus the question of the relative risk and benefit of repetitive courses of prenatal glucocorticoid administration is still open (Figure 1).

Furthermore, the effects of prenatal glucocorticoid administration in cases of congenital adrenal hyperplasia (CAH) that must begin early in the first trimester to be effective in preventing female genital ambiguity are not completely known. CAH is an inherited disease in which a disordered steroidogenic enzyme P450C21 diverts adrenal steroid synthesis away from cortisol toward androgen. As a consequence girls are masculinized, because the adrenal glands secrete large amounts of androgens during prenatal development. Dexamethasone treatment should be introduced very early in pregnancy, before the seventh week of gestation, with the aim to increase fetal glucocorticoid concentrations, thus suppressing the elevated ACTH level that drives adrenal androgen production [146, 163].

In obstetric practice different synthetic glucocorticoids are used: dexamethasone, betamethasone, or prednisolone. Synthetic glucocorticoids are slightly different from their endogenous equivalents in chemical structure. Dexamethasone and bethamethasone both have the additional 9α-fluoro groups, and 16β- or 16α-methyl groups, respectively [164]. Prednisolone differs from cortisol by a 1δ-dehydro configuration (Figure 2). The choice of the concrete drug use will depend on its biological half-life, which represents the time that passes until one half of the initial drug concentration has disappeared from the blood [165]. Physiological and synthetic glucocorticoids have been divided into short-, medium- and long-acting substances dependent on the duration of measurable biological half-life [165]. Cortisol belongs to the short-acting category with the biological half-life of 8–12 h, prednisolone belongs to the medium-acting category with the half-life of 12–36 h, while dexamethasone and betamethasone have long-acting properties, ranging between 36 and 54 h [165].

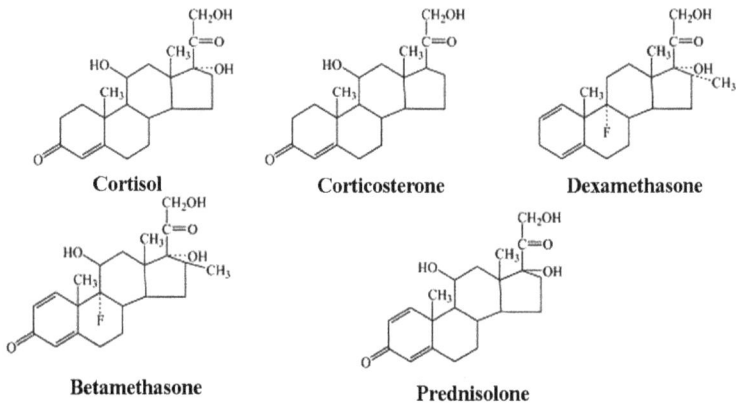

Figure 2. The structural formulas of natural (cortisol, cortocosterone) and synthetic glucocorticoids.

The biological activity of glucocorticoids is partly determined by the rate and selectivity of protein binding, because only the unbound glucocorticoids fraction is biologically active. Gayrard et al. [166] have found that the plasma free cortisol concentrations (6% to 14%), corticosteroid-binding globulin (CBG)-bound (67% to 87%) and albumin-bound (7% to 19%) concentrations are similar within species. Cortisol binding decreases as its concentration increases [167]. In human plasma, betamethasone and dexamethasone bind predominantly to albumin, which has high capacity but low affinity for ligating, while both steroids bind only marginally to CBG [167]. Dexamethasone displays higher protein affinity than betamethasone. The potency of glucocorticoids in a biological system also depends on its affinity for its receptor. Genomic potency of betamethasone was reported to be moderately higher than that of dexamethasone, while both steroids have a 25-fold higher affinity to the GR than cortisol [168].

4. Programming of endocrine axes

4.1. Programming of the fetal hypothalamic-pituitary-adrenal axis

The HPA axis is particularly sensitive to glucocorticoid levels. Fetal exposure to excessive glucocorticoids, natural or synthetic, can occur via a number of mechanisms including maternal stress, undernutrition as well as maternal antenatal treatment. As previously noted, synthetic glucocorticoids such as dexamethasone and betamethasone pass easily through the placental barrier avoiding the placental enzyme 11β-HSD2 [7], while maternal stress and undernutrition affect the same enzyme, resulting in increased fetal exposure to maternal glucocorticoids [18]. As the increased fetal exposure to glucocorticoids occurs during a critical period of the HPA axis development, when its control is just setting up, permanent alterations in the basal and stress induced HPA axis activity and regulation occur in the offspring, and sustain throughout life. Crucial changes that underlie the programming of the HPA axis will be presented below. Additionally, disturbances of the complex maturational process such as HPA axis development that have far-reaching immediate and delayed physiological effects will be discussed later.

The hippocampus represents a major inhibitory input to the HPA axis function. This is the point where glucocorticoid feedback, via GR an MR in the hippocampus and GR in the hypothalamic PVN and anterior pituitary, inhibits further HPA activity [169]. Thus, the balance between GR and MR in the hippocampus is an important factor in determining the HPA axis feedback sensitivity. Prenatal dexamethasone exposure alters GR and MR expression in the developing limbic system of guinea pig fetuses in both a region-specific and a sex-specific manner. After a single dexamethasone dose, female fetuses exhibited a significant increase in MR and GR mRNA levels in the CA1 and CA2 regions of the hippocampus and MR mRNA in the dentate gyrus [170]. Other results showed that multiple dexamethasone administration during pregnancy led to a marked increase in hippocampal GR and MR mRNA levels in male fetuses [171]. In mice, a single course of dexamethasone transiently reduced MR mRNA expression in the fetal hippocampus [172]. In addition, prenatal stress, or dexamethasone exposure are implicated in the development of rat hippocampal GR and MR in the offspring. In rat offspring exposed to glucocorticoid excess during late pregnancy permanently attenuated GR and MR mRNA expression in specific hippocampal regions reduced sensitivity to glucocorticoids [173]. The administration of betamethasone to pregnant sheep resulted in significant increases in MR and 11-βHSD2 gene expression in adult animals, reflecting a possible role for the locally produced glucocorticoids within the hippocampus, and the potential for long term alterations in HPA function [20].

At the level of the hypothalamic PVN, significantly decreased amounts of CRH mRNA were seen in male fetuses and female offspring after treatment of guinea pig mothers with dexamethasone or betamethasone, supporting the idea that synthetic glucocorticoids enter the fetal brain and inhibit central drive to the fetal HPA axis [171]. In addition, it has been shown that prenatal dexamethasone treatment induces a clear delay in increment of CRH in the external zone of the median eminence [174]. Morphometric analyses of rat PVN neurosecretory cells at eight distinct subdivisions indicate that dexamethasone given to pregnant dams causes significant changes in PVN neurosecretory cells in 20-day-old fetuses as well as in neonatal offspring. Significantly decreased neurosecretory cell nuclei volume and number in PVN, due to decreased proliferative activity, were found at the levels were parvocellular neurons are present, i.e. where CRH neurons are dominant [175, 176]. On the other hand, removal of maternal adrenals at day 16 of gestation significantly affected the size of neurosecretory cells in different subgroups of fetal PVN. These effects persisted during the neonatal period [177], confirming that prenatal glucocorticoid exposure alters the development and function of prenatal and neonatal PVN.

Prenatal glucocorticoid application alters the monoaminergic transmitter systems involved in the regulation of GR expression in the brain. Significant differences in the turnovers of serotonin, dopamine and noradrenaline contents between the weeks 3 and 14 of life were found in a wide area in the rat brain [54]. Thus, developmental alterations of monoaminergic neurons, that represent major modulators of the HPA axis function, influence endocrine response in the adult offspring. The data suggest that key targets for programming include GR gene expression and the CRH system [178].

Antenatal treatment with synthetic glucocorticoids affects pituitary development and the differentiation of hormone-producing cell types during the fetal period as well as after birth. A significant reduction in fetal ACTH cell volume and number was demonstrated in 19 and 21-day-old fetuses after multiple prenatal dexamethasone administration (Figure 3) [38, 42]. Dexamethasone decreased the rate of division of both immature cells and the existing fetal ACTH in the period when its proliferation was most intensive, on day 19 of fetal development [179], thus leaving long lasting consequences. Multiple dexamethasone exposure during pregnancy affects the ultrastructure of ACTH cells, which in the Golgi complex show much lower presence of specific granules as well as dilation of the endoplasmatic reticulum [180]. Decreased morphometric parameters of the ACTH cells and their changed ultrastructure resulted in significantly reduced plasma ACTH levels in fetuses and neonatal offspring after multiple dexamethasone administration during pregnancy [180, 181]. On the contrary, a single dose of dexamethasone, given to pregnant rats on day 16 of gestation, suppressed the synthetic activity of fetal ACTH cells, but in the early neonatal period this suppression was followed by stimulation of ACTH secretion and increased circulating ACTH levels [182]. Other results showed that following antenatal exposure to synthetic glucocorticoids in juvenile males POMC mRNA and CRH receptor mRNA on the pituitary level were increased [183].

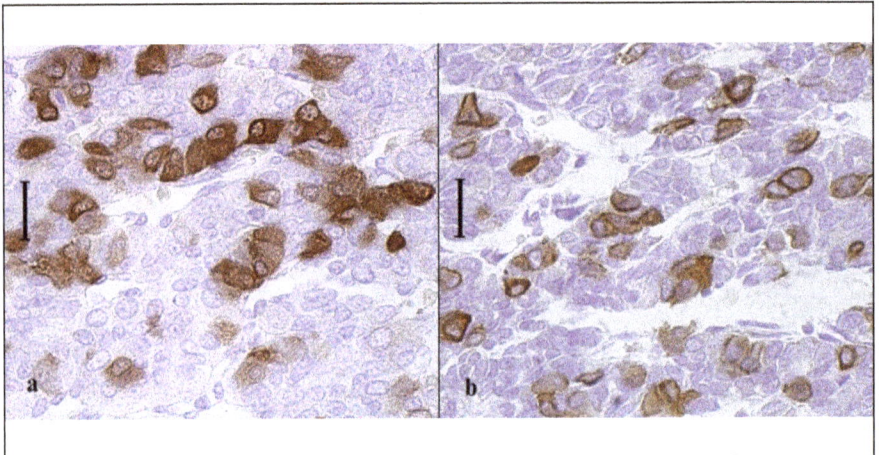

Figure 3. a) Intensive immunopositivity of ACTH cells located near the capillary network is characteristic for 21-day-old fetus. b) Decreased size, immunopositivity and number of ACTH cells in 21-day-old fetuses after maternal dexamethasone administration. Bar - 25 μm.

After maternal glucocorticoid exposure the absence of peaks in ACTH blood concentration in near term (19-day-old) fetuses reduces ACTH-trophic support and reflects on the adrenal glands structure and functional activity [42]. Administration of a single or multiple dexamethasone dose to pregnant rats induced a significant decrease in adrenal glands weight, volume of whole adrenal glands, as well as average volume and total number of cells in near term fetuses and neonatal rat offspring, a consequence of the decreased proliferative activity of adrenocortical cells [45, 46]. Interestingly, in 19-day-old fetuses the proliferative activity of adrenocortical cells that is most intensive in the outer portion of the fetal adrenal glands is markedly reduced in ZG. The proliferation rate of adrenocortical cells in IZ was not affected by prenatal dexamethasone application [42], suggesting that different sensitivity and/or responses of the proliferating cells in ZG and the outer portion of IZ to external stimuli could be a possible mechanism for the formation and maintenance of the zonal structure of the adrenal cortex [184].

In the rat adrenal glands of fetuses and pups of dexamethasone treated dams, during during the early neonatal period adrenocortical cells in various stages of degeneration were abundant, especially near the central part of the gland where zona reticularis (ZR) begins to differentiate. Resorption zones with lymphocytic infiltrations and presence of macrophages and multinuclear giant cells were observed, indicating that remodeling of the adrenal gland

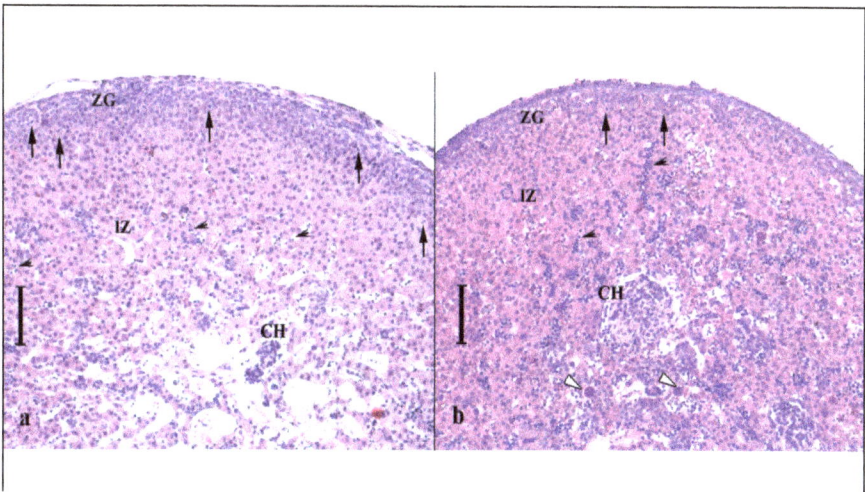

Figure 4. a) Zona glomerulosa (ZG) with numerous dividing cells (→), inner zone (IZ) with lymphocytes (black arrowheads), cellular interspaces, and centrally positioned group of chromoblasts (CH) are seen in adrenal gland of 21-day-old fetus. b) Decreased number of proliferating cells (→) in the adrenal gland of 21-day-old fetuses from gravid females treated with dexamethasone. Infiltration of lymphocytes (black arrowheads) and giant cells (white arrowheads) are indications of intensive tissue remodeling. Bar - 100 μm.

structure is affected by prenatal glucocorticoid exposure (Figure 4) [45, 46]. In the juvenile period, decreased expression of steroidogenic enzyme CYP17 after antenatal exposure to synthetic glucocorticoids has been established, reflecting the persistence of the adrenal glands functional changes [183].

The influence of a single dexamethasone treatment given to gravid females resulted in the decreased volume of adrenal medulla and the number of chromaffin cells that persisted during the fetal and neonatal period. Decreased proliferation of chromaffin cells during the fetal and early neonatal period was followed by significantly higher values in relation to controls during the second neonatal week, indicating the capacity of the adrenal gland medulla to recover [185]. Multiple dexamethasone doses applied during pregnancy exert a more potent inhibitory effect. A reduced number of chromaffin cells and significantly decreased adrenaline content in the adrenals were seen in 14-day-old neonatal offspring [181].

As pointed out, the consequences of fetal glucocorticoid exposure occur at the level of central regulation, pituitary ACTH cells and the adrenal gland, causing programming effects on HPA axis function in later life. In offspring HPA axis activity may be changed in different directions under basal conditions and after stress challenge [186]. Permanently elevated basal plasma glucocorticoid levels [178, 187], greater glucocorticoid response to stress [54] as well as blunted HPA axis response to stress [183] have been established in offspring following antenatal exposure to synthetic glucocorticoids. In addition, antenatal glucocorticoid treatment programs HPA function in the adult offspring in a sex-specific manner [188]. Programming of the fetal HPA axis, although it could have had an adverse postnatal outcome, actually demonstrated the amazing plasticity of the HPA axis.

Exposure to stress or glucocorticoids, exogenous or endogenous, causes fetal growth retardation and low birth weight in parallel with deregulation of the HPA axis during the life cycle [139]. Additionally, there is a correlation between the natural variation in body weight and the HPA axis function in offspring. In adult pigs that were low-weight at birth and remained small after birth altered HPA axis function has been recorded in later life, i.e. elevated adrenal responsiveness to insulin-induced hypoglycaemia [189]. Thus, it can be concluded that growth retardation and programming of the HPA axis are two mutually dependent processes that actually represent the modality by which prenatal environment influences adult stress-related diseases (Figure 1).

It has been shown that in rodents, effects of programming can be induced by insults even in neonatal period of life. One of the striking characteristics of the HPA axis is the stress hypo-responsive period during the first 2 weeks of life for species that are immature at birth, such as rats and mice. During the stress hypo-responsive period there is low basal corticosterone secretion and the inability to increase corticosterone in response to mild stressors, in order to protect the developing nervous system from glucocorticoid excess. Thus, neonatal glucocorticoid exposure and early life experience that activate the HPA axis have programming effects on HPA axis organization and functioning during the life cycle. Postnatal handling attenuated HPA response to stress in adult animals. Most likely this is an indirect effect, caused by altered maternal behavior which results in increased licking and grooming of pups by the dam. It is considered that serotonin plays a crucial role in the persistence of the handling effect through increased hippocampal GR levels [190]. Similarly, as adults, the offspring of mothers that exhibited more licking and grooming of pups during the first 10 days of life showed reduced HPA axis stress response due to increased hippocampal GR mRNA expression and decreased levels of hypothalamic CRH mRNA [191]. On the other hand, maternal separations during the critical periods of hippocampal development can disrupt hippocampal cytoarchitecture and neurogenesis in a stable manner, with stress hyper-responsiveness observed in these animals as adults [192, 193].

4.2. Programming of the somatotropic axis

Programming of the somatotropic axis (GH-IGF axis) is known to be induced by transient events in early postnatal life. The best described example is the effect of transient neonatal manipulation of sex steroids to permanently alter subsequent GH secretion to resemble the pattern of GH secretion of the opposite sex in rodents [194]. Intrauterine programming of the somatotropic (GH-IGF) axis is still not fully understood, despite its importance in postnatal growth and metabolism. Synthetic activity, storage, and proliferation of rat pituitary GH cells, indicated by the significant increase in GH cell immunopositivity, size, and number per volume and unit of area, rise markedly from the 19th till the 21st fetal day [195]. This corresponds with an increase in plasma corticosterone concentration in near term rat fetuses [46]. It has been shown that dexamethasone administered during the last week of pregnancy has a maturational effect on pituitary GH cells in rats [196]. Dexamethasone induced GHRHR mRNA expression and accumulation in the fetal rat pituitary gland [70] and amplified the stimulatory influence of GHRH. As a consequence, dexamethasone induced GH cells to synthesize and release more GH, leading to increases in GH cell size and immunopositivity (Figure 5) [196]. Corticosterone-induced GH cell differentiation involves GH expression in cells not expressing GH mRNA previously [197]. Moreover, dexamethasone can induce GH progenitors to start GH synthesis one day earlier than in normal fetuses. *In vitro* findings suggested that incubation of the pituitary gland with dexamethasone for 24 h increased GH mRNA on fetal day 18 to a level nearly identical to that in intact 19-day-old fetuses [70]. In humans, low-weight babies have high basal GH and low IGF-I concentrations at birth, with an increased GH response to GHRH [198]. These altered concentrations are maintained during early childhood and are accompanied by changes in the pattern of GH secretion. By early adulthood, urinary GH excretion, which reflects GH secretion, is low in men and women with low birth weights, but in old age birth weight is unrelated to either urinary GH excretion or the GH secretory profile [198]. Low birth weight is associated with decreased IGF-I, IGF-II and IGFBP-3, and elevated levels of IGFBP-1 [199].

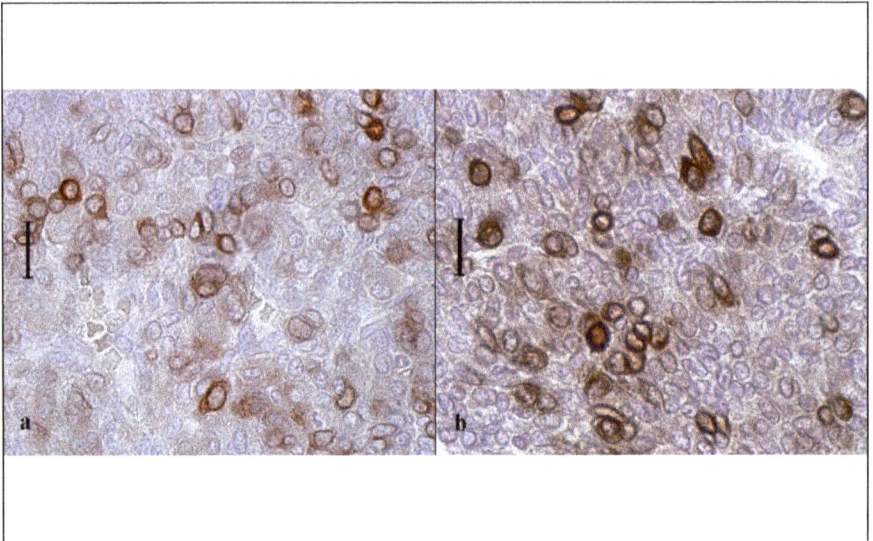

Figure 5. a) Pituitary GH cells of control 21-day-old fetus. b) Intensive immunostaining of GH cells in 21-day-old fetuses after maternal dexamethasone treatment. Bar - 25 μm.

In the fetus, IGF-I together with insulin, acts as a signal of nutrient plenty at the cellular level and promotes tissue growth in line with substrate availability in the fetus [24]. In fetal sheep, concentrations of insulin and IGF-I rise with increasing fetal concentrations of glucose over the normal range of values induced by variations in maternal nutritional state. The rise in fetal plasma IGF-I probably reflects overspill of IGF-I produced by a number of different fetal tissues, since IGF-I is primarily a paracrine growth factor *in utero*. In contrast, the concentrations of cortisol rise as fetal glucose levels decline [200]. Fetal undernutrition induced by maternal dietary manipulation, placental insufficiency and restriction of uterine blood flow, all reduce the circulating levels and tissue expression of IGF-I [200]. Glucocorticoids affect the expression of Igf1 and Igf2 genes, although their effects are tissue and Igf-specific. In fetal sheep, cortisol up- and down-regulates Igf1 gene expression in the liver and skeletal muscle, respectively, whereas it down-regulates Igf2 gene expression in these tissues. These changes in tissue expression occur both in response to exogenous cortisol infusion before term, and when fetal cortisol levels rise endogenously during the immediate prepartum period [200]. The cortisol-induced changes in tissue Igf gene expression are also accompanied by decreases in the fetal growth rate and, close to term, by a fall in plasma IGF-II levels [77, 201]. Cortisol, therefore, appears to initiate the switch from paracrine IGF production *in utero* to the hepatic production of endocrine IGF-I characteristic of the postnatal animal. Glucocorticoids may act on Igf gene expression either directly or indirectly, through changes in the GH receptor gene expression [79] and/or via other transcription factors or cortisol-dependent hormones, such as T3 [202]. This premature transition from IGF-II to

IGF-I production has beneficial effects on tissue differentiation, should delivery occur before full term. However, if delivery is not stimulated prematurely, the glucocorticoid-induced switch from the fetal to the adult mode of somatotrophic regulation may lead to inappropriate changes in cell proliferation and differentiation *in utero* with adverse sequelae both at birth and much later in life [200]. The reduced axial growth and reduced femur and tibia length reported in juvenile rats prenatally exposed to dexamethasone could serve as an illustration [203]. Altogether, the long-term consequences of such fetal changes in the GH-IGF axis are yet not fully understood in terms of functional adaptation or diseases. However, glucocorticoid-induced alterations might appear as potentially beneficial for short-term survival in an environment of shortage of nutritional resources. After birth, normalization of insulin, IGFs and IGFPs occurs. During this period, when suddenly exposed to increased concentrations of insulin and IGF-1, tissues chronically depleted of these two hormones during fetal life may counteract the hike by developing insulin resistance as a metabolic defense against developing hypoglycemia [204]. Therefore, infants with low birth weight who show early and complete growth recovery could be at higher risk for the occurrence of the metabolic syndrome in adulthood. Indeed, recent results in rats have shown permanent and sexually dimorphic changes in the expression of genes involved in the GH-IGF axis in animals that were weaned on to a high fat diet [203].

4.3. Programming of the hypothalamic-pituitary-thyroid axis

Glucocorticoid milieu strongly influences HPT axis activity during critical developmental periods. Prenatal alterations in glucocorticoid levels, caused by the application of synthetic glucocorticoids, maternal undernutrition or adrenalectomy, reflect on the fetal, neonatal and adult HPT axis structure and function.

Unbiased estimation of the cell number applying a design-based modern stereological approach revealed that maternal dexamethasone treatment significantly decreased pituitary TSH cell number in near term fetuses. This result together with the strong immunopositivity of TSH cells, and the fact that the decreased number of TSH cells sustains serum TSH concentrations at the control level, indicates that glucocorticoids exert a maturation-promoting effect on fetal TSH cells enhancing TSH synthesis (Figure 6) [205]. In sheep fetuses, antenatal glucocorticoid administration induced an increase in the circulating T3 concentration. Tissue-specific changes in deiodinase enzyme activities show stimulation of hepatic D1 activity with consequent increases in hepatic T3 production, as well as decreased T3 clearance by suppression of D3 enzymes in the kidney and placenta [206]. In the brain, glucocorticoid application stimulated TH activity during a period between gestational day 20 and neonatal day 12 that largely overlaps with the transient window in time during which brain development is TH sensitive [207]. On the contrary, maternal undernutrition during the gestational period results in lower serum T3 and higher serum reverse T3 concentrations in neonatal pups [208].

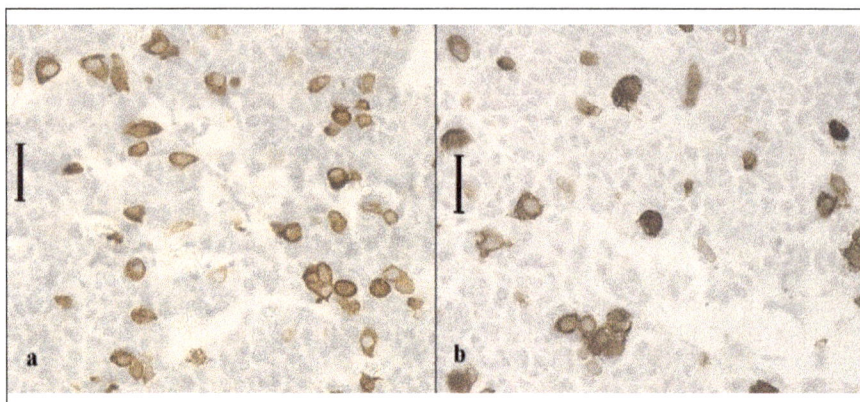

Figure 6. a) Numerous TSH cells characteristic for pituitary of 21-day-old fetus. b) Decreased number of TSH cells, with intense immunopositivity was observed in 21-day-old fetuses after maternal dexamethasone administration. Bar - 25 μm.

Alteration of the glucocorticoid milieu caused by maternal adrenalectomy influences HPT axis functioning in adult offspring. Decreased hypothalamic TRH mRNA levels and increased plasma TSH levels recorded in both male and female adult offspring of adrenalectomized dams were reversed by the administration of corticosterone to the pregnant adrenalectomized dam. The decreased plasma T3 concentrations in female offspring, which were reversed by the administration of higher levels of corticosterone to the adrenalectomized pregnant rats, suggest that the adult HPT axis responded to variations in maternal glucocorticoid milieu in a sex-specific manner [209].

Importantly, TH per se are potent programming factors. Fetal and neonatal hyperthyroidism or hypothyroidism results in programming of the HPT function. During critical periods, TSH secretion is suppressed by an excess of TH, but cannot be increased despite the marked lowering of circulating TH caused by perinatal propylthiouracil administration. More importantly, perinatal thyroid status "programs" its own future reactivity, so that early hypothyroidism results in reduced T4 and T3 levels in adulthood, despite normal levels of TSH [210].

TH influence the accretion, differentiation and metabolism of many tissues and cell types during development in a time-dependent manner. The effects of its deficiency during critical periods, when the tissues still have some plasticity and are in a higher proliferating and differentiating stage, are thus notable, often permanent. Fetal hypothyroidism leads to asymmetrical growth retardation, with reduction in muscle mass [211]. Fetal metabolism and utilization of oxygen, as well as bone tissue growth were adversely affected by TH deficiency in utero [211]. A well known example is that hypothyroidism during the period of thyroid-dependent brain development, in fetuses and during infancy, causes permanent mental retardation [212]. Thus, the structure and function of TH-dependent tissues, determined during critical periods by the striking effects of TH action [139], might be the cause of different (patho)physiological alterations which manifest during the life cycle. The potent influence of glucocorticoids on serum TH concentrations and the TH tissue bioavailability in the same period represents an important additional cause of the programming events recorded in different tissues.

4.4. Programming of endocrine pancreas

A number of epidemiological and clinical studies demonstrate an association between low birth weight and an increased incidence of metabolic, cardiovascular and other diseases in adult life. Adverse intrauterine environment caused by inadequate maternal nutrition status [13], poor placental function [17], maternal stress [15] or treatment with synthetic glucocorticoids [187] is linked with impaired intrauterine growth and increased rates of metabolic diseases such as type 2 diabetes in adulthood.

The increased fetal glucocorticoid exposure observed during and after suboptimal conditions, triggers cell differentiation in many of the tissues, resetting the set points of metabolic homeostasis and endocrine axes and in most individual fetal tissues leads to weight reduction, restricted fetal growth and decreased birth weight [24]. Glucocorticoids therefore switch the cell cycle from tissue accretion to tissue differentiation in preparation for delivery. At the same time, glucocorticoids are involved in the programming of the HPA axis during critical periods, causing structural and functional changes specified in the above section. Alterations in the feedback sensitivity of the fetal HPA axis, as adaptation to suboptimal conditions, mostly result in enhanced HPA axis activity postnatally, under basal conditions or after stress challenge, with elevated glucocorticoid levels [21]. These changes are in close association with the programming of susceptibility in the fetus to develop metabolic syndrome in later life. Indeed, hyperactivity of the HPA axis with chronically elevated glucocorticoids is positively correlated with the metabolic syndrome, which includes a cluster of symptoms such as hyperglycemia, hyperinsulinemia, or insulin resistance. Dyslipidemia, hyperleptinemia, raised serum triglycerides, lowered serum high-density lipoprotein cholesterol, and high blood pressure have also been recorded. All of those risk factors are a prelude to the development of diseases such as type 2 diabetes, atherosclerosis and cardio-vascular complications [28].

Suboptimal conditions *in utero* lead to changes in the endocrine environment which influence fetal development so that its nutrient requirements are decreased and a thrifty phenotype is produced to maximize its chances for survival. These short-term beneficial adaptations may be maladaptive in postnatal life, contributing to poor health outcomes [26]. If postnatal nutrient availability is better than predicted, metabolic dysfunctions occur, as the organism is not adapted to cope with excessive caloric intake in later life. The association of low birth weight with early postnatal catch-up growth, in situations where discrepancies between the pre- and postnatal environment are significant, adversely affects body composition, producing increased susceptibility to non-insulin dependent type 2 diabetes. But if environmental conditions remain unchanged, and the offspring of mothers on a low protein diet continue with the low protein diet during lactation, development of the metabolic phenotype is prevented. The "predictive adaptive response" hypothesis proposes that the degree of mismatch between the pre- and postnatal environments is a major determinant of subsequent disease, and leads to the premise that adult disease arises *in utero* [28, 213].

The thrifty phenotype is not able to respond to unexpected environmental conditions because the changes in metabolic tissues established during critical periods are directed towards low nutritional demands. The fetus adapts to an adverse intrauterine milieu through changes that permanently affect the pancreas, muscles, adipose tissue, and liver structure and function, which are involved in the pathogenesis of obesity and type 2 diabetes [25].

Progressive reduction in insulin-producing β-cell mass is observed in rats with restricted fetal growth [214]. There is evidence that prenatal caloric restriction during pregnancy causes alteration in pancreatic islet neogenesis by decreasing the β-cell precursor pool [215], while maternal protein restriction in rats lowers β-cell proliferation and/or increases apoptosis rates in the fetal endocrine pancreas [215, 216]. Permanent reductions in β-cell mass and its functional efficiency, although achieved by different mechanisms, result in glucose intolerance in adulthood [214]. Nutritional deprivation as severe stress induces a rise in both maternal and fetal corticosterone levels, which in turn are responsible for the observed effects [217].

Prenatal stress that induces a restriction in intrauterine growth in aged male rats causes hyperglycemia, glucose intolerance, and decreased basal leptin levels. Again, an adverse glucocorticoid environment during critical periods might be the underlying mechanism that mediates long-lasting disturbances in feeding behavior and dysfunctions related to type 2 diabetes [15].

Overexposure to exogenous glucocorticoids during different stages of development reduces β-cell mass in the fetal endocrine pancreas: impairment of β-cell commitment is recorded in fetuses exposed to glucocortiocoid during the last week of gestation, while glucocorticoids treatment throughout gestation lowers β-cell proliferation and impairs islet vascularization [218]. Glucocorticoid excess during the last week of gestation leads to lower levels of insulin expression in the β-cells of 3-week-old offspring via a mechanism that involves down-regulation of Pdx-1, the transcription factor that initiates and promotes β-cells development [219]. Programming of the functional capacity of pancreatic β-cell mass by adverse intrauterine conditions increases susceptibility to type 2 diabetes during adulthood that is especially evident if offspring when they are challenged with nutritional abundance. As during adulthood the majority of β-cells are formed through proliferation of the existing cells [220], smaller β-cell mass in the newborn means fewer β-cells will be available for renewal during life, which increases the risk of developing glucose intolerance or diabetes [221].

Impaired insulin action at the major sites of glucose utilization, such as skeletal muscles, liver and adipose tissue, further predisposes to a later diabetic state. Excess prenatal glucocorticoid exposure, uteroplacental insufficiency as well as maternal low protein diet in the perinatal period prepare skeletal muscle metabolism for poor metabolic conditions in later life [22, 25, 213]. These changes include up-regulation of GR expression that determines higher muscle glucocorticoid sensitivity, with the promotion of protein breakdown and blunted protein synthesis in muscles [222]. Prenatal growth restriction caused by adverse intrauterine conditions of different etiology has a long-term influence on adiposity. Redistribution of body fat from the periphery to the central or visceral deposits that have a relatively higher level of GR expression and are thus more sensitive to glucocorticoid action is established in adult rats and sheep prenatally exposed to glucocorticoid excess [223-225], contributing to decreased insulin sensitivity and blunted glucose intake [2]. Adipocytes from 15-month-old low-protein rat offspring are also resistant to the antilipolytic action of insulin and insulin-induced glucose uptake [25]. It can be concluded that adverse conditions during critical periods may program adipocyte metabolism to give rise to later obesity and type 2 diabetes, especially when challenged postnatally with a hypercaloric diet [226]. Suboptimal conditions during fetal development program an increased level of liver GR expression that enables much higher glucocorticoid impact in diabetic animals [227]. Down-regulation of glucokinase activity in parallel with decreased liver glucose uptake, and up-regulation of gluconeogenic enzyme activities, notably phosphoenolpyruvate carboxykinase which catalyzes a rate-limiting step in gluconeogenesis, have been established in rats exposed to excessive glucocorticoids in utero [25, 228]. The programming effects established in glucocorticoid overexposed fetuses with restricted growth are thus directed toward enhanced glucose production and reduced glucose utilization in the liver and other peripheral tissues in adulthood, and represent the structural and physiological basis of the development of type 2 diabetes [19].

4.5. Programming of hipothalamic-pituitary-gonadal axis

Steroid hormone excess during fetal life, including glucocorticoids and sex hormones, is well known to induce permanent alterations in the physiology of the adult HPG axis in both sexes [229]. The majority of data describing the effects of elevated levels of glucocorticoids on the HPG axis and possible mechanisms, come from studies in adults, and there are only limited data on fetal effects. It has been known that the HPA axis, when activated by stress, exerts an inhibitory effect on the female and male reproductive system. Reallocation of resources during the stress response suppresses the reproductive axis, which gives higher priority to an individual's survival rather than the maintenance of species. This effect is responsible for the "hypothalamic amenorrhea of stress" in females, which is observed in anxiety and depression, malnutrition, eating disorders and chronic excessive exercise, and the hypogonadism in Cushing's syndrome [230]. Stressors trigger a rise in glucocorticoids that suppress reproductive functions along the HPG axis [3]. Glucocorticoids decrease expression of GnRH mRNA [231] in the hypothalamus, and are associated with alterations in both FSH and LH cells [232, 233]. Glucocorticoids also affect gonads directly. It has been reported that dexamethasone inhibits ovarian function in immature female rats and the differentiation of granulosa cells by FSH [234]. In the testis, elevated levels of glucocorticoids suppress testosterone biosynthesis [3]. Additionally, dexamethasone induces apoptosis of tubules and germ cells in adult rat testis [235].

Elevation of maternal glucocorticoids induced by maternal stress, undernutrition or exogenously administered dexamethasone or betamethasone, along with IUGR cause alterations in HPG axis function in male and female offspring. The major alterations reported were related to changed sexual behavior, delayed puberty, and delayed development of the gonads. In rats, exposure to prenatal stress demasculinizes and feminizes the behavior of the male offspring. When dams are restrained under bright light from days 14 to 21 of gestation, the male offspring display reduced anogenital distance and lower testis weight at birth compared to controls [18, 236], which could predict impaired sexual activity at adulthood [237]. Prenatal treatment with glucocorticoids caused the disappearance of sexual dimorphism of aromatase activity in the brain preoptic area of rat pups in early postnatal life [238]. Prenatal bethamethasone treatment diminished the testosterone peak in male pups, a peak crucial for brain sexual differentiation. As a consequence, this prenatal treatment may have impaired the hypothalamus–pituitary axis, thus reducing production of testosterone in adulthood and altering the partner preference and sexual behavior [239].

It has been reported that maternal protein restriction altered the key components of pregnant maternal steroid endocrinology, as well as the endocrinology of the offspring. Maternal corticosterone and testosterone levels were elevated, which resulted in an increased anogenital distance in males [240]. In females exposed to protein restriction during development the onset of puberty was delayed and the cycle length was increased [241]. The decrease of LH and slight, but not significant, decrease of FSH levels was detected in adult females that experienced maternal protein restriction at some stage of development. Together with the increases in testosterone levels at 1 year, this presage potential reproductive problems, including changes in the ovarian cycle [241]. Maternal protein restriction leads to similar changes in reproductive hormones in the male offspring [240], indicating that a major effect of the challenge imposed on the developing offspring is to alter hypothalamic–pituitary endocrine function. The reproductive function aged more rapidly in females that had been exposed to protein restriction during development [241]. Testicular and ovarian growth was drastically retarded, and the onset of puberty was delayed in male and female rats prenatally exposed to maternal food restriction [242]. In addition, the ovulation rate in adulthood was reduced in female sheep that experienced undernutrition during the prenatal period [243]. The suggested main mechanism by which maternal calorie restriction induced delay of puberty in the female offspring is that decreased function of the kisspeptin system retards the development of reproductive function and the onset of puberty. Hypothalamic levels of Kiss1 mRNA were decreased in prenatally undernourished rats, and the replacement of kisspeptin normalized the timing of vaginal opening in these females [244]. However, this mechanism is not responsible for delaying puberty in dexamethasone-induced IUGR females, since the levels of Kiss1 mRNA were not altered [245]. On the other hand, alterations of ovarian functions found in dexamethasone-induced IUGR rats, can affect sexual maturation [246]. As ovarian weight in the dexamethasone-induced IUGR rats was lower than in the controls during the prepubertal period (postnatal day 28), but not on the day of vaginal opening, the retardation of ovarian function development might be involved in the delayed onset of puberty [245]. Smith and Waddell [247] have shown that variations in fetal glucocorticoid exposure across the normal physiological range are capable of influencing the timing of subsequent puberty. Puberty was substantially delayed by increased exposure to glucocorticoids, which was most clearly evident in female offspring. Of particular importance were the observations that increased exposure of the fetus to endogenous maternal glucocorticoids (via inhibition of placental 11β-HSD by carbenoxolone treatment) delayed puberty in the female offspring, whereas an experimental reduction in fetal glucocorticoid exposure (by maternal metyrapone treatment) advanced puberty in the male offspring [247].

When higher multiple doses of dexamethasone were administered to dams between the 16th and 18th day of gestation, a significant reduction in body weight was recorded in near-term fetuses that persisted till the peripubertal period of life. The volume of pituitaries of the exposed females were also significanly reduced till the peripubertal period. The absolute number of both types of gonadotropic cells, obtained by design-based stereological methods, was decreased in the pituitaries of exposed females (Figure 7). As the pituitaries, the ovaries of exposed females were smaller than that of controls (Figure 8). Significant decrease in healthy, but an increase in atretic primordial follicles was observed in neonatal period (at 5 days of age) [246]. Alterations in the number of healthy and degenerated germinative cells were evident in fetuses as well, and sustained till the peripubertal period of life. Since the puberty was delayed in females exposed prenatally to dexamethasone, no *corpora lutea* were seen in their ovaries. In contrast, 3-5 *corpora lutea* were present in the ovaries of control females (Figure 8). However, the process of folliculogenesis remained unchanged, since the follicles at all stages of development seen in the ovaries of control females in the neonatal [246], infantile and peripubertal period, were present in the ovaries of females prenatally exposed to high levels of glucocorticoids. Therefore, a clear programming effect of dexamethasone was detected in the female HPG axis. It has been shown that glucocorticoids mediate changes in the dynamic balance between mitosis and apoptosis [248], and may be a mechanism for the control of total cell number in developing tissues and organs [249, 250]. This could be one of the mechanisms by which glucocorticoid overexposure affects the hypothalamic–pituitary–ovarian axis.

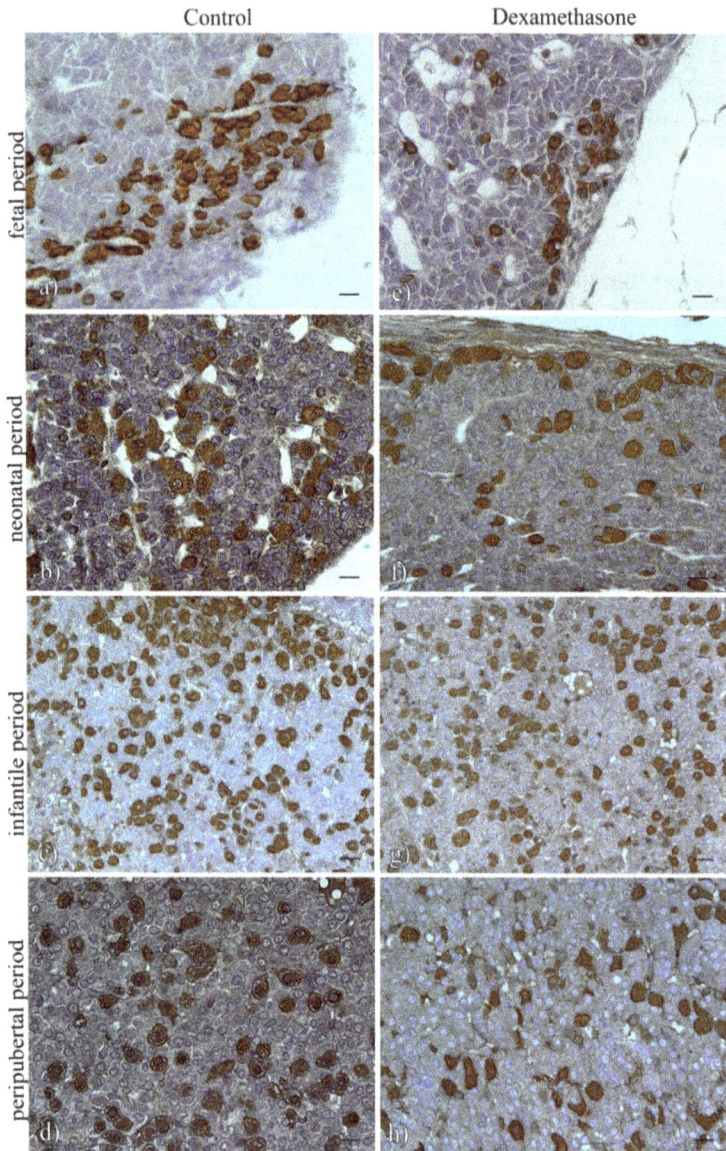

Figure 7. Immunohistochemically stained FSH cells in the pituitaries of control (a-d), and females prenatally exposed to dexamethasone (e-h). FSH cells were examined in different periods of life: in nearm-term fetal period (a, e), neonatal (b, f), infantile (c, g) and peripubertal period (d, h). In all examined periods the number of FSH cells was lower in the pituitaries of dexamethasone exposed females compared to controls. Bar - 20 μm.

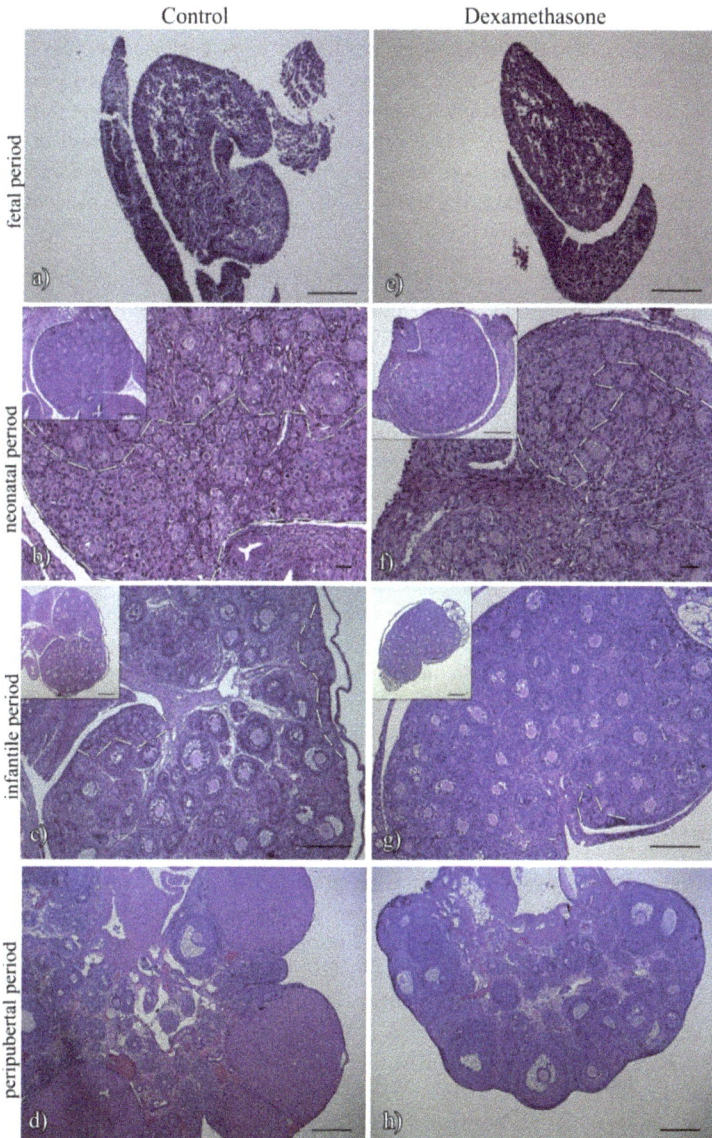

Figure 8. Ovaries of control (a-d), and females prenatally exposed to dexamethasone (e-h). Ovaries were examined in different periods of life: in nearm-term fetal period (a, e), neonatal (b, f), infantile (c, g) and peripubertal period (d, h) and they were smaller in dexamethasone exposed females. Numerous primordial follicles (dashed line) are present in the ovaries of control females, while they were fewer in number in the ovaries of dexamethasone exposed rats in all examined periods of life. Bar - 200 μm. In b) and f) bar - 20 μm.

Maternal bethamethasone administration affected the morphological development of the testes in male sheep fetuses, by reducing the length of testicular cords, the amount of interstitial tissue and testicular weight. Because interstitial tissue is primarily made up of Leydig cells, it is possible that betamethasone altered Leydig cell development. In contrast, there was no inhibitory effect on Sertoli cell number. This could be a result of the direct influence of the glucocorticoid used, since the presence of glucocorticoid receptor was demonstrated in ovine fetal Leydig cells, while the level of glucocorticoid receptor expression in Sertoli cells was low [251].

Fetal overexposure to glucocrticoids without any doubt has programming effects on the HPG axis, and reproduction in later life is thus impaired in both sexes. However, the mechanism of HPG programming is yet to be elucidated. The time interval between the exact insult and a fully functioning HPG axis is long, and prone to influences and interplay with other endocrine axes that are also altered by glucocrticoid overexposure. For example, an impaired somatotropic axis negatively affects reproduction. Somatostatin treatment inhibits pituitary gonadotropic cells and initial folliculogenesis in the ovaries of infant, peripubertal and adult females [252-257]. Polycystic ovary syndrome (PCOS) is of great importance, owing to its prevalence in up to 10% of the women population of reproductive age. Besides being characterized by perturbed gonadotropin secretion and excess production of androgens, PCOS shares a lot of commons with the metabolic syndrome. Metabolic syndrome is also believed to be of fetal origin and the result of programming in which glucocorticoids play a crucial role [213]. The short-term benefits of glucocorticoid exposure are also difficult to establish due to physiological dormancy of the system till puberty. The maturational effect of glucocorticoids is evident in the pituitary and in the ovary, since fetal overexposure induces a decreased volume of these glands, and of the absolute number of gonadotrops and ovarian somatic and germinative cells till puberty (Figure 1).

5. Conclusion

Glucocorticoids have a powerful influence on growth, maturation and tissue remodeling during fetal development. Their use in human pregnancies at risk of preterm delivery reduces neonatal mortality and morbidity. Glucocorticoids are also the key mediators between the maternal environment and the fetus, and their levels rise, in the mother and in the fetus, when the conditions are suboptimal. They reduce fetal growth, force maturational processes and provoke permanent changes in physiological systems in order to adapt the fetus to an adverse postnatal environment and ensure the maximum chances of survival at birth. These short-term beneficial effects of prenatal glucocorticoids are, at the same time, the ones that increase the long-term risks of dysregulation of the metabolic function and endocrine axes, including stress response, growth and reproduction.

Author details

Milica Manojlović-Stojanoski, Nataša Nestorović and Verica Milošević
University of Belgrade, Institute for Biological Research „Siniša Stanković", Serbia

Acknowledgments

This work was supported by the Ministry of Education and Science of the Republic of Serbia, Grant No. 173009

6. References

[1] Hayashi R, Wada H, Ito K, Adcock IM (2004) Effects of Glucocorticoids on Gene Transcription. Eur. j. pharmacol. 500: 51-62.

[2] Rose AJ, Vegiopoulos A, Herzig S (2010) Role of Glucocorticoids and the Glucocorticoid Receptor in Metabolism: Insights from Genetic Manipulations. J. steroid biochem. mol. biol. 122: 10-20.

[3] Whirledge S, Cidlowski JA (2010) Glucocorticoids, Stress, and Fertility. Minerva endocrinol. 35: 109-125.

[4] Mitani F, Mukai K, Miyamoto H, Suematsu M, Ishimura Y (1999) Development of Functional Zonation in the Rat Adrenal Cortex. Endocrinology. 140: 3342-3353.

[5] Condon J, Gosden C, Gardener D, Nickson P, Hewison M, Howie AJ, Stewart PM (1998) Expression of Type 2 11beta-Hydroxysteroid Dehydrogenase and Corticosteroid Hormone Receptors in Early Human Fetal Life. J. clin. endocrinol. metab. 83: 4490-4497.

[6] Kitraki E, Kittas C, Stylianopoulou F (1997) Glucocorticoid Receptor Gene Expression During Rat Embryogenesis. An in Situ Hybridization Study. Differentiation. 62: 21-31.

[7] Miller WL (1998) Steroid Hormone Biosynthesis and Actions in the Materno-Feto-Placental Unit. Clin. perinatol. 25: 799-817.

[8] Flagel SB, Vazquez DM, Watson SJ, Jr., Neal CR, Jr. (2002) Effects of Tapering Neonatal Dexamethasone on Rat Growth, Neurodevelopment, and Stress Response. Am. j. physiol. regul. integr. comp. physiol. 282: R55-63.

[9] Gesina E, Blondeau B, Milet A, Le Nin I, Duchene B, Czernichow P, Scharfmann R, Tronche F, Breant B (2006) Glucocorticoid Signalling Affects Pancreatic Development through Both Direct and Indirect Effects. Diabetologia. 49: 2939-2947.

[10] Fowden AL, Forhead AJ (2011) Adrenal Glands Are Essential for Activation of Glucogenesis During Undernutrition in Fetal Sheep near Term. Am. j. physiol. endocrinol. metab. 300: E94-102.

[11] Fowden AL, Li J, Forhead AJ (1998) Glucocorticoids and the Preparation for Life after Birth: Are There Long-Term Consequences of the Life Insurance? Proc. nutr. soc. 57: 113-122.

[12] Harris A, Seckl J (2011) Glucocorticoids, Prenatal Stress and the Programming of Disease. Horm. behav. 59: 279-289.

[13] Bloomfield FH, Oliver MH, Giannoulias CD, Gluckman PD, Harding JE, Challis JR (2003) Brief Undernutrition in Late-Gestation Sheep Programs the Hypothalamic-Pituitary-Adrenal Axis in Adult Offspring. Endocrinology. 144: 2933-2940.

[14] Belkacemi L, Jelks A, Chen CH, Ross MG, Desai M (2011) Altered Placental Development in Undernourished Rats: Role of Maternal Glucocorticoids. Reprod. biol. endocrinol. 9: 105.

[15] Lesage J, Del-Favero F, Leonhardt M, Louvart H, Maccari S, Vieau D, Darnaudery M (2004) Prenatal Stress Induces Intrauterine Growth Restriction and Programmes Glucose Intolerance and Feeding Behaviour Disturbances in the Aged Rat. J. endocrinol. 181: 291-296.

[16] Kapoor A, Leen J, Matthews SG (2008) Molecular Regulation of the Hypothalamic-Pituitary-Adrenal Axis in Adult Male Guinea Pigs after Prenatal Stress at Different Stages of Gestation. J. physiol. 586: 4317-4326.

[17] Godfrey KM (2002) The Role of the Placenta in Fetal Programming-a Review. Placenta. 23 Suppl A: S20-27.

[18] Mairesse J, Lesage J, Breton C, Breant B, Hahn T, Darnaudery M, Dickson SL, Seckl J, Blondeau B, Vieau D, Maccari S, Viltart O (2007) Maternal Stress Alters Endocrine Function of the Feto-Placental Unit in Rats. Am. j. physiol. endocrinol. metab. 292: E1526-1533.

[19] Seckl JR, Meaney MJ (2004) Glucocorticoid Programming. Ann. NY. acad. sci. 1032: 63-84.

[20] Sloboda DM, Moss TJ, Li S, Matthews SG, Challis JR, Newnham JP (2008) Expression of Glucocorticoid Receptor, Mineralocorticoid Receptor, and 11beta-Hydroxysteroid Dehydrogenase 1 and 2 in the Fetal and Postnatal Ovine Hippocampus: Ontogeny and Effects of Prenatal Glucocorticoid Exposure. J. endocrinol. 197: 213-220.

[21] Matthews SG (2002) Early Programming of the Hypothalamo-Pituitary-Adrenal Axis. Trends. endocrinol. metab. 13: 373-380.

[22] Fowden AL, Gardner DS, Ousey JC, Giussani DA, Forhead AJ (2005) Maturation of Pancreatic Beta-Cell Function in the Fetal Horse During Late Gestation. J. endocrinol. 186: 467-473.

[23] Barker DJ, Eriksson JG, Forsen T, Osmond C (2002) Fetal Origins of Adult Disease: Strength of Effects and Biological Basis. Int. j. epidemiol. 31: 1235-1239.

[24] Fowden AL, Forhead AJ (2009) Endocrine Regulation of Feto-Placental Growth. Horm. res. 72: 257-265.

[25] Ozanne SE, Hales CN (2002) Early Programming of Glucose-Insulin Metabolism. Trends. endocrinol. metab. 13: 368-373.

[26] Hales CN, Barker DJ (1992) Type 2 (Non-Insulin-Dependent) Diabetes Mellitus: The Thrifty Phenotype Hypothesis. Diabetologia. 35: 595-601.

[27] Langley-Evans S, Jackson A (1996) Intrauterine Programming of Hypertension: Nutrient-Hormone Interactions. Nutr. rev. 54: 163-169.

[28] Luo ZC, Xiao L, Nuyt AM (2010) Mechanisms of Developmental Programming of the Metabolic Syndrome and Related Disorders. World. j. diabetes. 1: 89-98.

[29] Vickers MH (2011) Developmental Programming of the Metabolic Syndrome - Critical Windows for Intervention. World. j. diabetes. 2: 137-148.

[30] Osamura RY, Egashira N, Recent Developments in Molecular Embryogenesis and Molecular Biology of the Pituitary, in: Loyd RV (Ed.), Endocrine Pathology Differential

Diagnosis and Molecular Advances, Springer, New York Dordrecht Heidelberg London, 2010. pp. 91-103.

[31] Nemeskeri A, Setalo G, Halasz B (1988) Ontogenesis of the Three Parts of the Fetal Rat Adenohypophysis. A Detailed Immunohistochemical Analysis. Neuroendocrinology. 48: 534-543.

[32] Chatelain A, Dupouy JP, Dubois MP (1979) Ontogenesis of Cells Producing Polypeptide Hormones (Acth, Msh, Lph, Gh, Prolactin) in the Fetal Hypophysis of the Rat: Influence of the Hypothalamus. Cell. tissue. res. 196: 409-427.

[33] Nemeskeri A, Halasz B (1989) Cultured Fetal Rat Pituitaries Kept in Synthetic Medium Are Able to Initiate Synthesis of Trophic Hormones. Cell. tissue. res. 255: 645-650.

[34] Pilavdzic D, Kovacs K, Asa SL (1997) Pituitary Morphology in Anencephalic Human Fetuses. Neuroendocrinology. 65: 164-172.

[35] Daikoku S, Okamura Y, Kawano H, Tsuruo Y, Maegawa M, Shibasaki T (1984) Immunohistochemical Study on the Development of Crf-Containing Neurons in the Hypothalamus of the Rat. Cell. tissue. res. 238: 539-544.

[36] Chatelain A, Dupouy JP (1981) Adrenocorticotrophic Hormone in the Anterior and Neurointermediate Lobes of the Fetal Rat Pituitary Gland. J. endocrinol. 89: 181-186.

[37] Challis JR, Sloboda D, Matthews SG, Holloway A, Alfaidy N, Patel FA, Whittle W, Fraser M, Moss TJ, Newnham J (2001) The Fetal Placental Hypothalamic-Pituitary-Adrenal (Hpa) Axis, Parturition and Post Natal Health. Mol. cell. endocrinol. 185: 135-144.

[38] Stojanoski MM, Nestorovic N, Filipovic B, Milosevic V (2004) Acth-Producing Cells of 21-Day-Old Rat Fetuses after Maternal Dexamethasone Exposure. Acta histochem. 106: 199-205.

[39] Muscatelli F, Strom TM, Walker AP, Zanaria E, Recan D, Meindl A, Bardoni B, Guioli S, Zehetner G, Rabl W, et al. (1994) Mutations in the Dax-1 Gene Give Rise to Both X-Linked Adrenal Hypoplasia Congenita and Hypogonadotropic Hypogonadism. Nature. 372: 672-676.

[40] Rogler LE, Pintar JE (1993) Expression of the P450 Side-Chain Cleavage and Adrenodoxin Genes Begins During Early Stages of Adrenal Cortex Development. Mol. endocrinol. 7: 453-461.

[41] Nussdorfer G, Mazzocchi G, Rebonato L (1971) Long-Term Trophic Effect of Acth on Rat Adrenocortical Cells. An Ultrastructural, Morphometric and Autoradiographic Study. Z. zellforsch. mikrosk. anat. 115: 30-45.

[42] Manolović-Stojanoski M, Nestorović N, Negić N, Filipović B, Šošić-Jurjević B, Milošević V, Sekulić M (2006) The Pituitary-Adrenal Axis of Fetal Rats after Maternal Dedxamethasone Exposure. Anat. embryol. 61-69.

[43] Wotus C, Levay-Young BK, Rogers LM, Gomez-Sanchez CE, Engeland WC (1998) Development of Adrenal Zonation in Fetal Rats Defined by Expression of Aldosterone Synthase and 11beta-Hydroxylase. Endocrinology. 139: 4397-4403.

[44] Mitani F, Mukai K, Ogawa T, Miyamoto H, Ishimura Y (1997) Expression of Cytochromes P450aldo and P45011 Beta in Rat Adrenal Gland During Late Gestational and Neonatal Stages. Steroids. 62: 57-61.

[45] Hristić M, Kalafatić D, Plećaš B, Jovanović V (1995) The Effect of Dexamethasone on the Adrenal Gland in Fetal and Neonatal Rats. J. exp. zool. 272: 281-290.

[46] Hristić M, Kalafatić D, Plećaš B, Manojlović M (1997) The Influence of Prolonged Dexamethasone Treatment of Pregnant Rats on the Perinatal Development of the Adrenal Gland of Their Offspring. J. exp. zool. 279: 54-61.

[47] Bolt RJ, van Weissenbruch MM, Lafeber HN, Delemarre-van de Waal HA (2002) Development of the Hypothalamic-Pituitary-Adrenal Axis in the Fetus and Preterm Infant. J. pediatr. endocrinol. metab. 15: 759-769.

[48] Mesiano S, Jaffe RB (1997) Developmental and Functional Biology of the Primate Fetal Adrenal Cortex. Endocr. rev. 18: 378-403.

[49] Blumenfeld Z, Jaffe RB (1986) Hypophysiotropic and Neuromodulatory Regulation of Adrenocorticotropin in the Human Fetal Pituitary Gland. J. clin. invest. 78: 288-294.

[50] Gluckman PD, Sizonenko SV, Bassett NS (1999) The Transition from Fetus to Neonate--an Endocrine Perspective. Acta. paediatr. suppl. 88: 7-11.

[51] Reichardt HM, Schutz G (1996) Feedback Control of Glucocorticoid Production Is Established During Fetal Development. Mol. med. 2: 735-744.

[52] Ducsay CA (1998) Fetal and Maternal Adaptations to Chronic Hypoxia: Prevention of Premature Labor in Response to Chronic Stress. Comp. biochem. physiol. a mol. integr. physiol. 119: 675-681.

[53] Slotkin TA, Lappi SE, McCook EC, Tayyeb MI, Eylers JP, Seidler FJ (1992) Glucocorticoids and the Development of Neuronal Function: Effects of Prenatal Dexamethasone Exposure on Central Noradrenergic Activity. Biol. neonate. 61: 326-336.

[54] Muneoka K, Mikuni M, Ogawa T, Kitera K, Kamei K, Takigawa M, Takahashi K (1997) Prenatal Dexamethasone Exposure Alters Brain Monoamine Metabolism and Adrenocortical Response in Rat Offspring. Am. j. physiol. 273: R1669-1675.

[55] Seidl K, Unsicker K (1989) The Determination of the Adrenal Medullary Cell Fate During Embryogenesis. Dev. biol. 136: 481-490.

[56] Michelsohn AM, Anderson DJ (1992) Changes in Competence Determine the Timing of Two Sequential Glucocorticoid Effects on Sympathoadrenal Progenitors. Neuron. 8: 589-604.

[57] Pratt L, Magness RR, Phernetton T, Hendricks SK, Abbott DH, Bird IM (1999) Repeated Use of Betamethasone in Rabbits: Effects of Treatment Variation on Adrenal Suppression, Pulmonary Maturation, and Pregnancy Outcome. Am. j. obstet. gynecol. 180: 995-1005.

[58] Pearce S, Mostyn A, Alves-Guerra MC, Pecqueur C, Miroux B, Webb R, Stephenson T, Symond ME (2003) Prolactin, Prolactin Receptor and Uncoupling Proteins During Fetal and Neonatal Development. Proc. nutr. soc. 62: 421-427.

[59] Gnanalingham MG, Mostyn A, Forhead AJ, Fowden AL, Symonds ME, Stephenson T (2005) Increased Uncoupling Protein-2 mRNA Abundance and Glucocorticoid Action in

Adipose Tissue in the Sheep Fetus During Late Gestation Is Dependent on Plasma Cortisol and Triiodothyronine. J. physiol. 567: 283-292.

[60] Myers DA, Hanson K, Mlynarczyk M, Kaushal KM, Ducsay CA (2008) Long-Term Hypoxia Modulates Expression of Key Genes Regulating Adipose Function in the Late-Gestation Ovine Fetus. Am. j. physiol. regul. integr. comp. physiol. 294: R1312-1318.

[61] Nakae J, Kido Y, Accili D (2001) Distinct and Overlapping Functions of Insulin and IGF-I Receptors. Endocr. rev. 22: 818-835.

[62] Lupu F, Terwilliger JD, Lee K, Segre GV, Efstratiadis A (2001) Roles of Growth Hormone and Insulin-Like Growth Factor 1 in Mouse Postnatal Growth. Dev. biol. 229: 141-162.

[63] Murakami S, Salmon A, Miller RA (2003) Multiplex Stress Resistance in Cells from Long-Lived Dwarf Mice. FASEB. J. 17: 1565-1566.

[64] Cella SG, Locatelli V, Broccia ML, Menegola E, Giavini E, De Gennaro Colonna V, Torsello A, Wehrenberg WB, Muller EE (1994) Long-Term Changes of Somatotrophic Function Induced by Deprivation of Growth Hormone-Releasing Hormone During the Fetal Life of the Rat. J. endocrinol. 140: 111-117.

[65] Baram TZ, Lerner SP (1991) Ontogeny of Corticotropin Releasing Hormone Gene Expression in Rat Hypothalamus--Comparison with Somatostatin. Int. j. dev. neurosci. 9: 473-478.

[66] Rodriguez-Garcia M, Jolin T, Santos A, Perez-Castillo A (1995) Effect of Perinatal Hypothyroidism on the Developmental Regulation of Rat Pituitary Growth Hormone and Thyrotropin Genes. Endocrinology. 136: 4339-4350.

[67] Savage JJ, Yaden BC, Kiratipranon P, Rhodes SJ (2003) Transcriptional Control During Mammalian Anterior Pituitary Development. Gene. 319: 1-19.

[68] Taniguchi Y, Yasutaka S, Kominami R, Shinohara H (2001) Proliferation and Differentiation of Thyrotrophs in the Pars Distalis of the Rat Pituitary Gland During the Fetal and Postnatal Period. Anat. embryol. (Berl). 203: 249-253.

[69] Korytko AI, Zeitler P, Cuttler L (1996) Developmental Regulation of Pituitary Growth Hormone-Releasing Hormone Receptor Gene Expression in the Rat. Endocrinology. 137: 1326-1331.

[70] Nogami H, Inoue K, Moriya H, Ishida A, Kobayashi S, Hisano S, Katayama M, Kawamura K (1999) Regulation of Growth Hormone-Releasing Hormone Receptor Messenger Ribonucleic Acid Expression by Glucocorticoids in Mtt-S Cells and in the Pituitary Gland of Fetal Rats. Endocrinology. 140: 2763-2770.

[71] Sanders EJ, Harvey S (2004) Growth Hormone as an Early Embryonic Growth and Differentiation Factor. Anat. embryol. (Berl). 209: 1-9.

[72] Rodier PM, Kates B, White WA, Phelps CJ (1990) Birthdates of the Growth Hormone Releasing Factor Cells of the Rat Hypothalamus: An Autoradiographic Study of Immunocytochemically Identified Neurons. J. comp. neurol. 291: 363-372.

[73] Mulchahey JJ, DiBlasio AM, Martin MC, Blumenfeld Z, Jaffe RB (1987) Hormone Production and Peptide Regulation of the Human Fetal Pituitary Gland. Endocr. rev. 8: 406-425.

[74] Hill DJ, Petrik J, Arany E (1998) Growth Factors and the Regulation of Fetal Growth. Diabetes care. 21 Suppl 2: B60-69.

[75] Daughaday WH, Parker KA, Borowsky S, Trivedi B, Kapadia M (1982) Measurement of Somatomedin-Related Peptides in Fetal, Neonatal, and Maternal Rat Serum by Insulin-Like Growth Factor (IGF) I Radioimmunoassay, IGF-II Radioreceptor Assay (Rra), and Multiplication-Stimulating Activity Rra after Acid-Ethanol Extraction. Endocrinology. 110: 575-581.

[76] Straus DS, Ooi GT, Orlowski CC, Rechler MM (1991) Expression of the Genes for Insulin-Like Growth Factor-I (IGF-I), IGF-II, and IGF-Binding Proteins-1 and -2 in Fetal Rat under Conditions of Intrauterine Growth Retardation Caused by Maternal Fasting. Endocrinology. 128: 518-525.

[77] Gluckman PD, Butler JH (1983) Parturition-Related Changes in Insulin-Like Growth Factors-I and -II in the Perinatal Lamb. J. endocrinol. 99: 223-232.

[78] Lee JE, Pintar J, Efstratiadis A (1990) Pattern of the Insulin-Like Growth Factor II Gene Expression During Early Mouse Embryogenesis. Development. 110: 151-159.

[79] Li J, Gilmour RS, Saunders JC, Dauncey MJ, Fowden AL (1999) Activation of the Adult Mode of Ovine Growth Hormone Receptor Gene Expression by Cortisol During Late Fetal Development. FASEB J. 13: 545-552.

[80] Allan GJ, Flint DJ, Patel K (2001) Insulin-Like Growth Factor Axis During Embryonic Development. Reproduction. 122: 31-39.

[81] Brown RS, Shalhoub V, Coulter S, Alex S, Joris I, De Vito W, Lian J, Stein GS (2000) Developmental Regulation of Thyrotropin Receptor Gene Expression in the Fetal and Neonatal Rat Thyroid: Relation to Thyroid Morphology and to Thyroid-Specific Gene Expression. Endocrinology. 141: 340-345.

[82] Oliver C, Eskay RL, Porter JC (1980) Developmental Changes in Brain Trh and in Plasma and Pituitary Tsh and Prolactin Levels in the Rat. Biol. neonate. 37: 145-152.

[83] Murakami M, Mori M, Kato Y, Kobayashi I (1991) Hypothalamic Thyrotropin-Releasing Hormone Regulates Pituitary Thyrotropin Beta- and Alpha-Subunit mRNA Levels in the Rat. Neuroendocrinology. 53: 276-280.

[84] Parlato R, Rosica A, Rodriguez-Mallon A, Affuso A, Postiglione MP, Arra C, Mansouri A, Kimura S, Di Lauro R, De Felice M (2004) An Integrated Regulatory Network Controlling Survival and Migration in Thyroid Organogenesis. Dev. biol. 276: 464-475.

[85] Kimura S, Hara Y, Pineau T, Fernandez-Salguero P, Fox CH, Ward JM, Gonzalez FJ (1996) The T/Ebp Null Mouse: Thyroid-Specific Enhancer-Binding Protein Is Essential for the Organogenesis of the Thyroid, Lung, Ventral Forebrain, and Pituitary. Genes dev. 10: 60-69.

[86] Mansouri A, Chowdhury K, Gruss P (1998) Follicular Cells of the Thyroid Gland Require Pax8 Gene Function. Nat. genet. 19: 87-90.

[87] Gereben B, Zavacki AM, Ribich S, Kim BW, Huang SA, Simonides WS, Zeold A, Bianco AC (2008) Cellular and Molecular Basis of Deiodinase-Regulated Thyroid Hormone Signaling. Endocr. rev. 29: 898-938.

[88] Kester MH, Martinez de Mena R, Obregon MJ, Marinkovic D, Howatson A, Visser TJ, Hume R, Morreale de Escobar G (2004) Iodothyronine Levels in the Human Developing Brain: Major Regulatory Roles of Iodothyronine Deiodinases in Different Areas. J. clin. endocrinol. metab. 89: 3117-3128.

[89] Obregon MJ, Escobar del Rey F, Morreale de Escobar G (2005) The Effects of Iodine Deficiency on Thyroid Hormone Deiodination. Thyroid. 15: 917-929.

[90] Obregon MJ, Calvo RM, Del Rey FE, de Escobar GM (2007) Ontogenesis of Thyroid Function and Interactions with Maternal Function. Endocr. dev. 10: 86-98.

[91] Patel J, Landers K, Li H, Mortimer RH, Richard K (2011) Thyroid Hormones and Fetal Neurological Development. J. endocrinol. 209: 1-8.

[92] Ashizawa S, Brunicardi FC, Wang XP (2004) Pdx-1 and the Pancreas. Pancreas. 28: 109-120.

[93] Gu G, Dubauskaite J, Melton DA (2002) Direct Evidence for the Pancreatic Lineage: Ngn3+ Cells Are Islet Progenitors and Are Distinct from Duct Progenitors. Development. 129: 2447-2457.

[94] Zaret KS (2008) Genetic Programming of Liver and Pancreas Progenitors: Lessons for Stem-Cell Differentiation. Nat. rev. genet. 9: 329-340.

[95] Lackie PM, Zuber C, Roth J (1994) Polysialic Acid of the Neural Cell Adhesion Molecule (N-Cam) Is Widely Expressed During Organogenesis in Mesodermal and Endodermal Derivatives. Differentiation. 57: 119-131.

[96] Stefan Y, Grasso S, Perrelet A, Orci L (1983) A Quantitative Immunofluorescent Study of the Endocrine Cell Populations in the Developing Human Pancreas. Diabetes. 32: 293-301.

[97] Bonal C, Avril I, Herrera PL (2008) Experimental Models of Beta-Cell Regeneration. Biochem. soc. trans. 36: 286-289.

[98] Aye T, Toschi E, Sharma A, Sgroi D, Bonner-Weir S (2010) Identification of Markers for Newly Formed Beta-Cells in the Perinatal Period: A Time of Recognized Beta-Cell Immaturity. J. histochem. cytochem. 58: 369-376.

[99] Cabrera-Vasquez S, Navarro-Tableros V, Sanchez-Soto C, Gutierrez-Ospina G, Hiriart M (2009) Remodelling Sympathetic Innervation in Rat Pancreatic Islets Ontogeny. BMC dev. biol. 9: 34.

[100] Ammon HP, Glocker C, Waldner RG, Wahl MA (1989) Insulin Release from Pancreatic Islets of Fetal Rats Mediated by Leucine B-Bch, Tolbutamide, Glibenclamide, Arginine, Potassium Chloride, and Theophylline Does Not Require Stimulation of Ca2+ Net Uptake. Cell calcium. 10: 441-450.

[101] Navarro-Tableros V, Fiordelisio T, Hernandez-Cruz A, Hiriart M (2007) Physiological Development of Insulin Secretion, Calcium Channels, and Glut2 Expression of Pancreatic Rat Beta-Cells. Am. j. physiol. endocrinol. metab. 292: E1018-1029.

[102] Jermendy A, Toschi E, Aye T, Koh A, Aguayo-Mazzucato C, Sharma A, Weir GC, Sgroi D, Bonner-Weir S (2011) Rat Neonatal Beta Cells Lack the Specialised Metabolic Phenotype of Mature Beta Cells. Diabetologia. 54: 594-604.

[103] Hoglund E, Mattsson G, Tyrberg B, Andersson A, Carlsson C (2009) Growth Hormone Increases Beta-Cell Proliferation in Transplanted Human and Fetal Rat Islets. JOP. 10: 242-248.

[104] Aubert ML, Begeot M, Winiger BP, Morel G, Sizonenko PC, Dubois PM (1985) Ontogeny of Hypothalamic Luteinizing Hormone-Releasing Hormone (Gnrh) and Pituitary Gnrh Receptors in Fetal and Neonatal Rats. Endocrinology. 116: 1565-1576.

[105] Jorgensen JS, Quirk CC, Nilson JH (2004) Multiple and Overlapping Combinatorial Codes Orchestrate Hormonal Responsiveness and Dictate Cell-Specific Expression of the Genes Encoding Luteinizing Hormone. Endocr. rev. 25: 521-542.

[106] Parker KL, Schimmer BP (1997) Steroidogenic Factor 1: A Key Determinant of Endocrine Development and Function. Endocr. rev. 18: 361-377.

[107] Zhu X, Gleiberman AS, Rosenfeld MG (2007) Molecular Physiology of Pituitary Development: Signaling and Transcriptional Networks. Physiol. rev. 87: 933-963.

[108] Wen S, Ai W, Alim Z, Boehm U (2010) Embryonic Gonadotropin-Releasing Hormone Signaling Is Necessary for Maturation of the Male Reproductive Axis. Proc. natl. acad. sci. U S A. 107: 16372-16377.

[109] Winter JS, Faiman C, Reyes FI (1977) Sex Steroid Production by the Human Fetus: Its Role in Morphogenesis and Control by Gonadotropins. Birth defects. orig. artic. ser. 13: 41-58.

[110] Ginsburg M, Snow MH, McLaren A (1990) Primordial Germ Cells in the Mouse Embryo During Gastrulation. Development. 110: 521-528.

[111] Edson MA, Nagaraja AK, Matzuk MM (2009) The Mammalian Ovary from Genesis to Revelation. Endocr. rev. 30: 624-712.

[112] Gubbay J, Collignon J, Koopman P, Capel B, Economou A, Munsterberg A, Vivian N, Goodfellow P, Lovell-Badge R (1990) A Gene Mapping to the Sex-Determining Region of the Mouse Y Chromosome Is a Member of a Novel Family of Embryonically Expressed Genes. Nature. 346: 245-250.

[113] Sekido R, Bar I, Narvaez V, Penny G, Lovell-Badge R (2004) Sox9 Is up-Regulated by the Transient Expression of Sry Specifically in Sertoli Cell Precursors. Dev. biol. 274: 271-279.

[114] Eicher EM, Shown EP, Washburn LL (1995) Sex Reversal in C57bl/6j-Ypos Mice Corrected by a Sry Transgene. Philos. trans. r. soc. lond. b. biol. sci. 350: 263-268; discussion 268-269.

[115] Lovell-Badge R, Robertson E (1990) Xy Female Mice Resulting from a Heritable Mutation in the Primary Testis-Determining Gene, Tdy. Development. 109: 635-646.

[116] Brennan J, Capel B (2004) One Tissue, Two Fates: Molecular Genetic Events That Underlie Testis Versus Ovary Development. Nat. rev. genet. 5: 509-521.

[117] Adams IR, McLaren A (2002) Sexually Dimorphic Development of Mouse Primordial Germ Cells: Switching from Oogenesis to Spermatogenesis. Development. 129: 1155-1164.

[118] Nef S, Parada LF (1999) Cryptorchidism in Mice Mutant for Insl3. Nat. genet. 22: 295-299.

[119] Warren DW, Huhtaniemi IT, Tapanainen J, Dufau ML, Catt KJ (1984) Ontogeny of Gonadotropin Receptors in the Fetal and Neonatal Rat Testis. Endocrinology. 114: 470-476.

[120] Sokka TA, Hamalainen TM, Kaipia A, Warren DW, Huhtaniemi IT (1996) Development of Luteinizing Hormone Action in the Perinatal Rat Ovary. Biol. reprod. 55: 663-670.

[121] Meijs-Roelofs HM, de Greef WJ, Uilenbroek JT (1975) Plasma Progesterone and Its Relationship to Serum Gonadotrophins in Immature Female Rats. J. endocrinol. 64: 329-336.

[122] Sokka T, Huhtaniemi I (1990) Ontogeny of Gonadotrophin Receptors and Gonadotrophin-Stimulated Cyclic Amp Production in the Neonatal Rat Ovary. J. endocrinol. 127: 297-303.

[123] Couse JF, Hewitt SC, Bunch DO, Sar M, Walker VR, Davis BJ, Korach KS (1999) Postnatal Sex Reversal of the Ovaries in Mice Lacking Estrogen Receptors Alpha and Beta. Science. 286: 2328-2331.

[124] Britt KL, Drummond AE, Dyson M, Wreford NG, Jones ME, Simpson ER, Findlay JK (2001) The Ovarian Phenotype of the Aromatase Knockout (Arko) Mouse. J. steroid. biochem. mol. biol. 79: 181-185.

[125] Baker TG (1963) A Quantitative and Cytological Study of Germ Cells in Human Ovaries. Proc. r. soc. lond. b. biol. sci. 158: 417-433.

[126] Fulton N, Martins da Silva SJ, Bayne RA, Anderson RA (2005) Germ Cell Proliferation and Apoptosis in the Developing Human Ovary. J. clin. endocrinol. metab. 90: 4664-4670.

[127] Hunt PA, Hassold TJ (2008) Human Female Meiosis: What Makes a Good Egg Go Bad? Trends. genet. 24: 86-93.

[128] George FW, Wilson JD (1978) Conversion of Androgen to Estrogen by the Human Fetal Ovary. J. clin. endocrinol. metab. 47: 550-555.

[129] Gurpide E, Schwers J, Welch MT, Vande Wiele RL, Lieberman S (1966) Fetal and Maternal Metabolism of Estradiol During Pregnancy. J. clin. endocrinol. metab. 26: 1355-1365.

[130] Ostrer H, Huang HY, Masch RJ, Shapiro E (2007) A Cellular Study of Human Testis Development. Sex. dev. 1: 286-292.

[131] Reyes FI, Boroditsky RS, Winter JS, Faiman C (1974) Studies on Human Sexual Development. 2. Fetal and Maternal Serum Gonadotropin and Sex Steroid Concentrations. J. clin. endocrinol. metab. 38: 612-617.

[132] Takagi S, Yoshida T, Tsubata K, Ozaki H, Fujii TK, Nomura Y, Sawada M (1977) Sex Differences in Fetal Gonadotropins and Androgens. J. steroid. biochem. 8: 609-620.

[133] Barker DJP, Mothers, Babies and Disease in Later Life, BMJ Publishing, London, 1994.

[134] Gluckman PD, Hanson MA (2004) The Developmental Origins of the Metabolic Syndrome. Trends. endocrinol. metab. 15: 183-187.

[135] Lucas A (1991) Programming by Early Nutrition in Man. Ciba. found. symp. 156: 38-50; discussion 50-35.

[136] Roseboom T, de Rooij S, Painter R (2006) The Dutch Famine and Its Long-Term Consequences for Adult Health. Early hum. dev. 82: 485-491.

[137] Weinstock M, Fride E, Hertzberg R (1988) Prenatal Stress Effects on Functional Development of the Offspring. Prog. brain. res. 73: 319-331.

[138] Nathanielsz PW (2006) Animal Models That Elucidate Basic Principles of the Developmental Origins of Adult Diseases. ILAR J. 47: 73-82.

[139] Fowden AL, Forhead AJ (2004) Endocrine Mechanisms of Intrauterine Programming. Reproduction. 127: 515-526.

[140] Cottrell EC, Holmes MC, Livingstone DE, Kenyon CJ, Seckl JR (2012) Reconciling the Nutritional and Glucocorticoid Hypotheses of Fetal Programming. FASEB J. doi: 10.1096/fj.1012-203489.

[141] Fowden AL, Forhead AJ (2009) Hormones as Epigenetic Signals in Developmental Programming. Exp. physiol. 94: 607-625.

[142] Seckl JR (2004) Prenatal Glucocorticoids and Long-Term Programming. Eur. j. endocrinol. 151 Suppl 3: U49-62.

[143] Edwards CR, Benediktsson R, Lindsay RS, Seckl JR (1996) 11 Beta-Hydroxysteroid Dehydrogenases: Key Enzymes in Determining Tissue-Specific Glucocorticoid Effects. Steroids. 61: 263-269.

[144] Waddell BJ, Benediktsson R, Brown RW, Seckl JR (1998) Tissue-Specific Messenger Ribonucleic Acid Expression of 11beta-Hydroxysteroid Dehydrogenase Types 1 and 2 and the Glucocorticoid Receptor within Rat Placenta Suggests Exquisite Local Control of Glucocorticoid Action. Endocrinology. 139: 1517-1523.

[145] Wyrwoll CS, Holmes MC, Seckl JR (2011) 11beta-Hydroxysteroid Dehydrogenases and the Brain: From Zero to Hero, a Decade of Progress. Front. neuroendocrinol. 32: 265-286.

[146] Seckl JR (1997) Glucocorticoids, Feto-Placental 11 Beta-Hydroxysteroid Dehydrogenase Type 2, and the Early Life Origins of Adult Disease. Steroids. 62: 89-94.

[147] Wyrwoll CS, Seckl JR, Holmes MC (2009) Altered Placental Function of 11beta-Hydroxysteroid Dehydrogenase 2 Knockout Mice. Endocrinology. 150: 1287-1293.

[148] Brown RW, Diaz R, Robson AC, Kotelevtsev YV, Mullins JJ, Kaufman MH, Seckl JR (1996) The Ontogeny of 11 Beta-Hydroxysteroid Dehydrogenase Type 2 and Mineralocorticoid Receptor Gene Expression Reveal Intricate Control of Glucocorticoid Action in Development. Endocrinology. 137: 794-797.

[149] Lindsay RS, Lindsay RM, Edwards CR, Seckl JR (1996) Inhibition of 11-Beta-Hydroxysteroid Dehydrogenase in Pregnant Rats and the Programming of Blood Pressure in the Offspring. Hypertension. 27: 1200-1204.

[150] Kajantie E, Dunkel L, Turpeinen U, Stenman UH, Wood PJ, Nuutila M, Andersson S (2003) Placental 11 Beta-Hydroxysteroid Dehydrogenase-2 and Fetal Cortisol/Cortisone Shuttle in Small Preterm Infants. J. clin. endocrinol. metab. 88: 493-500.

[151] Williams MT, Davis HN, McCrea AE, Hennessy MB (1999) Stress During Pregnancy Alters the Offspring Hypothalamic, Pituitary, Adrenal, and Testicular Response to Isolation on the Day of Weaning. Neurotoxicol. teratol. 21: 653-659.

[152] Sinha P, Halasz I, Choi JF, McGivern RF, Redei E (1997) Maternal Adrenalectomy Eliminates a Surge of Plasma Dehydroepiandrosterone in the Mother and Attenuates the Prenatal Testosterone Surge in the Male Fetus. Endocrinology. 138: 4792-4797.

[153] Barbazanges A, Piazza PV, Le Moal M, Maccari S (1996) Maternal Glucocorticoid Secretion Mediates Long-Term Effects of Prenatal Stress. J. neurosci. 16: 3943-3949.

[154] Langley-Evans SC (1997) Hypertension Induced by Foetal Exposure to a Maternal Low-Protein Diet, in the Rat, Is Prevented by Pharmacological Blockade of Maternal Glucocorticoid Synthesis. J. hypertens. 15: 537-544.

[155] Halasz I, Rittenhouse PA, Zorrilla EP, Redei E (1997) Sexually Dimorphic Effects of Maternal Adrenalectomy on Hypothalamic Corticotrophin-Releasing Factor, Glucocorticoid Receptor and Anterior Pituitary POMC mRNA Levels in Rat Neonates. Brain. res. dev. brain. res. 100: 198-204.

[156] Fujioka T, Sakata Y, Yamaguchi K, Shibasaki T, Kato H, Nakamura S (1999) The Effects of Prenatal Stress on the Development of Hypothalamic Paraventricular Neurons in Fetal Rats. Neuroscience. 92: 1079-1088.

[157] Barker DJ, Bull AR, Osmond C, Simmonds SJ (1990) Fetal and Placental Size and Risk of Hypertension in Adult Life. BMJ. 301: 259-262.

[158] Bertram C, Trowern AR, Copin N, Jackson AA, Whorwood CB (2001) The Maternal Diet During Pregnancy Programs Altered Expression of the Glucocorticoid Receptor and Type 2 11beta-Hydroxysteroid Dehydrogenase: Potential Molecular Mechanisms Underlying the Programming of Hypertension in Utero. Endocrinology. 142: 2841-2853.

[159] Crowley PA (1995) Antenatal Corticosteroid Therapy: A Meta-Analysis of the Randomized Trials, 1972 to 1994. Am. j. obstet. gynecol. 173: 322-335.

[160] NIH (1994) Effect of Corticosteroids for Fetal Maturation on Perinatal Outcomes. NIH Consens Statement. 12: 1-24.

[161] Miracle X, Di Renzo GC, Stark A, Fanaroff A, Carbonell-Estrany X, Saling E (2008) Guideline for the Use of Antenatal Corticosteroids for Fetal Maturation. J. Perinat. Med. 36: 191-196.

[162] Ain R, Canham LN, Soares MJ (2005) Dexamethasone-Induced Intrauterine Growth Restriction Impacts the Placental Prolactin Family, Insulin-Like Growth Factor-Ii and the Akt Signaling Pathway. J. Endocrinol. 185: 253-263.

[163] Lajic S, Nordenstrom A, Ritzen EM, Wedell A (2004) Prenatal Treatment of Congenital Adrenal Hyperplasia. Eur. j. endocrinol. 151 Suppl 3: U63-69.

[164] Diederich S, Eigendorff E, Burkhardt P, Quinkler M, Bumke-Vogt C, Rochel M, Seidelmann D, Esperling P, Oelkers W, Bahr V (2002) 11beta-Hydroxysteroid Dehydrogenase Types 1 and 2: An Important Pharmacokinetic Determinant for the

Activity of Synthetic Mineralo- and Glucocorticoids. J. clin. endocrinol. metab. 87: 5695-5701.

[165] Melby JC (1977) Clinical Pharmacology of Systemic Corticosteroids. Annu. rev. pharmacol. toxicol. 17: 511-527.

[166] Gayrard V, Alvinerie M, Toutain PL (1996) Interspecies Variations of Corticosteroid-Binding Globulin Parameters. Domest anim endocrinol. 13: 35-45.

[167] Peets EA, Staub M, Symchowicz S (1969) Plasma Binding of Betamethasone-3h, Dexamethasone-3h, and Cortisol-14c--a Comparative Study. Biochem. pharmacol. 18: 1655-1663.

[168] Buttgereit F, Burmester GR, Brand MD (2000) Bioenergetics of Immune Functions: Fundamental and Therapeutic Aspects. Immunol. today. 21: 192-199.

[169] de Kloet ER, Reul JM, Sutanto W (1990) Corticosteroids and the Brain. J. steroid. biochem. mol. biol. 37: 387-394.

[170] Dean F, Matthews SG (1999) Maternal Dexamethasone Treatment in Late Gestation Alters Glucocorticoid and Mineralocorticoid Receptor mRNA in the Fetal Guinea Pig Brain. Brain res. 846: 253-259.

[171] McCabe L, Marash D, Li A, Matthews SG (2001) Repeated Antenatal Glucocorticoid Treatment Decreases Hypothalamic Corticotropin Releasing Hormone mRNA but Not Corticosteroid Receptor mRNA Expression in the Fetal Guinea-Pig Brain. J. neuroendocrinol. 13: 425-431.

[172] Noorlander CW, De Graan PN, Middeldorp J, Van Beers JJ, Visser GH (2006) Ontogeny of Hippocampal Corticosteroid Receptors: Effects of Antenatal Glucocorticoids in Human and Mouse. J. comp. neurol. 499: 924-932.

[173] Levitt NS, Lindsay RS, Holmes MC, Seckl JR (1996) Dexamethasone in the Last Week of Pregnancy Attenuates Hippocampal Glucocorticoid Receptor Gene Expression and Elevates Blood Pressure in the Adult Offspring in the Rat. Neuroendocrinology. 64: 412-418.

[174] Bakker JM, Schmidt ED, Kroes H, Kavelaars A, Heijnen CJ, Tilders FJ, van Rees EP (1995) Effects of Short-Term Dexamethasone Treatment During Pregnancy on the Development of the Immune System and the Hypothalamo-Pituitary Adrenal Axis in the Rat. J. neuroimmunol. 63: 183-191.

[175] Hristić M, Kalafatić D, Plećaš B, Mićić Z, Manojlović M (1997) The Paraventricular and Supraoptic Nuclei of Fetal and Neonatal Offspring of Rats Treated with Dexamethasone During Gestation. Acta vet. 47: 95-106.

[176] Kalafatić D, Manojlović-Stojanoski M, Plećaš B, Hristić M (2000) Development and Differentiation of the Nucleus Paraventricularis and Nucleus Supraopticus of the Hypothalamus During the Perinatal Period in Rats. Arch. biol. sci. 52: 19-20.

[177] Kalafatić D, Plećaš B, Hristić M, Manojlović M (1998) Manipulation of Prenatal Blood Glucocorticoid Level Affects Development of the Hipothalamic Paraventricular Nuclei in Rats. Biomed. res. 19: 293-301.

[178] Welberg LA, Seckl JR, Holmes MC (2001) Prenatal Glucocorticoid Programming of Brain Corticosteroid Receptors and Corticotrophin-Releasing Hormone: Possible Implications for Behaviour. Neuroscience. 104: 71-79.

[179] Taniguchi Y, Kominami R, Yasutaka S, Shinohara H (2001) Mitoses of Existing Corticotrophs Contribute to Their Proliferation in the Rat Pituitary During the Late Fetal Period. Anat. embryol. (Berl). 203: 89-93.
[180] Kalafatić D, Plećaš B, Hristić M, Manojlović-Stojanoski M, Čakić M (2000) The Effect of Repeated Maternal Dexamethasone Treatment on Plasma Adrenocorticotropin Concentration and Acth-Cells During the Perinatal Period in Rats. Arch. biol. sci. 52: 159-164.
[181] Manojlović M, Kalafatić D, Hristić M, Plećaš B, Virag A, Čakić M (1998) Treatment of Pregnant Females with Dexamethasone Influences Postnatal Development of the Adrenal Medulla. Ann anat. 180: 131-135.
[182] Kalafatić D, Hristić M, Plećaš B, Manojlović-Stojanoski M (2000) The Effects of Dexamethasone Treatment of Pregnant Rats Neonatal Acth-Cells. Acta vet. 50: 195.
[183] Owen D, Matthews SG (2007) Prenatal Glucocorticoid Exposure Alters Hypothalamic-Pituitary-Adrenal Function in Juvenile Guinea Pigs. J. neuroendocrinol. 19: 172-180.
[184] Miyamoto H, Mitani F, Mukai K, Suematsu M, Ishimura Y (1999) Studies on Cytogenesis in Adult Rat Adrenal Cortex: Circadian and Zonal Variations and Their Modulation by Adrenocorticotropic Hormone. J. biochem. 126: 1175-1183.
[185] Manojlović M, Hristić M, Kalafatić D, Plećaš B, Urešić N (1998) The Influence of Dexamethasone Treatment of Pregnant Rats on the Development of Chromafin Tissue in Their Offspring During the Fetal and Neonatal Period. J. endocrinol. invest. 21: 211-218.
[186] Kapoor A, Petropoulos S, Matthews SG (2008) Fetal Programming of Hypothalamic-Pituitary-Adrenal (Hpa) Axis Function and Behavior by Synthetic Glucocorticoids. Brain. res. rev. 57: 586-595.
[187] Nyirenda MJ, Welberg LA, Seckl JR (2001) Programming Hyperglycaemia in the Rat through Prenatal Exposure to Glucocorticoids-Fetal Effect or Maternal Influence? J. endocrinol. 170: 653-660.
[188] Liu L, Li A, Matthews SG (2001) Maternal Glucocorticoid Treatment Programs Hpa Regulation in Adult Offspring: Sex-Specific Effects. Am. j. physiol. endocrinol. metab. 280: E729-739.
[189] Poore KR, Fowden AL (2003) The Effect of Birth Weight on Hypothalamo-Pituitary-Adrenal Axis Function in Juvenile and Adult Pigs. J physiol. 547: 107-116.
[190] Meaney MJ, Diorio J, Francis D, Weaver S, Yau J, Chapman K, Seckl JR (2000) Postnatal Handling Increases the Expression of Camp-Inducible Transcription Factors in the Rat Hippocampus: The Effects of Thyroid Hormones and Serotonin. J. neurosci. 20: 3926-3935.
[191] Liu D, Diorio J, Tannenbaum B, Caldji C, Francis D, Freedman A, Sharma S, Pearson D, Plotsky PM, Meaney MJ (1997) Maternal Care, Hippocampal Glucocorticoid Receptors, and Hypothalamic-Pituitary-Adrenal Responses to Stress. Science. 277: 1659-1662.
[192] Huot RL, Plotsky PM, Lenox RH, McNamara RK (2002) Neonatal Maternal Separation Reduces Hippocampal Mossy Fiber Density in Adult Long Evans Rats. Brain. res. 950: 52-63.
[193] Lajud N, Roque A, Cajero M, Gutierrez-Ospina G, Torner L (2012) Periodic Maternal Separation Decreases Hippocampal Neurogenesis without Affecting Basal Corticosterone

During the Stress Hyporesponsive Period, but Alters Hpa Axis and Coping Behavior in Adulthood. Psychoneuroendocrinology. 37: 410-420.

[194] Jansson JO, Ekberg S, Isaksson O, Mode A, Gustafsson JA (1985) Imprinting of Growth Hormone Secretion, Body Growth, and Hepatic Steroid Metabolism by Neonatal Testosterone. Endocrinology. 117: 1881-1889.

[195] Manojlović-Stojanoski M, Nestorović N, Negić N, Trifunović S, Sekulić M, Milošević V (2007) Development of Pituitary Acth and Gh Cells in near Term Rat Fetuses. Arch. biol. sci. 59: 37-44.

[196] Manojlović-Stojanoski M, Nestorović N, Negić N, Filipović B, Šošic-Jurjević B, Sekulić M, Milošević V (2007) Influence of Maternal Dexamethasone Treatment on Morphometric Characteristics of Pituitary Gh Cells and Body Weight in near-Term Rat Fetuses. Folia histochem. cytobiol. 45: 51-56.

[197] Porter TE, Dean CE, Piper MM, Medvedev KL, Ghavam S, Sandor J (2001) Somatotroph Recruitment by Glucocorticoids Involves Induction of Growth Hormone Gene Expression and Secretagogue Responsiveness. J. endocrinol. 169: 499-509.

[198] Holt RI (2002) Fetal Programming of the Growth Hormone-Insulin-Like Growth Factor Axis. Trends endocrinol metab. 13: 392-397.

[199] Boyne MS, Thame M, Bennett FI, Osmond C, Miell JP, Forrester TE (2003) The Relationship among Circulating Insulin-Like Growth Factor (IGF)-I, IGF-Binding Proteins-1 and -2, and Birth Anthropometry: A Prospective Study. J. clin. endocrinol. metab. 88: 1687-1691.

[200] Fowden AL (2003) The Insulin-Like Growth Factors and Feto-Placental Growth. Placenta. 24: 803-812.

[201] Fowden AL, Szemere J, Hughes P, Gilmour RS, Forhead AJ (1996) The Effects of Cortisol on the Growth Rate of the Sheep Fetus During Late Gestation. J. endocrinol. 151: 97-105.

[202] Forhead AJ, Li J, Gilmour RS, Fowden AL (1998) Control of Hepatic Insulin-Like Growth Factor Ii Gene Expression by Thyroid Hormones in Fetal Sheep near Term. Am. j. physiol. 275: E149-156.

[203] Carbone DL, Zuloaga DG, Hiroi R, Foradori CD, Legare ME, Handa RJ (2012) Prenatal Dexamethasone Exposure Potentiates Diet-Induced Hepatosteatosis and Decreases Plasma IGF-I in a Sex-Specific Fashion. Endocrinology. 153: 295-306.

[204] Cianfarani S, Germani D, Branca F (1999) Low Birthweight and Adult Insulin Resistance: The "Catch-up Growth" Hypothesis. Arch. dis. child. fetal. neonatal ed. 81: F71-73.

[205] Manojlović-Stojanoski M, Nestorović N, Ristić N, Trifunović S, Filipović B, Šošic-Jurjević B, Sekulić M (2010) Unbiased Stereological Estimation of the Rat Fetal Pituitary Volume and of the Total Number and Volume of Tsh Cells after Maternal Dexamethasone Application. Microsc. res. tech. 73: 1077-1085.

[206] Forhead AJ, Jellyman JK, Gardner DS, Giussani DA, Kaptein E, Visser TJ, Fowden AL (2007) Differential Effects of Maternal Dexamethasone Treatment on Circulating Thyroid Hormone Concentrations and Tissue Deiodinase Activity in the Pregnant Ewe and Fetus. Endocrinology. 148: 800-805.

[207] Van der Geyten S, Darras VM (2005) Developmentally Defined Regulation of Thyroid Hormone Metabolism by Glucocorticoids in the Rat. J. endocrinol. 185: 327-336.

[208] Oberkotter LV, Rasmussen KM (1992) Changes in Plasma Thyroid Hormone Concentrations in Chronically Food-Restricted Female Rats and Their Offspring During Suckling. J. nutr. 122: 435-441.

[209] Slone-Wilcoxon J, Redei EE (2004) Maternal-Fetal Glucocorticoid Milieu Programs Hypothalamic-Pituitary-Thyroid Function of Adult Offspring. Endocrinology. 145: 4068-4072.

[210] Pracyk JB, Seidler FJ, McCook EC, Slotkin TA (1992) Pituitary-Thyroid Axis Reactivity to Hyper- and Hypothyroidism in the Perinatal Period: Ontogeny of Regulation of Regulation and Long-Term Programming of Responses. J. dev. physiol. 18: 105-109.

[211] Fowden AL, Silver M (1995) The Effects of Thyroid Hormones on Oxygen and Glucose Metabolism in the Sheep Fetus During Late Gestation. J. physiol. 482 (Pt 1): 203-213.

[212] Mansourian AR (2011) A Review on the Metabolic Disorders of Iodine Deficiency. Pak. j. biol. sci. 14: 412-424.

[213] Xita N, Tsatsoulis A (2010) Fetal Origins of the Metabolic Syndrome. Ann. NY acad. sci. 1205: 148-155.

[214] Schwitzgebel VM, Somm E, Klee P (2009) Modeling Intrauterine Growth Retardation in Rodents: Impact on Pancreas Development and Glucose Homeostasis. Mol. cell. endocrinol. 304: 78-83.

[215] Dumortier O, Blondeau B, Duvillie B, Reusens B, Breant B, Remacle C (2007) Different Mechanisms Operating During Different Critical Time-Windows Reduce Rat Fetal Beta Cell Mass Due to a Maternal Low-Protein or Low-Energy Diet. Diabetologia. 50: 2495-2503.

[216] Ranta F, Avram D, Berchtold S, Dufer M, Drews G, Lang F, Ullrich S (2006) Dexamethasone Induces Cell Death in Insulin-Secreting Cells, an Effect Reversed by Exendin-4. Diabetes. 55: 1380-1390.

[217] Blondeau B, Lesage J, Czernichow P, Dupouy JP, Breant B (2001) Glucocorticoids Impair Fetal Beta-Cell Development in Rats. Am. j. physiol. endocrinol. metab. 281: E592-599.

[218] Dumortier O, Theys N, Ahn MT, Remacle C, Reusens B (2011) Impairment of Rat Fetal Beta-Cell Development by Maternal Exposure to Dexamethasone During Different Time-Windows. PLoS One. 6: e25576.

[219] Shen CN, Seckl JR, Slack JM, Tosh D (2003) Glucocorticoids Suppress Beta-Cell Development and Induce Hepatic Metaplasia in Embryonic Pancreas. Biochem j. 375: 41-50.

[220] Zhou Q, Brown J, Kanarek A, Rajagopal J, Melton DA (2008) In Vivo Reprogramming of Adult Pancreatic Exocrine Cells to Beta-Cells. Nature. 455: 627-632.

[221] Ackermann AM, Gannon M (2007) Molecular Regulation of Pancreatic Beta-Cell Mass Development, Maintenance, and Expansion. J. mol. endocrinol. 38: 193-206.

[222] Vegiopoulos A, Herzig S (2007) Glucocorticoids, Metabolism and Metabolic Diseases. Mol. cell. endocrinol. 275: 43-61.

[223] Bjorntorp P (1991) Adipose Tissue Distribution and Function. Int. j. obes. 15 Suppl 2: 67-81.

[224] Whorwood CB, Firth KM, Budge H, Symonds ME (2001) Maternal Undernutrition During Early to Midgestation Programs Tissue-Specific Alterations in the Expression of

the Glucocorticoid Receptor, 11beta-Hydroxysteroid Dehydrogenase Isoforms, and Type 1 Angiotensin Ii Receptor in Neonatal Sheep. Endocrinology. 142: 2854-2864.

[225] Cleasby ME, Kelly PA, Walker BR, Seckl JR (2003) Programming of Rat Muscle and Fat Metabolism by in Utero Overexposure to Glucocorticoids. Endocrinology. 144: 999-1007.

[226] Fetita LS, Sobngwi E, Serradas P, Calvo F, Gautier JF (2006) Consequences of Fetal Exposure to Maternal Diabetes in Offspring. J. clin. endocrinol. metab. 91: 3718-3724.

[227] Liu Y, Nakagawa Y, Wang Y, Sakurai R, Tripathi PV, Lutfy K, Friedman TC (2005) Increased Glucocorticoid Receptor and 11{Beta}-Hydroxysteroid Dehydrogenase Type 1 Expression in Hepatocytes May Contribute to the Phenotype of Type 2 Diabetes in Db/Db Mice. Diabetes. 54: 32-40.

[228] Nyirenda MJ, Lindsay RS, Kenyon CJ, Burchell A, Seckl JR (1998) Glucocorticoid Exposure in Late Gestation Permanently Programs Rat Hepatic Phosphoenolpyruvate Carboxykinase and Glucocorticoid Receptor Expression and Causes Glucose Intolerance in Adult Offspring. J. Clin. Invest. 101: 2174-2181.

[229] Davies MJ, Norman RJ (2002) Programming and Reproductive Functioning. Trends. endocrinol. metab. 13: 386-392.

[230] Kalantaridou SN, Makrigiannakis A, Zoumakis E, Chrousos GP (2004) Stress and the Female Reproductive System. J. reprod. immunol. 62: 61-68.

[231] Gore AC, Attardi B, DeFranco DB (2006) Glucocorticoid Repression of the Reproductive Axis: Effects on Gnrh and Gonadotropin Subunit mRNA Levels. Mol. cell. endocrinol. 256: 40-48.

[232] Negić N, Nestorović N, Manojlović-Stojanoski M, Filipović B, Šošić-Jurjević B, Milosević V, Sekulić M (2006) Multiple Dexamethasone Treatment Affects Morphometric Parameters of Gonadotrophic Cells in Adult Female Rats. Folia histochem. cytobiol. 44: 87-92.

[233] Negić N, Nestorović N, Manojlović-Stojanoski M, Filipović B, Šošić-Jurjevic B, Trifunović S, Milosević V, Sekulić M (2007) Pregnancy and Dexamethasone: Effects on Morphometric Parameters of Gonadotropic Cells in Rats. Acta histochem. 109: 185-192.

[234] Tohei A, Kogo H (1999) Dexamethasone Increases Follicle-Stimulating Hormone Secretion Via Suppression of Inhibin in Rats. Eur. j. pharmacol. 386: 69-74.

[235] Yazawa H, Sasagawa I, Nakada T (2000) Apoptosis of Testicular Germ Cells Induced by Exogenous Glucocorticoid in Rats. Hum. reprod. 15: 1917-1920.

[236] Shishkina GT, Bykova TS (1989) [the Postnatal Development of the Genital System in Male Rats Following the Prenatal Administration of Corticosterone]. Ontogenez. 20: 431-434.

[237] Keshet GI, Weinstock M (1995) Maternal Naltrexone Prevents Morphological and Behavioral Alterations Induced in Rats by Prenatal Stress. Pharmacol. biochem. behav. 50: 413-419.

[238] Castellano JM, Bentsen AH, Sanchez-Garrido MA, Ruiz-Pino F, Romero M, Garcia-Galiano D, Aguilar E, Pinilla L, Dieguez C, Mikkelsen JD, Tena-Sempere M (2011) Early Metabolic Programming of Puberty Onset: Impact of Changes in Postnatal Feeding and Rearing Conditions on the Timing of Puberty and Development of the Hypothalamic Kisspeptin System. Endocrinology. 152: 3396-3408.

[239] Piffer RC, Garcia PC, Pereira OC (2009) Adult Partner Preference and Sexual Behavior of Male Rats Exposed Prenatally to Betamethasone. Physiol. behav. 98: 163-167.

[240] Zambrano E, Rodriguez-Gonzalez GL, Guzman C, Garcia-Becerra R, Boeck L, Diaz L, Menjivar M, Larrea F, Nathanielsz PW (2005) A Maternal Low Protein Diet During Pregnancy and Lactation in the Rat Impairs Male Reproductive Development. J. physiol. 563: 275-284.

[241] Guzman C, Cabrera R, Cardenas M, Larrea F, Nathanielsz PW, Zambrano E (2006) Protein Restriction During Fetal and Neonatal Development in the Rat Alters Reproductive Function and Accelerates Reproductive Ageing in Female Progeny. J. physiol. 572: 97-108.

[242] Leonhardt M, Lesage J, Croix D, Dutriez-Casteloot I, Beauvillain JC, Dupouy JP (2003) Effects of Perinatal Maternal Food Restriction on Pituitary-Gonadal Axis and Plasma Leptin Level in Rat Pup at Birth and Weaning and on Timing of Puberty. Biol. reprod. 68: 390-400.

[243] Rae MT, Kyle CE, Miller DW, Hammond AJ, Brooks AN, Rhind SM (2002) The Effects of Undernutrition, in Utero, on Reproductive Function in Adult Male and Female Sheep. Anim. reprod. sci. 72: 63-71.

[244] Iwasa T, Matsuzaki T, Murakami M, Fujisawa S, Kinouchi R, Gereltsetseg G, Kuwahara A, Yasui T, Irahara M (2010) Effects of Intrauterine Undernutrition on Hypothalamic Kiss1 Expression and the Timing of Puberty in Female Rats. J. physiol. 588: 821-829.

[245] Iwasa T, Matsuzaki T, Murakami M, Kinouchi R, Gereltsetseg G, Yamamoto S, Kuwahara A, Yasui T, Irahara M (2011) Delayed Puberty in Prenatally Glucocorticoid Administered Female Rats Occurs Independently of the Hypothalamic Kiss1-Kiss1r-Gnrh System. Int. j. dev. neurosci. 29: 183-188.

[246] Ristić N, Nestorović N, Manojlović-Stojanoski M, Filipović B, Šošić-Jurjević B, Milosević V, Sekulić M (2008) Maternal Dexamethasone Treatment Reduces Ovarian Follicle Number in Neonatal Rat Offspring. J. microsc. 232: 549-557.

[247] Smith JT, Waddell BJ (2000) Increased Fetal Glucocorticoid Exposure Delays Puberty Onset in Postnatal Life. Endocrinology. 141: 2422-2428.

[248] Gao HB, Tong MH, Hu YQ, Guo QS, Ge R, Hardy MP (2002) Glucocorticoid Induces Apoptosis in Rat Leydig Cells. Endocrinology. 143: 130-138.

[249] Evan GI, Brown L, Whyte M, Harrington E (1995) Apoptosis and the Cell Cycle. Curr. opin. cell. biol. 7: 825-834.

[250] King KL, Cidlowski JA (1998) Cell Cycle Regulation and Apoptosis. Annu. rev. physiol. 60: 601-617.

[251] Pedrana G, Sloboda DM, Perez W, Newnham JP, Bielli A, Martin GB (2008) Effects of Pre-Natal Glucocorticoids on Testicular Development in Sheep. Anat. histol. embryol. 37: 352-358.

[252] Nestorović N, Lovren M, Sekulić M, Filipović B, Milošević V (2001) Effects of Multiple Somatostatin Treatment on Rat Gonadotrophic Cells and Ovaries. Histochem. j. 33: 695-702.

[253] Milosević V, Nestorović N, Filipović B, Velkovski S, Startcević V (2004) Centrally Applied Somatostatin Influences Morphology of Pituitary Fsh Cells but Not Fsh Release. Gen physiol biophys. 23: 375-380.

[254] Nestorović N, Lovren M, Sekulić M, Negić N, Šošic-Jurjević B, Filipović B, Milošević V (2004) Chronic Somatostatin Treatment Affects Pituitary Gonadotrophs, Ovaries and Onset of Puberty in Rats. Life sci. 74: 1359-1373.

[255] Nestorović N, Lovren M, Sekulić M, Negić N, Šošić-Jurjević B, Manojlović-Stojanoski M, Filipović B, Milošević V (2004) Effects of Intracerebroventricularly Administered Octreotide on Gonadotrophic Cells in Female Rats. Jugoslov. med. biohem. 23.

[256] Nestorović N, Manojlović-Stojanoski M, Ristić N, Sekulić M, Šošić-Jurjević B, Filipović B, Milošević V (2008) Somatostatin-14 Influences Pituitary-Ovarian Axis in Peripubertal Rats. Histochem. cell. biol. 130: 699-708.

[257] Nestorović N, Ristić N, Manojlović-Stojanoski M, Šošić-Jurjevic B, Trifunović S, Savin S, Milošević V (2011) Somatostatin 14 Affects the Pituitary-Ovarian Axis in Infant Rats. Histol. histopathol. 26: 157-166.

Chapter 2

The Effects of Glucocorticoids on Fetal and Placental Development

Emin Turkay Korgun, Aslı Ozmen, Gozde Unek and Inanc Mendilcioglu

Additional information is available at the end of the chapter

1. Introduction

Glucocorticoids (GCs), steroid hormones produced predominantly by the adrenal gland, are key mediators of stress responses. Whilst the acute and chronic effects of pharmacological glucocorticoid excess are well-recognized (including induction of hyperglycemia, insulin resistance, hyperlipidemia, hypertension and dysphoria, with suppression of immune, inflammatory and cognitive processes), their role in the biology of the response to stress is more nuanced, with balanced homeostatic effects to facilitate short-term survival and recovery from challenge [1, 2]. In addition, glucocorticoids play an essential role in normal fetal development and are important for the development and maturation of various fetal tissues including the liver, lungs, gut, skeletal muscle and adipose tissue in preparation for extrauterine life. Glucocorticoids most notably act during late gestation to stimulate surfactant production by the lung. This action is critical to prepare the fetus for extrauterine life, and it is for this reason that synthetic glucocorticoid treatment is so widely used in preterm pregnancies where lung immaturity threatens neonatal viability. Although these treatments greatly improve survival [3], they are not without adverse effects.

Glucocorticoids regulate many of the processes required for successful embryo implantation, as well as for the subsequent growth and development of the fetus and placenta. In utero, the endometrium, placenta and embryo/fetus are each exposed to physiological glucocorticoids arising from either maternal or fetal adrenal glands. It has been shown that glucocorticoids have several roles in improving the intrauterine environment. For example, in uterus, glucocorticoids regulate the synthesis of prostaglandins that have been implicated to play critical roles during implantation by increasing stromal vascular permeability [4] and in the initiation of parturition [5]. The peri-implantation secretion of human chorionic gonadotrophin (hCG) from human term trophoblasts can be stimulated by up to 10-fold by treatment for 24 to 72 h with synthetic glucocorticoids dexamethasone and triamcinolone [6, 7]. Glucocorticoids have several anti-inflammatory actions required for implantation. In first trimester human cytotrophoblasts, cortisol can suppress the synthesis of the pro-inflammatory interleukin (IL)-1b [8]. Similarly, in term human placental cytotrophoblasts, physiological concentrations of cortisol and numerous synthetic glucocorticoids can inhibit secretion of pro-inflammatory cytokines tumor necrosis factor (TNF)-α, IL-6 and IL-8 without affecting the expression of anti-inflammatory cytokine IL-10 [9-11]. Glucocorticoids contribute to preventing immunological rejection of the fetal semiallograft in the pregnant uterus by inhibiting eosinophil infiltration [12]. Moreover, glucocorticoids profoundly and specifically suppress expression of fibronectin and laminin, two extracellular matrix proteins that are important mediators of uterine–placental adherence [6].

Furthermore, glucocorticoids activate many of the biochemical processes in these tissues such as altering expression of numerous receptors, enzymes, ion channels, transporters, growth factors, cytoskeleton proteins, binding proteins, clotting factors, gap and tight junction proteins and intracellular signaling pathways' components involved in growth. Taken together, these glucocorticoid-induced changes in cell physiology combine to produce functional alterations at the systemic level [13].

In pregnancy, glucocorticoid administration is used mainly in the management of women at risk of preterm labor and in the antenatal treatment of fetuses at risk of congenital adrenal hyperplasia. It is recommended that, for pregnant women who are at risk of preterm delivery within 7 days between 24 weeks and 34 weeks of gestation, a single course of corticosteroid administration should be performed. And a single course of antenatal corticoids should be administered to women with premature rupture of membranes before 32 weeks gestation to reduce the risks of respiratory distress syndrome, perinatal mortality and other morbidities [14]. Numerous evidence indicates that increased exposure of the fetus to glucocorticoids in mid- to late pregnancy may result in adverse outcomes including intrauterine growth restriction (IUGR) [15-18], postnatal hypertension [15, 19], postnatal cardiovascular disease [20], postnatal glucose intolerance [20], increased postnatal activity in the hypothalamo–pituitary–adrenal axis [21-24], effects on fetal brain development [21, 25, 26].

Glucocorticoid actions within the cell are regulated by Glucocorticoid Receptor (GR) [27]. On hormone binding, activated GR translocates from the cytoplasm to the nucleus as a dimer to associate with specific DNA sequences termed glucocorticoid response elements (GREs) and acts as a ligand-dependent transcription factor [28]. GR-mediated transcriptional activation is modulated by phosphorylation [29]. GRs are highly expressed in decidua, chorion, amnion, stromal fibroblasts, vascular smooth muscle cells and endothelial cells of human term placentas, with moderate expression in cytotrophoblasts and negligible expression in syncytiotrophoblast [30-34]. Because the significance of glucocorticoids to the early mammalian embryo is clear and glucocorticoid action within the cell is regulated by GR, we investigated GR expression during the course of rat embryogenesis until day 12 of gestation. The demonstrated ontogenetic pattern of GR expression indicates the potential sites of biological action of the glucocorticoids, providing supportive evidence for its critical importance during the course of embryogenesis in rats [35].

The intracellular enzyme 11β-hydroxysteroid dehydrogenase (11β-HSD) catalyzes the interconversion of bioactive glucocorticoids (cortisol and corticosterone) and their inactive metabolites (cortisone and 11-dehydrocorticosterone). Thus, it is an important modulator of glucocorticoid bioavailability in both glucocorticoid and mineralocorticoid target organs [36]. To date, two 11β-HSD isoenzymes (known as 11β-HSD1 and 11β-HSD2) have been identified, characterized and cloned [37]. The conversion of cortisone to active cortisol is catalyzed by 11β-HSD1, whereas the metabolism of cortisol to cortisone is mediated via both 11β-HSD1 and 11β-HSD2 [38]. In placenta, 11β-HSD1 protein is expressed specifically in the placental villous endothelial cells, amnion, chorionic and extravillous trophoblasts (EVTs). 11β-HSD1 expression increases throughout pregnancy in response to progesterone [39]. As the placenta differentiates, there is an up-regulation in the expression of 11β-HSD2 enzyme that becomes the major placental isoenzyme [40]. 11β-HSD2 protein is localized exclusively in the syncytiotrophoblast and invasive extravillous trophoblasts with no expression in the chorion or amnion [41-43]. The distinct pattern of 11β-HSD1 and -2 localizations may indicate having different physiological functions. In normal pregnancy, maternal glucocorticoid levels are markedly higher than those in the fetal circulation. It has been stated that the role of placental 11β-HSD is to protect the fetus from adverse effects of maternal glucocorticoids. 11β-HSD2 is better suitable for this role because of its location (the site of maternal–fetal exchange) and its enzymatic properties (higher affinity for cortisol). This enzyme acts as a 'barrier' to prevent premature or inappropriate action at glucocorticoid-responsive tissues during fetal development [44]. It has been suggested that a reduction in the expression or activity of placental 11β-HSD2, by leading to increased transplacental passage of active glucocorticoids, reduces fetal growth. 11β-HSD2 knockout (11β-HSD2−/−) mice exhibit reduced birth weight and heightened anxiety in adulthood [45]. Numerous studies have shown that inhibition of 11β-HSD2 during pregnancy leads to a reduction in birth weight and the development of later hypertension and glucose intolerance [46-48], as well as programming increased HPA axis activity and anxiety-related behaviors [49]. Moreover, placentas from 11β-HSD2 knockout mice fetuses have impaired labyrinth zone capillary development accompanied by a decline in vascular endothelial growth factor (VEGF)-A mRNA expression and altered transport of nutrients by system A amino acid transporter (SNAT) [50]. Furthermore, a correlation between decreased activity of 11β-HSD2 in the human placenta and IUGR has been reported [15, 51, 52]. In addition, mutations in the HSD11B2 gene in humans, although rare, markedly reduce birth weight [53]. It was found that while maternal administration of glucocorticoids caused IUGR, glucocorticoid administration directly into the fetal circulation did not restrict fetal growth, which suggests that the growth limiting effects of glucocorticoids are mediated via actions in the utero-placental unit rather than effects on fetal tissues [54]

Placental development is a critical determinant of fetal growth and glucocorticoids affect growth and development of the fetus indirectly by affecting placental development and function. The actions of glucocorticoids on fetal growth are mediated, in part, by changes in the placenta. In sheep, rats, mice and non-human primates, administration of synthetic glucocorticoids during late gestation reduces placental weight. In most of these species, the effect of glucocorticoids on the placenta is greater than that on the fetus [13]. Glucocorticoids have been implicated in the fusion of cytotrophoblast cells to form the syncytiotrophoblast and associated with morphological (accelerated apical microvilli formation, nuclear maturation, and increase in cell organelle number) and functional (elevated hCG secretion and increased 11β-HSD2 mRNA expression) markers of syncytiotrophoblast differentiation. These findings suggest that glucocorticoids stimulate syncytiotrophoblast differentiation and maturation [55-57].

Microarray analysis showed that maternal glucocorticoid administration leads to marked changes in the gene expression profile in the placenta. Dexamethasone (Dex) caused a decrease in expression of genes involved in cell division such as cyclins A2, B1, D2, CDK 2, CDK 4 and M-phase protein kinase along with growth-promoting genes such as epidermal growth factor receptor, bone morphogenetic protein 4 and insulin-like growth factor-binding protein 3. In addition, Dex treatment led to down-regulation of genes involved in protein biosynthesis, skeletal development, and collagen metabolism. There was also decreased expression of genes involved in cell division, DNA replication, chromosome segregation, DNA alkylation, nucleotide and nucleoside biosynthesis, microtubule-based processes, B-cell activation and differentiation processes, innate immune response, antigen processing and presentation, and complement system [58]. Treatment of rats with glucocorticoids restricts placental vascular development via inhibition of the VEGF-A and peroxisome proliferator-activated receptor γ (PPARγ) which is regulated by VEGF-A expression [59, 60]. In addition, in response to glucocorticoid treatment of either the mother or fetus, there are changes in the placental handling of certain amino acids such as alanine, glutamine and glutamate. However, there have been few studies on the effects of glucocorticoids on amino acid transporters in the placenta of any species to date [61, 62]. Additionally, glucocorticoids change the production and metabolism of hormones by the placenta such as prostaglandins, placental lactogen, leptin, corticotrophin-releasing hormone (CRH), estrogens, progesterone and other progestagens [63, 64]. Glucocorticoids also alter the placental activity of various enzymes involved in the synthesis and inactivation of steroids and thyroid hormones such as 17,20-lyase, 17α-hydroxylase, aromatase, renin and endothelial nitric oxide synthase [63].

2. The effects of glucocorticoids on placental cell cycle

Glucocorticoids play a fundamental role in pregnancy with effects on decidualization, implantation, placental development, fetal brain development, lung maturation and parturition but fetal-placental exposure to maternally administered glucocorticoids may lead to abnormalities of fetal and placental growth [15, 19, 65]. The mode of action of glucocorticoids in placental growth inhibition has not been determined.

Human placental development is established by trophoblast invasion into the uterine endometrium and its vasculature. The resulting changes will facilitate an increase in intervillous blood flow and, hence, the exchange of nutrients and molecules between maternal and fetal blood. The transports as well as metabolic and endocrine functions of the placenta reside primarily in the floating villi covered by the syncytiotrophoblast, a tissue that results from terminal differentiation of underlying villous cytotrophoblasts and their subsequent fusion. Anchoring villi establish physical connection of the placenta with the decidua predominantly by a subpopulation of cytotrophoblasts known as EVT. They accumulate at the tips of the anchoring villi and form cell columns. Both villous and extravillous cytotrophoblast subpopulations arise by proliferation and differentiation from stem cells located within the cytotrophoblast layer of the chorionic villi [66].

On the basis of the immunostaining of the Ki67 antigen, a cell cycle regulator with yet unknown role, EVTs have been categorized as the proliferative phenotype, which is primarily located in the proximal part, and the invasive phenotype that is located mainly in the distal part of cell columns [66]. Current understanding assumes that EVT can differentiate, thereby acquiring an invasive phenotype, which eventually enables them to invade the maternal decidua and spiral arteries. Thus placental development involves proliferation and differentiation of the cytotrophoblasts in a manner that is tightly regulated in time and space.

Eukaryotic cell cycle consists of four phases, G1, S, G2 and M. G1 and G2 are preparation phases for DNA synthesis (S) and mitosis (M) phases respectively. During G1 and G2 phases cell growth, doubling of the amount of protein and organelles and preparation for the next phase occurs. If the conditions are not appropriate, cells in G1 phase stop cell cycle progression and enter into a resting state, known as G0 phase, where they continue biological functions but do not go through the rest of the cell cycle. When growth signals are received, cells in G0 phase can continue the cycle through the G1 phase [67, 68].

The eukaryotic cell cycle is regulated by the coordinated activity of a family of cyclin-dependent kinases (CDKs). These are positively and negatively regulated by the cyclin and CDK inhibitor families [69, 70]. Based on the timing of their appearance in the cell cycle, cyclins can be divided into two groups, i.e. the mitotic cyclins A and B and the G1 cyclins of the D and E families [71]. Cyclin A promotes both G1/S and G2/M transitions, whereas cyclin B1 accumulates in the cytosol during late S phase and G2 and enters the nucleus at the onset of mitosis [72].

In mammalian cells, there are at least two distinct families of CDK inhibitors: the INK4 and the Cip/Kip inhibitors (p21, p27, p57). Both families play regulatory roles during the G1/S cell cycle checkpoint [73]. Because of their broader panel of CDKs with which they interact [74], the inhibitors of the Cip/Kip family control other checkpoints as well. p21 plays a role during the G2/M phase transition [75] and may also mediate S phase [76] and G2 arrest [77]. Overall it is correlated with cell cycle arrest before terminal differentiation [78]. Also, p27 has the capacity to arrest cells in G2 [77]. p57 inhibits cyclin A- and E-associated CDKs and therefore regulates G1/S transition and completion of S phase [79] and is primarily expressed in terminally differentiated cells [80].

Despite the importance in understanding the mechanisms controlling proliferation, little is known about how cytotrophoblast proliferation is coordinated with differentiation and what factors determine whether cytotrophoblast cells divide or differentiate and syncytialize. A few studies localized cell cycle regulators that are specifically expressed during key transitions and phases [81-83].

The hypothesis that the coordinated expression of cell cycle progression and inhibition factors will determine whether cytotrophoblasts proliferate or undergo cell cycle arrest or cell cycle exit allowing subsequent differentiation was tested by our team. The cell cycle promoters cyclin A, cyclin B1, proliferating cell nuclear antigen (PCNA), Ki67 and the cell cycle inhibitors p21, p27 and p57 were immunolocalized in tissue sections of first trimester pregnancies (weeks 6 and 9-12). Villous cytotrophoblasts were immunolabelled for Ki67 and cyclin A but only few were stained with anti-cyclin B1. The syncytiotrophoblast was devoid of immunoreactivity for any of the cell cycle progression factors. It expressed especially p21, whereas p27 and p57 were predominantly found in villous cytotrophoblasts. PCNA, Ki67, cyclin A and cyclin B1 were immunolocalized in proximal and distal EVTs of anchoring villi and in EVT which had invaded the upper decidual segments. All EVTs strongly expressed p27 and p57, but not p21. These data clearly suggest different functions for p21, p27 and p57 in placental development with distinct roles for p21 and p57 in syncytiotrophoblast and EVT differentiation, respectively. p27 appears to be involved in both the processes. The results may also challenge the concept of differential mitotic activity in the proximal and distal parts of the first trimester cytotrophoblast cell column, but more functional studies are clearly needed. The presence of p27 and p57 in EVT cells, which invade the deciduas deeply, may account for the loss of mitogenic potential of these cells [84].

Although the architecture of the human and rodent placentas differs, their anatomical structures and molecular mechanisms have been compared [85, 86] and analogies drawn between the various cell types; furthermore, the molecular mechanisms of placental development are thought to be very similar between the two species. Thus, the rodent placenta is increasingly used as a model to study mechanisms underlying placental development [85, 87].

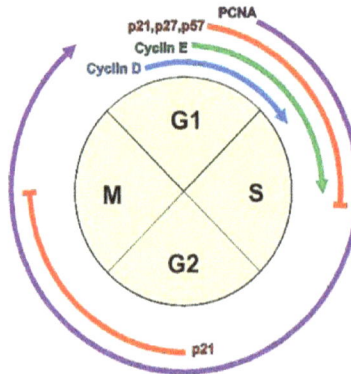

Figure 1. Schematic representation of cell cycle related proteins in rat placenta of our study [88].

We have been used to localize G1 cyclins (D1, D3, E), which are major determinants of proliferation, Cip/Kip inhibitors, p53 as a master regulator and proliferating cell nuclear antigen in all cell types of the rat term placenta. Schematic representation of cell cycle related proteins studied is showed in Figure 1. The proportion of each cell type immunolabeled was counted. Cyclin D1 and cyclin D3 were present mostly in cells of the fetal aspect of the placenta, whereas the G1/S cyclin E was present only in the spongio- and labyrinthine trophoblast populations. Among the Cip/Kip inhibitors, p21 was present only in cells of the fetal aspect whereas p27 and p57 were found in all cell types studied. p53 was only found in a small proportion of cells with no co-localization of p53 and p21 [88]. Schematic representation of our immunohistochemistry results in the rat placenta is showed in Figure 2. The data suggest that the cells of the fetal side of the rat placenta still have some proliferation potential which is kept in check by expression of the Cip/Kip cell cycle inhibitors, whereas cells of the maternal aspect have lost this potential. Apoptosis is only marginal in the term rat placenta. In conclusion, proliferation and apoptosis in rat placental cells appears controlled mostly by the Cip/Kip inhibitors in late pregnancy. It is still not known how coordination mechanisms of proliferation and differentiation are influenced by glucocorticoid induced IUGR in the placenta.

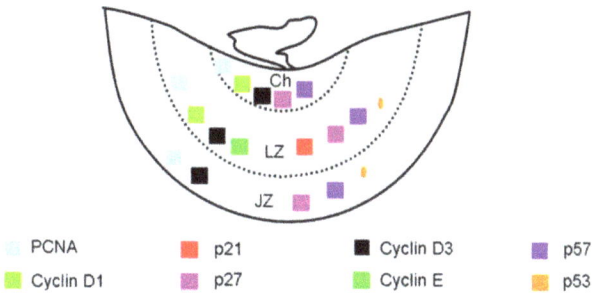

Ch: Chorion, LZ: Labyrinth Zone (fetal placenta), JZ: Junctional Zone (maternal placenta) [88].

Figure 2. Schematic representation of our immunohistochemistry results in the rat placenta.

We aimed to investigate the effects of maternally administered synthetic glucocorticoid Dex on cell proliferation, cell cycle arrest or apoptosis of placental development. We investigated the spatial and temporal immunolocalization of PCNA, Ki67, p27 and p57 in normal and Dex-induced IUGR placental development in pregnant rats. PCNA immunolabeling intensity in placentas of the control group was statistically significantly higher than that in the Dex-induced IUGR group placentas on all days in junctional and labyrinth zones (JZ and LZ, respectively). We observed decreased Ki67 staining intensity in the labyrinth trophoblasts of Dex-induced IUGR placentas compared to controls on day 21. Ki67 immunolabeling intensity was higher in the control group than that in the IUGR group placentas on all days in both zones except for day 21 in the junctional zone. These differences were statistically significant on days 15, 17 and 19 in the junctional zone and on days 13, 15, 17 and 21 in the labyrinth zone. Ki67 staining intensity decreased gradually after day 15 in both zones of control and

IUGR placentas. Ki67 immunostaining intensities were stronger in the labyrinth zone compared to the junctional zone in both groups. Moreover, after day 17, scarcely any Ki67 immunostaining was obtained in the IUGR placentas in the junctional zone. We found stronger p27 immunolabeling intensity in Dex-induced IUGR placentas when compared to control placentas in both junctional and labyrinth zones for all gestational days (Table 1) [89]. In accordance with this, in another study, it was observed that in the Dex-induced human choriocarcinoma JEG-3 cells p27 mRNAs were upregulated [90]. We observed that p57 immunostaining intensities in Dex-induced IUGR placentas were stronger compared to controls in both zones for all gestational days. We found that Dex-induction results in p57 upregulation in rat placental development [89]. In contrast to our results, p57 was not expressed in Dex-induced JEG-3 cells [90]. In another study, we wanted to determine the Ser/Thr protein kinase Akt and a MAPK (Mitogen-Activated Protein Kinase) ERK1/2 related proliferation and apoptosis mechanisms are influenced by Dex-induced IUGR placentas. Thus, we investigated the expression levels and spatio-temporal immunolocalization of Akt, p-Akt, ERK1/2 and p-ERK1/2 proteins in normal and Dex treated placental development of rats. We found that maternal Dex treatment led to a decrease in ERK1/2 and Akt activation during rat placental development together with placental and fetal weight loss. Akt activation was significant at junctional zones of the rat placenta, especially at spongiotrophoblast cells and giant cells, and reduced after dexamethasone treatment. On the other hand, ERK1/2 activation was seen in both junctional and labyrinth zones of the rat placentas and was weaker in labyrinth zones of IUGR group placentas. The decrease in ERK1/2 and Akt activation may result in cell survival inhibition or apoptosis stimulation. Consequently, Dex induced placental and embryonal developmental abnormalities could be associated with reduction of Akt and ERK1/2 activation [91]. In another study, decreased levels of placental Akt phosphorylation was observed after in utero exposure to Dex [92].

Antenatal Dex use is associated with reduction in fetal and placental weight with morphological changes in the placenta. Dex-treated mouse placentas showed swollen trophoblast cells in both the junctional and labyrinth zones and increased apoptosis of trophoblast cells in the junctional zone. Moreover, Dex-treated placentas were hydropic, friable and pale [58]. Increasing antenatal corticosteroid exposure was associated with villous fibrosis, stromal mineralization, and less frequent villous infarction [93]. In addition, treatment with Dex prevented the normal rise in VEGF expression and the associated increase in labyrinthine vascularity over the final third of pregnancy. Therefore, Dex appears to reduce labyrinth zone growth by preventing the normal development of the fetal vasculature within the labyrinth zone [59]. Moreover, microarray analysis showed that Dex caused a decrease in expression of genes involved in cell division such as cyclins A2, B1, D2, CDK 2, CDK 4 and M-phase protein kinase along with growth-promoting genes such as epidermal growth factor receptor, bone morphogenetic protein 4 and insulin-like growth factor-binding protein 3 [58]. In addition, 3H-thymidine incorporation assay revealed that proliferation of trophoblast cell lines JEG-3 and HTR-8/SV neo and human first-trimester primary trophoblasts was time- and dose-dependently inhibited by glucocorticoids [94]. Impaired growth in Dex-treated placentas was also characterized by decreased expression of both prolactin-like protein-B and insulin-like growth factor (IGF)-II, particularly in the junctional zone of the rat placenta [92]. Dex-treatment increased apoptosis of trophoblast cells in mouse and rat placentas. Dex-induced trophoblast apoptosis was mediated through activation of caspases 1 and 3 [58, 95]. Apoptosis was also induced in primary cultures of third trimester human decidual cells when treated with cortisol, cortisone, or dexamethasone [34]. Likewise, Dex was shown to induce both apoptosis and necrosis in primary cultures of term human placental trophoblast, in an in vitro model of syncytialization and in the SGH-PL4 cell line derived from human extravillous trophoblasts by measuring the cytokines TNF-alpha and IFN-gamma using the TUNEL technique, Annexin V binding, fluorescence microscopy and ATP/ADP measurements [96]. In another study, using a human in vitro term placental explant model, Dex treatment was shown to be associated with morphological (accelerated apical microvilli formation, nuclear maturation,

Gestational days	Junctional Zone	Labyrinth Zone	Cell cycle protein
13	↓	↓	
15	↓	↓	
17	↓	↓	PCNA
19	↓	↓	
21	↓	↓	
13	–	↓	
15	↓	↓	
17	↓	↓	Ki67
19	↓	–	
21	–	↓	
13	↑	↑	
15	↑	↑	
17	↑	↑	p27
19	–	↑	
21	↑	↑	
13	↑	–	
15	↑	↑	
17	↑	↑	p57
19	–	–	
21	↑	↑	

Table 1. Immunolabeling intensity changes of PCNA, Ki67, p27 and p57 in the junctional and labyrinth zones of placentas of the IUGR group rat placentas compared to control of given gestational day (p=<0.05). –, statistically significantly unchanged; ↑, statistically significantly increased; ↓, statistically significantly decreased.

and increased cell organelle number) and functional (elevated hCG secretion, increased 11β-HSD2 mRNA expression and reduced cytotrophoblast proliferation markers) of syncytiotrophoblast differentiation. These findings suggest that Dex stimulates syncytiotrophoblast differentiation and maturation [57]. In another study, BeWo and JEG-3 choriocarcinoma cell lines used as models for human trophoblast were cultured with another synthetic glucocorticoid triamcinolone acetonide (TA). TA altered the number of viable and dead cells as well as cyclin B1 expression levels shown by Western blotting and to a lesser extent, invasion of BeWo and JEG-3 cell lines determined by Matrigel invasion assay and by measuring the secretion (ELISA) of matrix-metalloproteinases (MMP-2, MMP-9) [97].

3. The effects of glucocorticoids on fetal and placental angiogenesis mechanisms

Angiogenesis is a complex process that may be initiated by a large number of stimuli and that is performed through multiple biologic pathways and a variety of molecules. With the increased understanding of angiogenesis, it has become clear that many of its pathways are parallel and redundant, greatly complicating efforts to interrupt the process. The disruption of one pathway most likely does not abolish completely the formation of new blood vessels, which may explain the less than perfect clinical results achieved when treating neovascular processes with currently available regimens. Combination therapies and drugs that target more than one pathway have become more popular and intensively explored.

Angiogenesis is required for the cyclic processes of endometrial growth, breakdown, and repair during the menstrual cycle, and it provides a richly vascularized tissue receptive for implantation and placentation [98]. Besides, the formation of new blood vessels is essential for organogenesis and successful embryonic and fetal development.

For many years glucocorticoids have been used in pregnant women for several reasons such as risk of premature deliveries or treatment of a variety of medical disorders like bronchial asthma, systemic lupus erythematosous etc.. The dosages and types of glucocorticoids changes depending on the severity of the symptoms and treatment procedure [99].

It is reviewed by Hadoka et al. [100] that endogenous GCs contribute to physiological angiogenesis mechanisms by regulating the new vessel formation processes. Endothelial cells are seem to be a target of glucocorticoid effect as they both express glucocorticoid and mineralocorticoid receptors [101, 102]. But overexposure to glucocorticoids during pregnancy has adverse effects on placental angiogenesis mechanisms. Therefore these steroids should be carefully used in pregnancy.

Hewitt et al. [59] investigated the impact of increased glucocorticoid exposure on the spatial and temporal expression of the endothelial cell-specific mitogen; VEGF and associated placental vascularization over the final third of rat pregnancy. They showed that treatment with dexamethasone prevented the normal rise in VEGF expression as a LZ specific manner. Their data suggest that glucocorticoid induced restriction of fetal and placental growth is mediated, in part, via inhibition of placental VEGF expression and associated reduction in placental vascularization. Therefore, dexamethasone appears to reduce LZ growth by preventing the normal development of the fetal vasculature within the LZ.

As it is mentioned in the study above, GCs have adverse effect on placental angiogenesis mechanisms. This effect would be related with both angiogenic activity of the endothelial cells or maybe related with proliferation or cell survival processes. It was reported in a previous study that GCs inhibit tube formation of cultured endothelial cells [103] but the molecular mechanisms underlying this effect hasn't been clearly understood [104].

Recently, Logie et al. [105] reported that GCs do not affect the endothelial cell viability or proliferation but tube formation capacity. This investigation addressed the hypothesis that the potent antiangiogenic action of glucocorticoids is due to prevention of tube formation by endothelial cells. Cultured human umbilical vein endothelial cells (HUVEC) and aortic endothelial cells (HAoEC) were used to determine the influence of glucocorticoids on tube-like structure (TLS) formation, and on cellular proliferation, viability and migration. Dexamethasone or cortisol (at physiological concentrations) inhibited both basal and prostaglandinF-2α -induced and VEGF stimulated TLS formation in endothelial cells cultured on Matrigel, effects which were blocked with the glucocorticoid receptor antagonist RU38486. Glucocorticoids had no effect on endothelial cell viability, migration or proliferation. Time-lapse imaging showed that cortisol blocked VEGF-stimulated cytoskeletal reorganization and initialization of tube formation. Exposure to glucocorticoids reduced the formation of cell-cell contacts rather than increasing degradation of existing tubes. They concluded that glucocorticoids interact directly with glucocorticoid receptors on vascular endothelial cells (ECs) to inhibit TLS formation. This action, which was conserved in ECs from two distinct vascular territories, was due to alterations in cell morphology rather than inhibition of EC viability, migration or proliferation. These findings provide important insights into the anti angiogenic action of endogenous glucocorticoids in health and disease [105].

According to the results of an ongoing study of us, Triamcinolone treatment decreased VEGF expression in HUVECs. In this study, we tested the hypothesis that IUGR could be observed in fetuses as a result of insufficient nutrient transport depending on the glucocorticoid effect on placental angiogenesis mechanism that leads to inadequate vessel development. HUVECs were cultured at different concentrations (0.5, 5, 50 µmol/L) of the synthetic glucocorticoid triamnicinolone acetonide for 48 and 72 hours. After culture, RT-PCR, ELISA, Western blot and Matrigel experiments were performed. On the other hand, dexamethasone was injected to rats during gestation. Placenta and blood samples were taken from rats on gestational days 14, 16, 18 and 20. RT-PCR and Western blot analyses were performed on placentas while ELISA test was applied to sera and HUVEC culture media. We found that in HUVECs; VEGF, VEGFR1, VEGFR2, Placental Growth Factor (PIGF) and Fibroblast Growth Factor (FGF) gene levels on 48 and 72 hours decreased in 50 mM TA groups compared to control. VEGF protein amount on 48 and 72 hours decreased in TA groups compared to control. VEGFR1 protein quantity decreased and VEGFR2 protein quantity increased in a dose- and time-dependent manner. According to ELISA results, VEGFR1 secreted by HUVEC cells decreased while VEGFR2 and FGF increased. In Matrigel experiments, decreased vessel tube structures were created by HUVEC cells exposed for 72 hours to 50 mM TA. The amount of VEGF in Dex treated rat sera statistically significantly decreased on days 14, 16 and 20, while there is no difference on day 18 compared to control. VEGF protein amount showed a decrease in all gestational days of IUGR group compared to control in rat placentas. VEGFR1 decreased in advancing pregnancy days of control group while increased in parallel to pregnancy days of IUGR group. VEGF and VEGFR1 gene level was lower at term rat placentas compared to control group at gestational day 20. In conclusion our results showed that glucocorticoids had a negative effect on angiogenesis mechanism (Figure 3) via altering the angiogenesis related protein and gene expression, and tube formation capacity and angiogenesis related proteins in sera (A.Ozmen, G.Unek, D.K. Korgun, I.Mendilcioğlu and E.T.Korgun unpublished).

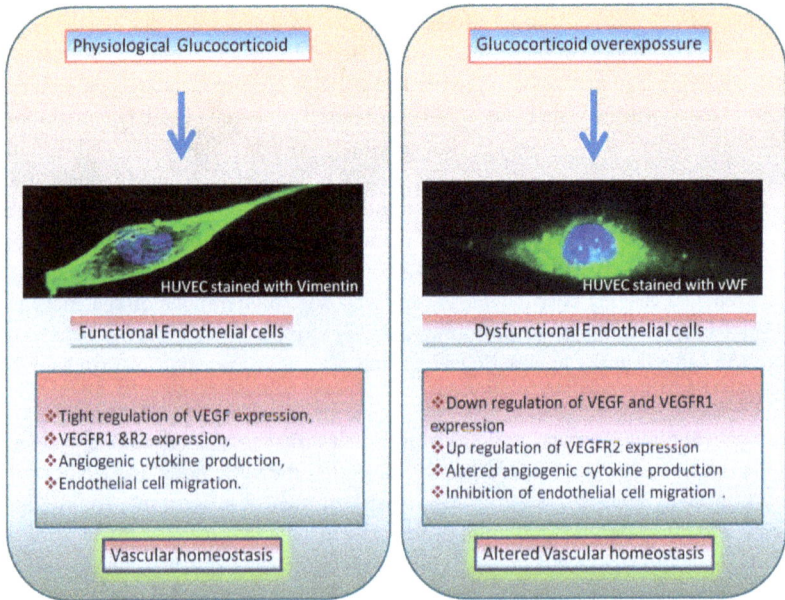

Figure 3. A possible model for glucocorticoid effect on endothelial cells. In physiological conditions; in the case of moderate GC concentrations (left picture), vascular homeostasis is tightly regulated. VEGF, VEGFR1&R2 expression, angiogenic cytokine production, endothelial cell migration, blood flow velocity etc… is maintained in a balance in functional endothelial cells. But when GC concentration is increased (right picture), endothelial cell are subjected to excess GC. And this GC overexposure results with endothelial dysfunction by downregulating VEGF and VEGFR1 expression, upregulating VEGFR2 expression, altering angiogenic cytokine production and by inhibiting endothelial cell migration etc… (vWF: Von Willebrand Factor)

In another study of ours, we investigated the effects of glucocorticoids on rat placental development depending on the PI3K/Akt and MAPK-ERK1/2 pathways [91]. It was observed that, the IUGR group had significantly smaller embryos on day 20 of gestation and had smaller placentas on day 14, 16, 18 and 20 compared with control. Maternal dexamethasone treatment led to a significant decrease in Akt activation on day 16, 18, and 20. Total Akt protein expression was not significantly affected by the treatment. There was a significant decrease in ERK1/2 activation on day 18 in IUGR group; on the other hand there was a significant increase on day 16. Total ERK1/2 protein expression didn't show any significant difference between groups. We observed that phospho-Akt immunolabelings were remarkable in junctional zone in control groups and weaker in IUGR groups. Phospho-ERK1/2 immunolabelings were considerable in the junctional and labyrinth zones in the control groups and weaker in IUGR groups. We found that ERK1/2 activity was decreased in the dexamethasone treated IUGR groups. This decrease was especially seen in the LZ of the rat placenta. Concerning the importance of Erk1/2 on placental vasculature development [106-109], it could be said that the decrease in ERK1/2 activity might be related with vascular failure and this could result with abnormal placental development. Besides it is mentioned in the literature that the PI3K/Akt pathway modulates the expression of some angiogenic factors such as nitric oxide and angiopoietins. Numerous inhibitors targeting the PI3K/Akt pathway have been developed, and these agents have been shown to decrease VEGF secretion and angiogenesis. [110]. Therefore, dexamethasone induced decreased Akt phosphorylation may negatively affect the placental angiogenesis mechanisms. There are some other studies [111, 112] mentioning the effect of GCs on fetal/placental vasculature during pregnancy. These studies report that GCs alter the physiological condition of the vasculature and leads pathological conditions. Aida et al. [111] determined a significant depression of total placental eNOS protein measured by ELISA (betamethasone treated vs control) and immunohistochemistry in both syncytiotrophoblast and vascular endothelium. In conclusion, maternally administered betamethasone produces a consistent decrease in several indices of placental eNOS function that may play a role in the altered cardiovascular dynamics and fetal growth retardation produced by betamethasone administration in late pregnancy.

Angiogenesis is tightly regulated by hormones. Hormones regulate blood vessel growth by controlling the production of local chemical mediators, often other hormones, but also growth factors, cytokines, enzymes, receptors, adhesion molecules, and metabolic factors. As mentioned above, GCs may show their effects directly on endothelial cells or indirectly for example by altering cytokine production that may affect placental vasculature. Xu et al. 2005, [9] studied the effects of GCs on placental cytokine production. Villous explants were cultured with increasing concentrations of glucocorticoids (betamethasone and methyl-prednisolone, 0.0025 mM, 0.25 mM and 25 mM). The dose effect of glucocorticoids on cytokine (TNF-α, IL-6 and IL-10) production was examined using ELISA. There was a stepwise reduction of TNF-α and IL-6 with increasing doses of betamethasone and methyl-prednisolone from placentas of women with preeclampsia and normal pregnancy.

However, IL-10 was not altered in conditioned medium by increasing doses of glucocorticoids. In pregnancy, TNF-α can cause direct damage to endothelial cells, increase endothelial cell permeability, up-regulate endothelial adhesion molecules (ICAM-1, VCAM-1, E-Selectin) and promote vasoconstriction, all of which are identified in the pathogenesis of preeclampsia [113]. IL-10 is an immunosuppressive Th2-type cytokine which is produced by immune cells including T-cells, monocytes, macrophages, granulocytes and NK cells and also trophoblasts. IL-10 has been also shown to be a potent inhibitor of Th1 cell proliferation and the production of Th1-type cytokines such as TNF-α [114].

To observe the influence of maternal betamethasone administration for fetal lung maturation on the arterial, venous and intracardiac blood flow of the fetus and the uterine arteries; twenty-seven women with singleton pregnancies were examined before the first, and 30 min and 8, 24, 48 and 72 h after the second of two single doses of 8 mg of betamethasone. The blood flow velocity waveforms of the umbilical artery (UA), the middle cerebral artery, the uterine arteries, the ductus venosus, the inferior vena cava and the right hepatic vein, the pulmonary trunk, the ductus arteriosus and the right and left intraventricular inflow of the heart was recorded. The resistance index of the UA showed a significant transient decrease 30 min after the second betamethasone dose. The peak systolic velocity of the ductus arteriosus increased significantly 30 min after the 2nd dose and then returned to non-significant values. No significant change was observed in any of the other vessels. So it could be said that Betamethasone causes short-term changes in fetal blood flow. However, this effect seems to be mild and reversible and does not appear to contraindicate the use of corticosteroids to promote fetal lung maturation [115]. Therefore, it could be mentioned that long term dexamethasone usage my result with decreased maternal blood velocity which would negatively affect angiogenesis mechanisms as maternal blood itself contains angiogenesis related proteins.

It is reviewed by Oliver et al. [116] that corticosteroids are believed to act at multiple levels of angiogenesis by regulating growth factors, proteases, and blood cell behavior, and have shown significant promise in clinical studies of neovascularization secondary to diabetes, age-related macular degeneration (AMD), and ocular histoplasmosis syndrome [117-121]. Angiostatic steroids have been proposed to inhibit angiogenesis by altering the capillary basement membrane composition, suppressing its dissolution, and inhibiting endothelial cell migration, in addition to their capacity of regulating the participation of inflammatory cells in the neovascular process [122-124]. There is a growing body of evidence that reports inhibitive effects of glucocorticoids on angiogenesis mechanisms [105, 125-128] but there is limited data about the impact of glucocorticoids on placental angiogenesis mechanisms. Glucocorticoid-mediated inhibition of angiogenesis is important in physiology, pathophysiology and therapy. However, the mechanisms through which glucocorticoids inhibit growth of new blood vessels have not been established. Over-exposure to GCs may alter intracellular signaling pathways such as MAPK/ERK1/2 and PI3K/Akt with a processes mediated by GR and finally expression of angiogenic proteins could be altered (Figure 4).

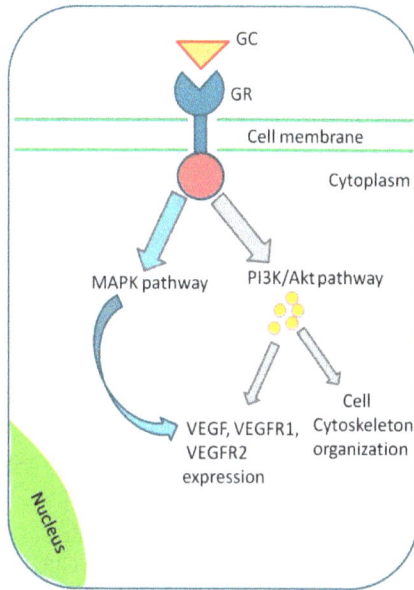

Figure 4. Glucocorticoids might show their effects on angiogenesis mechanisms by altering intracellular signal transduction pathways. GCs affect cellular processes via binding Glucocorticoid receptor. MAPK and PI3K/Akt (by phosphorylation of several downstream molecules; yellow dots in the picture) pathways mediate GC action on placental angiogenesis mechanisms like VEGF, VEGFR1&2 expression and endothelial cell cytoskeleton organization etc... (GC; Glucocorticoid, GR; Glucocorticoid Receptor)

4. The effects of glucocorticoids on placental glucose transporters

The Glut protein family belongs to the Major Facilitator Superfamily (MFS) of membrane transporters [129]. Most Glut proteins catalyze the facilitative (energy-independent) bidirectional transfer of their substrates across membranes. Up to now, 14 functional mammalian-facilitated hexose carriers (GLUTs) have been characterized by molecular cloning [130]. The Glut family members can be grouped into three (Class I, Class II and Class III) different classes based on their sequence similarities [131]. The isoforms GLUT1, 3 and 4 are included in Class I and represent high-affinity transport facilitators.

The existence of glucose transporters in the placenta have been known for many years. GLUT1 protein is present in placental endothelial cells [132, 133] and in the basal [132], or microvillous membranes of the syncytiotrophoblast [133-135]. GLUT3 mRNA is distributed throughout the cells of villous tissue; GLUT3 protein appears to be expressed only in the vascular endothelium and, is not expressed in the syncytiotrophoblast layer of the placenta. A strong GLUT4 signal was observed in intravillous stromal cells, appearing to co-localize with insulin receptors [136], a discovery which complements the observation of GLUT4 in fibroblasts from amnion and chorion [137].

GLUT proteins' cell surface expression level, greatly influences the rate of glucose uptake into the cells [131]. Uptake of glucose by the placenta is facilitated primarily by GLUT1 and in part by GLUT3 transporters [133, 138-140]. A possible major glucose transfer mechanism in the human placental villi may be depicted as follows. Glucose in the maternal bloodstream passes the apical microvillous plasma membrane of syncytiotrophoblast cells by means of GLUT1. Glucose moves through the cytoplasm of the syncytiotrophoblast by simple diffusion and leaves the cytoplasm via GLUT1 in the basal plasma membrane. GLUT1 and GLUT3 proteins contribute to the uptake of glucose by placental endothelial cells, as well as facilitate the transfer of glucose into and out of the fetal blood vessels in the villous core [133, 138-140]. About 25% of glucose entering the placenta is metabolized within this tissue; the majority of glucose is passed to the fetus through placental endothelial cells [141].

Efficient placental (maternal to fetal) transport of glucose is crucial to sustain the normal development and survival of the fetus in utero because its own glucose production is minimal [142]. The factors regulating transplacental glucose transfer are largely unknown.

In our recent study [143], we showed that Triamcinolone administration at doses of 0.5, 5 and 50μmol/L, led to a significant up-regulation of placental GLUT1 and GLUT3 transcripts and protein levels in Human Placental Endothelial Cells (HPECs). After several passages, the endothelial cells were cultured in the presence or absence (controls) of 0.5, 5 and 50μmol/L of TA. The lower (0.5 mmol) dose is a concentration in the lower range of doses generally used in previous cell culture studies [7] and considered comparable to the doses used to promote lung maturation in rats [144]. Other doses (5 and 50 mmol) were used to investigate the potentially detrimental effects of glucocorticoid excess. The highest TA dose administered to the endothelial cell cultures corresponds to the TA concentration in blood resulting after intravenous injection of a dose recommended by the manufacturers for therapy in humans. Our Western blot results showed that GC overexposure significantly increased placental GLUT1 and GLUT3 protein levels in all experimental groups of HPECs. RT-PCR analysis of placental GLUT expressions indicated that both GLUT1 and GLUT3 mRNA levels were affected by the GC induction. It was supposed that GCs caused an increase in placental GLUT proteins and mRNA expression.

The human placenta is a GC responsive organ consisting of multiple cell types including endothelial cells, fibroblasts and trophoblasts that demonstrate changes in gene expression after hormone treatment. However, little is known about the relative expression or activity of the Glucocorticoid Receptor among the various placental cell types. Previous studies have documented that placental endothelial cells expressed GR and Mineralocorticoid Receptor (MR) [101, 102] but the GR regulation of glucose transport have not been studied. We found that GR mRNA and protein expression down-regulated after 24-h cell culture of HPECs. Our results suggest that GC-mediated down-regulation of GR levels occurs through changes in protein and mRNA stability in HPECs after TA treatment. The data from the cell culture strengthens the hypothesis that increased GC levels specifically modulate GLUT expression via the GR.

Collectively, we conclude that TA is a potent regulator of HPECs' GLUT1 and GLUT3 expression (Figure 5). This effect is mediated by GR. We speculate that GC-induced up-regulation of the placental glucose transporter systems contributes to the retarded fetal and placental growth observed with GC treatment.

Similarly in a previous study [18], it is reported that exposure to excess glucocorticoids from day 15 of gestation modified rodent placental glucose transporter protein expression at day 21 of gestation in a concentration-dependent manner.

Dexamethasone treatment from day 15 to day 21 of pregnancy led to fetal hypoglycaemia. GLUT1 and GLUT3 protein expression were detectable in the rat placenta during late gestation, and dexamethasone treatment from day 15 to day 21 of pregnancy significantly decreased placental weight and up-regulated the placental protein expression of both glucose transporters during late gestation in a dose-dependent manner.

Dexamethasone administration at the lower dose (100µg/kg) led to modest up-regulation of placental GLUT1 protein expression, in the absence of any significant change in the protein expression of GLUT3. Dexamethasone at the higher dose (200µg/kg) led to significant up-regulation of the placental expression of both GLUT1 and GLUT3 in rats, with a slightly more marked effect on GLUT3 [18]. It is concluded that, depending on the dose administered, either maturational glucose transporter isoform switching might be accelerated by dexamethasone treatment during late pregnancy or, at a higher dose, placental glucose transporter expression would be down-regulated.

In another study of ours, the glucocorticoid effect on the glucose transporters in the diabetic rat placenta was questioned. It was hypothesized that GCs regulate placental glucose transport in many cell types and tissues and depending on this hypothesis the relationship between glucose transport and the glucocorticoid metabolism in rat placental development of normal and diabetic pregnancy was investigated. The immunohistochemical results indicated that GR and GLUT1 are expressed ubiquitously in the trophoblast and endothelial cells of the labyrinthine zone. Amounts of GR and GLUT1 proteins increased towards the end of gestation both in the control and the diabetic placenta. However, at days 17 and 19 of gestation, only the placental GR protein was significantly increased in the streptozotocin-induced diabetic rats compared to control rats. It is mentioned in this study that there might be a relationship between GR and GLUT1 expressions at the cellular level. GLUT1 does not play a pivotal role in diabetic pregnancies. However, placental growth abnormalities during diabetic pregnancy may be related with the amount of GR [145].

It was previously reported by Hahn et al. for the first time, that both GLUT1 and GLUT3 transcripts and protein were significantly down-regulated in isolated human trophoblast cells and in rat placentas by GCs, suggesting regulation at the transcriptional level [7]. Hyperglycemia is one of the well known systemic effects following GC treatment. Thus, elevated glucose concentrations might have affected placental GLUT expression [146]. However, in the rat model, a single injection of TA resulted in only short term hyperglycemia, followed by hypoglycemia. This hypoglycemia may be the reason for the smaller fetuses and placentas as well as for the markedly reduced weight gain of TA-treated rats during gestational days 16 and 21.The human trophoblast cells were cultured under physiological glucose concentrations, yet their GLUTs were down-regulated similar to those in TA-treated rats. Collectively, the investigators concluded that the synthetic GC Triamcinolone is a potent regulator of human and rodent placental GLUT1 and GLUT3 expression. This effect is mediated by the GR. They speculate that GC-induced down-regulation of the placental glucose transporter systems contributes to the retarded fetal and placental growth observed with GC treatment. This would represent a pathogenetic mechanism different from that leading to intrauterine growth retardation in the absence of GC treatment, in which trophoblast GLUT1 is not altered [134]. However, it is difficult to determine the cause and effect relationships, and the growth restriction could occur first, followed by an appropriate down-regulation of the transporters so as to match fetal size.

Consistent with this study, it was also reported that GLUT1 and GLUT3 mRNA levels were decreased in the dexamethasone treated group in the caruncles of the caw placenta [147]. In this study, plasma glucose concentrations of cows carrying a somatic cell clone fetus during late pregnancy and GLUT mRNA levels at parturition were examined. Parturition was induced by using dexamethasone and some other molecules. Cotyledon and caruncle tissues were removed just after parturition and were used for mRNA extraction. In the caruncules of the Dex induced parturition group GLUT1 and GLUT3 mRNA levels were decreased according to the Clone Pregnancy.

In another rat model, female pregnant rats were subjected to % 50 food restrictions in order to investigate the effect of maternal nutrient on placental GLUTs. In this model fetuses were overexposured to glucocorticoids as maternal protein restriction induces it. At day 21 of pregnancy plasma corticosterone levels were increased. Correspondingly, placental GLUT3 protein was decreased, GLUT1 and GLUT4 protein levels were not affected by maternal feeding regimen and therefore enhanced corticosterone level [148].

Besides placenta, GCs affect glucose transport in a variety of peripheral tissues, such as skeletal muscle, adipocytes, and endothelial cells [149-160]. High affinity low capacity GRs have been identified in the placenta of various species, including man, rat, and mouse [17, 35, 161, 162]. This would have important clinical implications, because GC-induced down-regulation of the placental glucose transport system(s) may contribute to the deleterious side-effects of GC treatment during pregnancy, such as the higher incidence of growth-retarded fetuses [46, 163-165].

Corticosteroids have also been shown to have major effects on fetal glucose homeostasis resulting in long-term persistence of these changes after birth in sheep and rats [166-172]. Prenatal corticosteroid exposure of mice resulted in programming of the fetus such that the adult progeny exhibited glucose intolerance [170, 171]. In addition, repeated courses of maternal corticosteroid administration have been shown to alter fetal glucose homeostasis and hepatic enzyme activity in rats [157, 173].

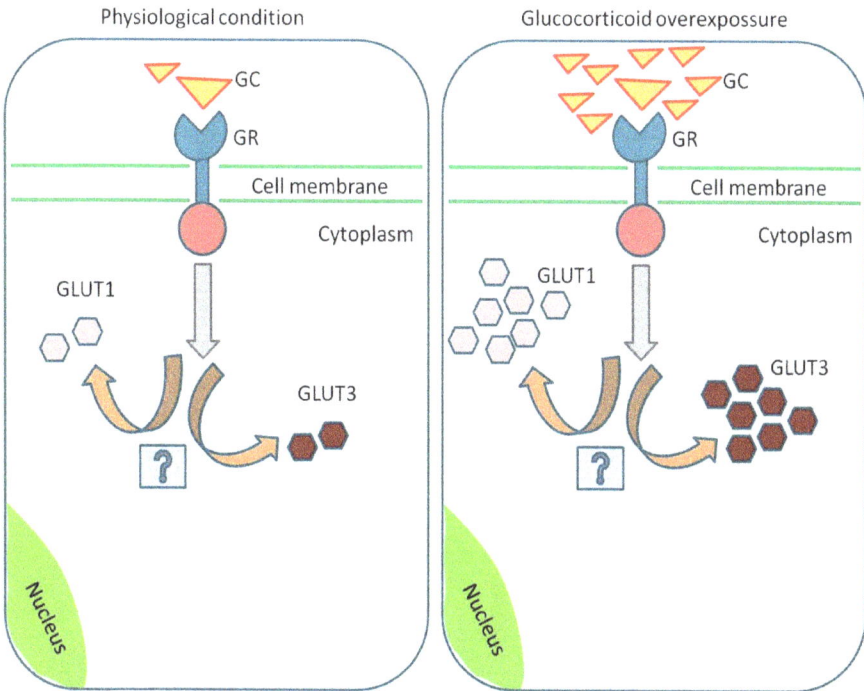

Figure 5. Effect of glucocorticoid overexposure on GLUT1 and GLUT3 expression in placental endothelial cells. GCs bind to GR and activate cellular signal transduction pathways. These molecular mechanisms remain to be unknown. As a result of GC overexposure GLUT1 and GLUT3 mRNA and proteins are increased in placental endothelial cells. Left panel refers possible physiological conditions and right panel refers effects of GC overexposure on GLUTs. (GC; Glucocorticoid, GR; Glucocorticoid Receptor, GLUT; Glucose Transporter)

In summary, the effects of glucocorticoids in placental glucose transport mechanisms in not fully understood. Further studies are needed to explain this issue.

5. Conclusion

Placental and fetal development is effected from glucocorticoids. Physiological glucocorticoid concentrations are necessary for healthy implantation, and pregnancy processes. On the other hand, glucocorticoid overexposure results with fetal and placental defects. Placentas of dexamethasone treated animals are smaller than healthy ones. In IUGR group placentas reduced placental proliferation and induced apoptosis seem to be a reason for decreased placental weigths. Dexamethasone caused a decrease in expression of genes involved in cell division such as cyclins A2, B1, D2, CDK 2, CDK 4 and M-phase protein kinase along with growth-promoting genes such as epidermal growth factor receptor. Moreover, in IUGR placentas cell cycle promoter proteins PCNA, Ki67 is decreased and cell cycle inhibitor proteins p27 and 57 are increased. Altered MAPK and Akt pathways are also unfavorably affected from glucocorticoid treatment. Decreased Akt and MAPK activations would result with reduced proliferation and/or induced apoptosis and reduced angiogenesis. GCs may affect placental angiogenesis by altering VEGF, VEGFR1 and VEGFR2 expression both at protein and gene levels with a direct effect on endothelial cells. Besides, without effecting endothelial cell viability and proliferation, GCs may affect endothelial cell migration and/or capacity of tube formation. The indirect effects of GCs seem to be via altering placental cytokine production processes which have negative effects on angiogenesis mechanisms. Another mechanism by which GCs may alter placental development is glucose transport mechanisms. It seems that GCs affect Glucose transporters via cell type dependent manner. In human endothelial cells GCs will up-regulate GLUT1 and GLUT3 expression but in trophoblast cells GCs adversely down regulates GLUT1 and GLUT3 expression in vitro.

In summary glucocorticoid overexposure may alter fetal development by altering, in part, placental development and function. It is clearly reviewed that placental development, proliferation, angiogenesis and glucose transport mechanisms are negatively affected from excess maternal glucocorticoid.

Author details

Emin Turkay Korgun*, Aslı Ozmen, Gozde Unek
Akdeniz University, Medical Faculty, Histology and Embryology Department, Antalya, Turkey

Inanc Mendilcioglu
Akdeniz University, Medical Faculty, Obstetrics and Gynecology Department, Antalya, Turkey

6. References

[1] Munck A, Naray-Fejes-Toth A (1994) Glucocorticoids and stress: permissive and suppressive actions. Ann N Y Acad Sci 746: 115-30; discussion 131-3.

[2] McEwen BS (2007) Physiology and neurobiology of stress and adaptation: central role of the brain. Physiol Rev 87: 873-904.

[3] Roberts D, Dalziel S (2006) Antenatal corticosteroids for accelerating fetal lung maturation for women at risk of preterm birth. Cochrane Database Syst Rev 3: CD004454.

[4] Kennedy TG (1983) Prostaglandin E2, adenosine 3':5'-cyclic monophosphate and changes in endometrial vascular permeability in rat uteri sensitized for the decidual cell reaction. Biol Reprod 29: 1069-76.

[5] Lopez Bernal A, Rivera J, Europe-Finner GN, Phaneuf S, Asboth G (1995) Parturition: activation of stimulatory pathways or loss of uterine quiescence? Adv Exp Med Biol 395: 435-51.

---

* Corresponding Author

[6] Guller S, Markiewicz L, Wozniak R, Burnham JM, Wang EY, Kaplan P, Lockwood CJ (1994) Developmental regulation of glucocorticoid-mediated effects on extracellular matrix protein expression in the human placenta. Endocrinology 134: 2064-71.

[7] Hahn T, Barth S, Graf R, Engelmann M, Beslagic D, Reul JM, Holsboer F, Dohr G, Desoye G (1999) Placental glucose transporter expression is regulated by glucocorticoids. J Clin Endocrinol Metab 84: 1445-52.

[8] Librach CL, Feigenbaum SL, Bass KE, Cui TY, Verastas N, Sadovsky Y, Quigley JP, French DL, Fisher SJ (1994) Interleukin-1 beta regulates human cytotrophoblast metalloproteinase activity and invasion in vitro. J Biol Chem 269: 17125-31.

[9] Xu B, Makris A, Thornton C, Hennessy A (2005) Glucocorticoids inhibit placental cytokines from cultured normal and preeclamptic placental explants. Placenta 26: 654-60.

[10] Ma Y, Kadner SS, Guller S (2004) Differential effects of lipopolysaccharide and thrombin on interleukin-8 expression in syncytiotrophoblasts and endothelial cells: implications for fetal survival. Ann N Y Acad Sci 1034: 236-44.

[11] Rosen T, Krikun G, Ma Y, Wang EY, Lockwood CJ, Guller S (1998) Chronic antagonism of nuclear factor-kappaB activity in cytotrophoblasts by dexamethasone: a potential mechanism for antiinflammatory action of glucocorticoids in human placenta. J Clin Endocrinol Metab 83: 3647-52.

[12] Tchernitchin A, Rooryck J, Tchernitchin X, Vandenhende J, Galand P (1975) Effects of cortisol on uterine eosinophilia and other oestrogenic responses. Mol Cell Endocrinol 2: 331-7.

[13] Fowden AL, Li J, Forhead AJ (1998) Glucocorticoids and the preparation for life after birth: are there long-term consequences of the life insurance? Proc Nutr Soc 57: 113-22.

[14] (2011) ACOG Committee Opinion No. 475: Antenatal corticosteroid therapy for fetal maturation. Obstet Gynecol 117: 422-4.

[15] Benediktsson R, Lindsay RS, Noble J, Seckl JR, Edwards CR (1993) Glucocorticoid exposure in utero: new model for adult hypertension. Lancet 341: 339-41.

[16] Levitt NS, Lindsay RS, Holmes MC, Seckl JR (1996) Dexamethasone in the last week of pregnancy attenuates hippocampal glucocorticoid receptor gene expression and elevates blood pressure in the adult offspring in the rat. Neuroendocrinology 64: 412-8.

[17] Bloom SL, Sheffield JS, McIntire DD, Leveno KJ (2001) Antenatal dexamethasone and decreased birth weight. Obstet Gynecol 97: 485-90.

[18] Langdown ML, Sugden MC (2001) Enhanced placental GLUT1 and GLUT3 expression in dexamethasone-induced fetal growth retardation. Mol Cell Endocrinol 185: 109-17.

[19] Sugden MC, Langdown ML, Munns MJ, Holness MJ (2001) Maternal glucocorticoid treatment modulates placental leptin and leptin receptor expression and materno-fetal leptin physiology during late pregnancy, and elicits hypertension associated with hyperleptinaemia in the early-growth-retarded adult offspring. Eur J Endocrinol 145: 529-39.

[20] Barker DJ (1997) Fetal nutrition and cardiovascular disease in later life. Br Med Bull 53: 96-108.

[21] Uno H, Eisele S, Sakai A, Shelton S, Baker E, DeJesus O, Holden J (1994) Neurotoxicity of glucocorticoids in the primate brain. Horm Behav 28: 336-48.

[22] Lesage J, Blondeau B, Grino M, Breant B, Dupouy JP (2001) Maternal undernutrition during late gestation induces fetal overexposure to glucocorticoids and intrauterine growth retardation, and disturbs the hypothalamo-pituitary adrenal axis in the newborn rat. Endocrinology 142: 1692-702.

[23] Bertram CE, Hanson MA (2002) Prenatal programming of postnatal endocrine responses by glucocorticoids. Reproduction 124: 459-67.

[24] de Vries A, Holmes MC, Heijnis A, Seier JV, Heerden J, Louw J, Wolfe-Coote S, Meaney MJ, Levitt NS, Seckl JR (2007) Prenatal dexamethasone exposure induces changes in nonhuman primate offspring cardiometabolic and hypothalamic-pituitary-adrenal axis function. J Clin Invest 117: 1058-67.

[25] Matthews SG (2000) Antenatal glucocorticoids and programming of the developing CNS. Pediatr Res 47: 291-300.

[26] Kranendonk G, Hopster H, Fillerup M, Ekkel ED, Mulder EJ, Taverne MA (2006) Cortisol administration to pregnant sows affects novelty-induced locomotion, aggressive behaviour, and blunts gender differences in their offspring. Horm Behav 49: 663-72.

[27] Funder JW (1997) Glucocorticoid and mineralocorticoid receptors: biology and clinical relevance. Annu Rev Med 48: 231-40.

[28] Li X, Wong J, Tsai SY, Tsai MJ, O'Malley BW (2003) Progesterone and glucocorticoid receptors recruit distinct coactivator complexes and promote distinct patterns of local chromatin modification. Mol Cell Biol 23: 3763-73.

[29] Wang Z, Frederick J, Garabedian MJ (2002) Deciphering the phosphorylation "code" of the glucocorticoid receptor in vivo. J Biol Chem 277: 26573-80.

[30] Yang Z, Guo C, Zhu P, Li W, Myatt L, Sun K (2007) Role of glucocorticoid receptor and CCAAT/enhancer-binding protein alpha in the feed-forward induction of 11beta-hydroxysteroid dehydrogenase type 1 expression by cortisol in human amnion fibroblasts. J Endocrinol 195: 241-53.

[31] Sun K, Myatt L (2003) Enhancement of glucocorticoid-induced 11beta-hydroxysteroid dehydrogenase type 1 expression by proinflammatory cytokines in cultured human amnion fibroblasts. Endocrinology 144: 5568-77.

[32] Sun M, Ramirez M, Challis JR, Gibb W (1996) Immunohistochemical localization of the glucocorticoid receptor in human fetal membranes and decidua at term and preterm delivery. J Endocrinol 149: 243-8.

[33] Chan CC, Lao TT, Ho PC, Sung EO, Cheung AN (2003) The effect of mifepristone on the expression of steroid hormone receptors in human decidua and placenta: a randomized placebo-controlled double-blind study. J Clin Endocrinol Metab 88: 5846-50.

[34] Chan J, Rabbitt EH, Innes BA, Bulmer JN, Stewart PM, Kilby MD, Hewison M (2007) Glucocorticoid-induced apoptosis in human decidua: a novel role for 11beta-hydroxysteroid dehydrogenase in late gestation. J Endocrinol 195: 7-15.

[35] Korgun ET, Dohr G, Desoye G, Demir R, Kayisli UA, Hahn T (2003) Expression of insulin, insulin-like growth factor I and glucocorticoid receptor in rat uterus and

embryo during decidualization, implantation and organogenesis. Reproduction 125: 75-84.

[36] Monder C, Shackleton CH (1984) 11 beta-Hydroxysteroid dehydrogenase: fact or fancy? Steroids 44: 383-417.

[37] Seckl JR (1993) 11 beta-hydroxysteroid dehydrogenase isoforms and their implications for blood pressure regulation. Eur J Clin Invest 23: 589-601.

[38] Seckl JR, Walker BR (2001) Minireview: 11beta-hydroxysteroid dehydrogenase type 1- a tissue-specific amplifier of glucocorticoid action. Endocrinology 142: 1371-6.

[39] Alfaidy N, Li W, MacIntosh T, Yang K, Challis J (2003) Late gestation increase in 11beta-hydroxysteroid dehydrogenase 1 expression in human fetal membranes: a novel intrauterine source of cortisol. J Clin Endocrinol Metab 88: 5033-8.

[40] Hardy DB, Yang K (2002) The expression of 11 beta-hydroxysteroid dehydrogenase type 2 is induced during trophoblast differentiation: effects of hypoxia. J Clin Endocrinol Metab 87: 3696-701.

[41] Krozowski Z, MaGuire JA, Stein-Oakley AN, Dowling J, Smith RE, Andrews RK (1995) Immunohistochemical localization of the 11 beta-hydroxysteroid dehydrogenase type II enzyme in human kidney and placenta. J Clin Endocrinol Metab 80: 2203-9.

[42] Sun K, Yang K, Challis JR (1997) Differential expression of 11 beta-hydroxysteroid dehydrogenase types 1 and 2 in human placenta and fetal membranes. J Clin Endocrinol Metab 82: 300-5.

[43] Driver PM, Kilby MD, Bujalska I, Walker EA, Hewison M, Stewart PM (2001) Expression of 11 beta-hydroxysteroid dehydrogenase isozymes and corticosteroid hormone receptors in primary cultures of human trophoblast and placental bed biopsies. Mol Hum Reprod 7: 357-63.

[44] Alfaidy N, Gupta S, DeMarco C, Caniggia I, Challis JR (2002) Oxygen regulation of placental 11 beta-hydroxysteroid dehydrogenase 2: physiological and pathological implications. J Clin Endocrinol Metab 87: 4797-805.

[45] Holmes MC, Abrahamsen CT, French KL, Paterson JM, Mullins JJ, Seckl JR (2006) The mother or the fetus? 11beta-hydroxysteroid dehydrogenase type 2 null mice provide evidence for direct fetal programming of behavior by endogenous glucocorticoids. J Neurosci 26: 3840-4.

[46] Edwards CR, Benediktsson R, Lindsay RS, Seckl JR (1993) Dysfunction of placental glucocorticoid barrier: link between fetal environment and adult hypertension? Lancet 341: 355-7.

[47] Lindsay RS, Lindsay RM, Waddell BJ, Seckl JR (1996) Prenatal glucocorticoid exposure leads to offspring hyperglycaemia in the rat: studies with the 11 beta-hydroxysteroid dehydrogenase inhibitor carbenoxolone. Diabetologia 39: 1299-305.

[48] Langley-Evans SC (1997) Maternal carbenoxolone treatment lowers birthweight and induces hypertension in the offspring of rats fed a protein-replete diet. Clin Sci (Lond) 93: 423-9.

[49] Welberg LA, Seckl JR, Holmes MC (2000) Inhibition of 11beta-hydroxysteroid dehydrogenase, the foeto-placental barrier to maternal glucocorticoids, permanently

programs amygdala GR mRNA expression and anxiety-like behaviour in the offspring. Eur J Neurosci 12: 1047-54.

[50] Wyrwoll CS, Seckl JR, Holmes MC (2009) Altered placental function of 11beta-hydroxysteroid dehydrogenase 2 knockout mice. Endocrinology 150: 1287-93.

[51] Stewart PM, Rogerson FM, Mason JI (1995) Type 2 11 beta-hydroxysteroid dehydrogenase messenger ribonucleic acid and activity in human placenta and fetal membranes: its relationship to birth weight and putative role in fetal adrenal steroidogenesis. J Clin Endocrinol Metab 80: 885-90.

[52] Kajantie E, Dunkel L, Turpeinen U, Stenman UH, Andersson S (2006) Placental 11beta-HSD2 activity, early postnatal clinical course, and adrenal function in extremely low birth weight infants. Pediatr Res 59: 575-8.

[53] Dave-Sharma S, Wilson RC, Harbison MD, Newfield R, Azar MR, Krozowski ZS, Funder JW, Shackleton CH, Bradlow HL, Wei JQ, Hertecant J, Moran A, Neiberger RE, Balfe JW, Fattah A, Daneman D, Akkurt HI, De Santis C, New MI (1998) Examination of genotype and phenotype relationships in 14 patients with apparent mineralocorticoid excess. J Clin Endocrinol Metab 83: 2244-54.

[54] Newnham JP, Evans SF, Godfrey M, Huang W, Ikegami M, Jobe A (1999) Maternal, but not fetal, administration of corticosteroids restricts fetal growth. J Matern Fetal Med 8: 81-7.

[55] Malassine A, Cronier L (2002) Hormones and human trophoblast differentiation: a review. Endocrine 19: 3-11.

[56] Morrish DW, Dakour J, Li H (1998) Functional regulation of human trophoblast differentiation. J Reprod Immunol 39: 179-95.

[57] Audette MC, Greenwood SL, Sibley CP, Jones CJ, Challis JR, Matthews SG, Jones RL (2010) Dexamethasone stimulates placental system A transport and trophoblast differentiation in term villous explants. Placenta 31: 97-105.

[58] Baisden B, Sonne S, Joshi RM, Ganapathy V, Shekhawat PS (2007) Antenatal dexamethasone treatment leads to changes in gene expression in a murine late placenta. Placenta 28: 1082-90.

[59] Hewitt DP, Mark PJ, Waddell BJ (2006) Glucocorticoids prevent the normal increase in placental vascular endothelial growth factor expression and placental vascularity during late pregnancy in the rat. Endocrinology 147: 5568-74.

[60] Hewitt DP, Mark PJ, Waddell BJ (2006) Placental expression of peroxisome proliferator-activated receptors in rat pregnancy and the effect of increased glucocorticoid exposure. Biol Reprod 74: 23-8.

[61] Timmerman M, Teng C, Wilkening RB, Fennessey P, Battaglia FC, Meschia G (2000) Effect of dexamethasone on fetal hepatic glutamine-glutamate exchange. Am J Physiol Endocrinol Metab 278: E839-45.

[62] Ward JW, Wooding FB, Fowden AL (2004) Ovine feto-placental metabolism. J Physiol 554: 529-41.

[63] Fowden AL, Forhead AJ (2009) Hormones as epigenetic signals in developmental programming. Exp Physiol 94: 607-25.

[64] Fowden AL, Forhead AJ, Coan PM, Burton GJ (2008) The placenta and intrauterine programming. J Neuroendocrinol 20: 439-50.

[65] McDonald TJ, Franko KL, Brown JM, Jenkins SL, Nathanielsz PW, Nijland MJ (2003) Betamethasone in the last week of pregnancy causes fetal growth retardation but not adult hypertension in rats. J Soc Gynecol Investig 10: 469-73.

[66] Kaufmann P, Castelluci M (1997) Extravillous trophoblast in the human placenta: A review. Trophoblast Research 18: 21-65.

[67] Lodish H, Berk A, Kaiser A, Krieger M, Scott P, Bretscher A, Ploegh H, Matsudaira P, *Molecular Cell Biology.* 5th ed. 2002, New York: W H Freeman.

[68] Alberts B, Johnson A, Lewis J, Raff M, Roberts K, Walter P, *Molecular Biology of the Cell.* 4th ed. 2002, New York Garland Science.

[69] Sherr CJ, Roberts JM (1995) Inhibitors of mammalian G1 cyclin-dependent kinases. Genes Dev 9: 1149-63.

[70] Xiong Y (1996) Why are there so many CDK inhibitors? Biochim Biophys Acta 1288: 01-5.

[71] Lew DJ, Dulic V, Reed SI (1991) Isolation of three novel human cyclins by rescue of G1 cyclin (Cln) function in yeast. Cell 66: 1197-206.

[72] Bailly E, Pines J, Hunter T, Bornens M (1992) Cytoplasmic accumulation of cyclin B1 in human cells: association with a detergent-resistant compartment and with the centrosome. J Cell Sci 101 (Pt 3): 529-45.

[73] Hunter T, Pines J (1994) Cyclins and cancer. II: Cyclin D and CDK inhibitors come of age. Cell 79: 573-82.

[74] Harper JW, Elledge SJ (1996) Cdk inhibitors in development and cancer. Curr Opin Genet Dev 6: 56-64.

[75] Dulic V, Stein GH, Far DF, Reed SI (1998) Nuclear accumulation of p21Cip1 at the onset of mitosis: a role at the G2/M-phase transition. Mol Cell Biol 18: 546-57.

[76] Ogryzko VV, Wong P, Howard BH (1997) WAF1 retards S-phase progression primarily by inhibition of cyclin-dependent kinases. Mol Cell Biol 17: 4877-82.

[77] Niculescu AB, 3rd, Chen X, Smeets M, Hengst L, Prives C, Reed SI (1998) Effects of p21(Cip1/Waf1) at both the G1/S and the G2/M cell cycle transitions: pRb is a critical determinant in blocking DNA replication and in preventing endoreduplication. Mol Cell Biol 18: 629-43.

[78] Parker SB, Eichele G, Zhang P, Rawls A, Sands AT, Bradley A, Olson EN, Harper JW, Elledge SJ (1995) p53-independent expression of p21Cip1 in muscle and other terminally differentiating cells. Science 267: 1024-7.

[79] Lee MH, Reynisdottir I, Massague J (1995) Cloning of p57KIP2, a cyclin-dependent kinase inhibitor with unique domain structure and tissue distribution. Genes Dev 9: 639-49.

[80] Yan Y, Frisen J, Lee MH, Massague J, Barbacid M (1997) Ablation of the CDK inhibitor p57Kip2 results in increased apoptosis and delayed differentiation during mouse development. Genes Dev 11: 973-83.

[81] Genbacev O, McMaster MT, Fisher SJ (2000) A repertoire of cell cycle regulators whose expression is coordinated with human cytotrophoblast differentiation. Am J Pathol 157: 1337-51.

[82] DeLoia JA, Burlingame JM, Krasnow JS (1997) Differential expression of G1 cyclins during human placentogenesis. Placenta 18: 9-16.

[83] Ichikawa N, Zhai YL, Shiozawa T, Toki T, Noguchi H, Nikaido T, Fujii S (1998) Immunohistochemical analysis of cell cycle regulatory gene products in normal trophoblast and placental site trophoblastic tumor. Int J Gynecol Pathol 17: 235-40.

[84] Korgun ET, Celik-Ozenci C, Acar N, Cayli S, Desoye G, Demir R (2006) Location of cell cycle regulators cyclin B1, cyclin A, PCNA, Ki67 and cell cycle inhibitors p21, p27 and p57 in human first trimester placenta and deciduas. Histochem Cell Biol 125: 615-24.

[85] Rossant J, Cross JC (2001) Placental development: lessons from mouse mutants. Nat Rev Genet 2: 538-48.

[86] Georgiades P, Ferguson-Smith AC, Burton GJ (2002) Comparative developmental anatomy of the murine and human definitive placentae. Placenta 23: 3-19.

[87] Pijnenborg R, Robertson WB, Brosens I, Dixon G (1981) Review article: trophoblast invasion and the establishment of haemochorial placentation in man and laboratory animals. Placenta 2: 71-91.

[88] Korgun ET, Unek G, Herrera E, Jones CJ, Wadsack C, Kipmen-Korgun D, Desoye G (2011) Mapping of CIP/KIP inhibitors, G1 cyclins D1, D3, E and p53 proteins in the rat term placenta. Histochem Cell Biol 136: 267-78.

[89] Unek G, Ozmen A, Kipmen-Korgun D, Korgun ET (2012) Immunolocalization of PCNA, Ki67, p27 and p57 in normal and dexamethasone-induced intrauterine growth restriction placental development in rat. Acta Histochem 114: 31-40.

[90] Kim ST, Lee SK, Gye MC (2005) The expression of Cdk inhibitors p27kip1 and p57kip2 in mouse placenta and human choriocarcinoma JEG-3 cells. Placenta 26: 73-80.

[91] Ozmen A, Unek G, Kipmen-Korgun D, Korgun ET (2011) The expression of Akt and ERK1/2 proteins decreased in dexamethasone-induced intrauterine growth restricted rat placental development. J Mol Histol 42: 237-49.

[92] Ain R, Canham LN, Soares MJ (2005) Dexamethasone-induced intrauterine growth restriction impacts the placental prolactin family, insulin-like growth factor-II and the Akt signaling pathway. J Endocrinol 185: 253-63.

[93] Ghidini A, Pezzullo JC, Sylvestre G, Lembet A, Salafia CM (2001) Antenatal corticosteroids and placental histology in preterm birth. Placenta 22: 412-7.

[94] Gennari-Moser C, Khankin EV, Schuller S, Escher G, Frey BM, Portmann CB, Baumann MU, Lehmann AD, Surbek D, Karumanchi SA, Frey FJ, Mohaupt MG (2011) Regulation of placental growth by aldosterone and cortisol. Endocrinology 152: 263-71.

[95] Waddell BJ, Hisheh S, Dharmarajan AM, Burton PJ (2000) Apoptosis in rat placenta is zone-dependent and stimulated by glucocorticoids. Biol Reprod 63: 1913-7.

[96] Crocker IP, Barratt S, Kaur M, Baker PN (2001) The in-vitro characterization of induced apoptosis in placental cytotrophoblasts and syncytiotrophoblasts. Placenta 22: 822-30.

[97] Mandl M, Ghaffari-Tabrizi N, Haas J, Nohammer G, Desoye G (2006) Differential glucocorticoid effects on proliferation and invasion of human trophoblast cell lines. Reproduction 132: 159-67.

[98] Clapp C, Thebault S, Jeziorski MC, Martinez De La Escalera G (2009) Peptide hormone regulation of angiogenesis. Physiol Rev 89: 1177-215.

[99] Lunghi L, Pavan B, Biondi C, Paolillo R, Valerio A, Vesce F, Patella A (2010) Use of glucocorticoids in pregnancy. Curr Pharm Des 16: 3616-37.

[100] Hadoke PW, Iqbal J, Walker BR (2009) Therapeutic manipulation of glucocorticoid metabolism in cardiovascular disease. Br J Pharmacol 156: 689-712.

[101] Oberleithner H, Schneider SW, Albermann L, Hillebrand U, Ludwig T, Riethmuller C, Shahin V, Schafer C, Schillers H (2003) Endothelial cell swelling by aldosterone. J Membr Biol 196: 163-72.

[102] Yang S, Zhang L (2004) Glucocorticoids and vascular reactivity. Curr Vasc Pharmacol 2: 1-12.

[103] Rae M, Mohamad A, Price D, Hadoke PW, Walker BR, Mason JI, Hillier SG, Critchley HO (2009) Cortisol inactivation by 11beta-hydroxysteroid dehydrogenase-2 may enhance endometrial angiogenesis via reduced thrombospondin-1 in heavy menstruation. J Clin Endocrinol Metab 94: 1443-50.

[104] Carmeliet P (2000) Mechanisms of angiogenesis and arteriogenesis. Nat Med 6: 389-95.

[105] Logie JJ, Ali S, Marshall KM, Heck MM, Walker BR, Hadoke PW (2010) Glucocorticoid-mediated inhibition of angiogenic changes in human endothelial cells is not caused by reductions in cell proliferation or migration. PLoS One 5: e14476.

[106] Giroux S, Tremblay M, Bernard D, Cardin-Girard JF, Aubry S, Larouche L, Rousseau S, Huot J, Landry J, Jeannotte L, Charron J (1999) Embryonic death of Mek1-deficient mice reveals a role for this kinase in angiogenesis in the labyrinthine region of the placenta. Curr Biol 9: 369-72.

[107] Hatano N, Mori Y, Oh-hora M, Kosugi A, Fujikawa T, Nakai N, Niwa H, Miyazaki J, Hamaoka T, Ogata M (2003) Essential role for ERK2 mitogen-activated protein kinase in placental development. Genes Cells 8: 847-56.

[108] Mikula M, Schreiber M, Husak Z, Kucerova L, Ruth J, Wieser R, Zatloukal K, Beug H, Wagner EF, Baccarini M (2001) Embryonic lethality and fetal liver apoptosis in mice lacking the c-raf-1 gene. EMBO J 20: 1952-62.

[109] Qian X, Esteban L, Vass WC, Upadhyaya C, Papageorge AG, Yienger K, Ward JM, Lowy DR, Santos E (2000) The Sos1 and Sos2 Ras-specific exchange factors: differences in placental expression and signaling properties. EMBO J 19: 642-54.

[110] Karar J, Maity A (2011) PI3K/AKT/mTOR Pathway in Angiogenesis. Front Mol Neurosci 4: 51.

[111] Aida K, Wang XL, Wang J, Li C, McDonald TJ, Nathanielsz PW (2004) Effect of betamethasone administration to the pregnant baboon at 0.75 gestation on placental eNOS distribution and activity. Placenta 25: 780-7.

[112] Schwab M, Coksaygan T, Nathanielsz PW (2006) Betamethasone effects on ovine uterine and umbilical placental perfusion at the dose used to enhance fetal lung maturation. Am J Obstet Gynecol 194: 572-9.

[113] Hunt JS, Chen HL, Miller L (1996) Tumor necrosis factors: pivotal components of pregnancy? Biol Reprod 54: 554-62.

[114] Moore KW, de Waal Malefyt R, Coffman RL, O'Garra A (2001) Interleukin-10 and the interleukin-10 receptor. Annu Rev Immunol 19: 683-765.

[115] Kahler C, Schleussner E, Moller A, Seewald HJ (2004) Doppler measurements in fetoplacental vessels after maternal betamethasone administration. Fetal Diagn Ther 19: 52-7.

[116] Oliver A, Ciulla TA (2006) Corticosteroids as antiangiogenic agents. Ophthalmol Clin North Am 19: 345-51, v.

[117] Challa JK, Gillies MC, Penfold PL, Gyory JF, Hunyor AB, Billson FA (1998) Exudative macular degeneration and intravitreal triamcinolone: 18 month follow up. Aust N Z J Ophthalmol 26: 277-81.

[118] Danis RP, Ciulla TA, Pratt LM, Anliker W (2000) Intravitreal triamcinolone acetonide in exudative age-related macular degeneration. Retina 20: 244-50.

[119] Martidis A, Miller DG, Ciulla TA, Danis RP, Moorthy RS (1999) Corticosteroids as an antiangiogenic agent for histoplasmosis-related subfoveal choroidal neovascularization. J Ocul Pharmacol Ther 15: 425-8.

[120] Penfold PL, Gyory JF, Hunyor AB, Billson FA (1995) Exudative macular degeneration and intravitreal triamcinolone. A pilot study. Aust N Z J Ophthalmol 23: 293-8.

[121] Zein WM, Noureddin BN, Jurdi FA, Schakal A, Bashshur ZF (2006) Panretinal photocoagulation and intravitreal triamcinolone acetonide for the management of proliferative diabetic retinopathy with macular edema. Retina 26: 137-42.

[122] Ingber DE, Madri JA, Folkman J (1986) A possible mechanism for inhibition of angiogenesis by angiostatic steroids: induction of capillary basement membrane dissolution. Endocrinology 119: 1768-75.

[123] Stokes CL, Weisz PB, Williams SK, Lauffenburger DA (1990) Inhibition of microvascular endothelial cell migration by beta-cyclodextrin tetradecasulfate and hydrocortisone. Microvasc Res 40: 279-84.

[124] Tokida Y, Aratani Y, Morita A, Kitagawa Y (1990) Production of two variant laminin forms by endothelial cells and shift of their relative levels by angiostatic steroids. J Biol Chem 265: 18123-9.

[125] Greenberger S, Boscolo E, Adini I, Mulliken JB, Bischoff J (2010) Corticosteroid suppression of VEGF-A in infantile hemangioma-derived stem cells. N Engl J Med 362: 1005-13.

[126] Kluetz PG, Figg WD, Dahut WL (2010) Angiogenesis inhibitors in the treatment of prostate cancer. Expert Opin Pharmacother 11: 233-47.

[127] Weinstein RS, Wan C, Liu Q, Wang Y, Almeida M, O'Brien CA, Thostenson J, Roberson PK, Boskey AL, Clemens TL, Manolagas SC (2010) Endogenous glucocorticoids decrease skeletal angiogenesis, vascularity, hydration, and strength in aged mice. Aging Cell 9: 147-61.

[128] Yano A, Fujii Y, Iwai A, Kageyama Y, Kihara K (2006) Glucocorticoids suppress tumor angiogenesis and in vivo growth of prostate cancer cells. Clin Cancer Res 12: 3003-9.

[129] Pao SS, Paulsen IT, Saier MH, Jr. (1998) Major facilitator superfamily. Microbiol Mol Biol Rev 62: 1-34.

[130] Thorens B, Mueckler M (2010) Glucose transporters in the 21st Century. Am J Physiol Endocrinol Metab 298: E141-5.

[131] Joost HG, Bell GI, Best JD, Birnbaum MJ, Charron MJ, Chen YT, Doege H, James DE, Lodish HF, Moley KH, Moley JF, Mueckler M, Rogers S, Schurmann A, Seino S, Thorens B (2002) Nomenclature of the GLUT/SLC2A family of sugar/polyol transport facilitators. Am J Physiol Endocrinol Metab 282: E974-6.

[132] Farrell CL, Yang J, Pardridge WM (1992) GLUT-1 glucose transporter is present within apical and basolateral membranes of brain epithelial interfaces and in microvascular endothelia with and without tight junctions. J Histochem Cytochem 40: 193-9.

[133] Takata K, Kasahara T, Kasahara M, Ezaki O, Hirano H (1992) Localization of erythrocyte/HepG2-type glucose transporter (GLUT1) in human placental villi. Cell Tissue Res 267: 407-12.

[134] Jansson T, Wennergren M, Illsley NP (1993) Glucose transporter protein expression in human placenta throughout gestation and in intrauterine growth retardation. J Clin Endocrinol Metab 77: 1554-62.

[135] Illsley NP (2000) Glucose transporters in the human placenta. Placenta 21: 14-22.

[136] Xing AY, Challier JC, Lepercq J, Cauzac M, Charron MJ, Girard J, Hauguel-de Mouzon S (1998) Unexpected expression of glucose transporter 4 in villous stromal cells of human placenta. J Clin Endocrinol Metab 83: 4097-101.

[137] Wolf HJ, Desoye G (1993) Immunohistochemical localization of glucose transporters and insulin receptors in human fetal membranes at term. Histochemistry 100: 379-85.

[138] Hahn D, Blaschitz A, Korgun ET, Lang I, Desoye G, Skofitsch G, Dohr G (2001) From maternal glucose to fetal glycogen: expression of key regulators in the human placenta. Mol Hum Reprod 7: 1173-8.

[139] Hauguel-de Mouzon S, Challier JC, Kacemi A, Cauzac M, Malek A, Girard J (1997) The GLUT3 glucose transporter isoform is differentially expressed within human placental cell types. J Clin Endocrinol Metab 82: 2689-94.

[140] Korgun ET, Celik-Ozenci C, Seval Y, Desoye G, Demir R (2005) Do glucose transporters have other roles in addition to placental glucose transport during early pregnancy? Histochem Cell Biol 123: 621-9.

[141] Hauguel-de Mouzon S, Shafrir E (2001) Carbohydrate and fat metabolism and related hormonal regulation in normal and diabetic placenta. Placenta 22: 619-27.

[142] Kalhan SC, D'Angelo LJ, Savin SM, Adam PA (1979) Glucose production in pregnant women at term gestation. Sources of glucose for human fetus. J Clin Invest 63: 388-94.

[143] Kipmen-Korgun D, Ozmen A, Unek G, Simsek M, Demir R, Korgun ET (2011) Triamcinolone up-regulates GLUT 1 and GLUT 3 expression in cultured human placental endothelial cells. Cell Biochem Funct.

[144] Anderson GG, Lamden MP, Cidlowski JA, Ashikaga T (1981) Comparative pulmonary surfactant-inducing effect of three corticosteroids in the near-term rat. Am J Obstet Gynecol 139: 562-4.

[145] Korgun ET, Acar N, Sati L, Kipmen-Korgun D, Ozen A, Unek G, Ustunel I, Demir R (2011) Expression of glucocorticoid receptor and glucose transporter-1 during placental development in the diabetic rat. Folia Histochem Cytobiol 49: 325-34.

[146] Hahn T, Barth S, Weiss U, Mosgoeller W, Desoye G (1998) Sustained hyperglycemia in vitro down-regulates the GLUT1 glucose transport system of cultured human term placental trophoblast: a mechanism to protect fetal development? FASEB J 12: 1221-31.

[147] Hirayama H, Sawai K, Hirayama M, Hirai T, Kageyama S, Onoe S, Minamihashi A, Moriyasu S (2011) Prepartum maternal plasma glucose concentrations and placental glucose transporter mRNA expression in cows carrying somatic cell clone fetuses. J Reprod Dev 57: 57-61.

[148] Lesage J, Hahn D, Leonhardt M, Blondeau B, Breant B, Dupouy JP (2002) Maternal undernutrition during late gestation-induced intrauterine growth restriction in the rat is associated with impaired placental GLUT3 expression, but does not correlate with endogenous corticosterone levels. J Endocrinol 174: 37-43.

[149] Boyett JD, Hofert JF (1972) Studies concerning the inhibition of glucose metabolism in thymus lymphocytes by cortisol and epinephrine. Endocrinology 91: 233-9.

[150] Garvey WT, Huecksteadt TP, Monzon R, Marshall S (1989) Dexamethasone regulates the glucose transport system in primary cultured adipocytes: different mechanisms of insulin resistance after acute and chronic exposure. Endocrinology 124: 2063-73.

[151] Haber RS, Weinstein SP (1992) Role of glucose transporters in glucocorticoid-induced insulin resistance. GLUT4 isoform in rat skeletal muscle is not decreased by dexamethasone. Diabetes 41: 728-35.

[152] Hajduch E, Hainault I, Meunier C, Jardel C, Hainque B, Guerre-Millo M, Lavau M (1995) Regulation of glucose transporters in cultured rat adipocytes: synergistic effect of insulin and dexamethasone on GLUT4 gene expression through promoter activation. Endocrinology 136: 4782-9.

[153] Langdown ML, Holness MJ, Sugden MC (2001) Early growth retardation induced by excessive exposure to glucocorticoids in utero selectively increases cardiac GLUT1 protein expression and Akt/protein kinase B activity in adulthood. J Endocrinol 169: 11-22.

[154] Olgemoller B, Schon J, Wieland OH (1985) Endothelial plasma membrane is a glucocorticoid-regulated barrier for the uptake of glucose into the cell. Mol Cell Endocrinol 43: 165-71.

[155] Weinstein SP, Wilson CM, Pritsker A, Cushman SW (1998) Dexamethasone inhibits insulin-stimulated recruitment of GLUT4 to the cell surface in rat skeletal muscle. Metabolism 47: 3-6.

[156] Ewart HS, Somwar R, Klip A (1998) Dexamethasone stimulates the expression of GLUT1 and GLUT4 proteins via different signalling pathways in L6 skeletal muscle cells. FEBS Lett 421: 120-4.

[157] Gray S, Stonestreet BS, Thamotharan S, Sadowska GB, Daood M, Watchko J, Devaskar SU (2006) Skeletal muscle glucose transporter protein responses to antenatal glucocorticoids in the ovine fetus. J Endocrinol 189: 219-29.

[158] Hernandez R, Teruel T, Lorenzo M (2003) Insulin and dexamethasone induce GLUT4 gene expression in foetal brown adipocytes: synergistic effect through CCAAT/enhancer-binding protein alpha. Biochem J 372: 617-24.

[159] Lundgren M, Buren J, Ruge T, Myrnas T, Eriksson JW (2004) Glucocorticoids down-regulate glucose uptake capacity and insulin-signaling proteins in omental but not subcutaneous human adipocytes. J Clin Endocrinol Metab 89: 2989-97.

[160] Tortorella LL, Pilch PF (2002) C2C12 myocytes lack an insulin-responsive vesicular compartment despite dexamethasone-induced GLUT4 expression. Am J Physiol Endocrinol Metab 283: E514-24.

[161] Costedoat-Chalumeau N, Amoura Z, Le Thi Hong D, Wechsler B, Vauthier D, Ghillani P, Papo T, Fain O, Musset L, Piette JC (2003) Questions about dexamethasone use for the prevention of anti-SSA related congenital heart block. Ann Rheum Dis 62: 1010-2.

[162] Matthews SG, Owen D, Kalabis G, Banjanin S, Setiawan EB, Dunn EA, Andrews MH (2004) Fetal glucocorticoid exposure and hypothalamo-pituitary-adrenal (HPA) function after birth. Endocr Res 30: 827-36.

[163] Garvey D, Scott J (1981) Placental and fetal contraindications of dexamethasone administration to pregnant rats. Experientia 37: 757-9.

[164] Katz VL, Thorp JM, Jr., Bowes WA, Jr. (1990) Severe symmetric intrauterine growth retardation associated with the topical use of triamcinolone. Am J Obstet Gynecol 162: 396-7.

[165] Reinisch JM, Simon NG, Karow WG, Gandelman R (1978) Prenatal exposure to prednisone in humans and animals retards intrauterine growth. Science 202: 436-8.

[166] Gatford KL, Wintour EM, De Blasio MJ, Owens JA, Dodic M (2000) Differential timing for programming of glucose homoeostasis, sensitivity to insulin and blood pressure by in utero exposure to dexamethasone in sheep. Clin Sci (Lond) 98: 553-60.

[167] Gurrin LC, Moss TJ, Sloboda DM, Hazelton ML, Challis JR, Newnham JP (2003) Uising WinBUGS to fit nonlinear mixed models with an application to pharmacokinetic modelling of insulin response to glucose challenge in sheep exposed antenatally to glucocorticoids. J Biopharm Stat 13: 117-39.

[168] Kutzler MA, Molnar J, Schlafer DH, Kuc RE, Davenport AP, Nathanielsz PW (2003) Maternal dexamethasone increases endothelin-1 sensitivity and endothelin a receptor expression in ovine foetal placental arteries. Placenta 24: 392-402.

[169] Moss TJ, Sloboda DM, Gurrin LC, Harding R, Challis JR, Newnham JP (2001) Programming effects in sheep of prenatal growth restriction and glucocorticoid exposure. Am J Physiol Regul Integr Comp Physiol 281: R960-70.

[170] Nyirenda MJ, Lindsay RS, Kenyon CJ, Burchell A, Seckl JR (1998) Glucocorticoid exposure in late gestation permanently programs rat hepatic phosphoenolpyruvate carboxykinase and glucocorticoid receptor expression and causes glucose intolerance in adult offspring. J Clin Invest 101: 2174-81.

[171] Nyirenda MJ, Welberg LA, Seckl JR (2001) Programming hyperglycaemia in the rat through prenatal exposure to glucocorticoids-fetal effect or maternal influence? J Endocrinol 170: 653-60.

[172] Sloboda DM, Newnham JP, Challis JR (2000) Effects of repeated maternal betamethasone administration on growth and hypothalamic-pituitary-adrenal function of the ovine fetus at term. J Endocrinol 165: 79-91.
[173] Drake AJ, Walker BR, Seckl JR (2005) Intergenerational consequences of fetal programming by in utero exposure to glucocorticoids in rats. Am J Physiol Regul Integr Comp Physiol 288: R34-8.

Chapter 3

Sex-Specific Effects of Prenatal Glucocorticoids on Placental Development

Hayley Dickinson, Bree A. O'Connell, David W. Walker and Karen M. Moritz

Additional information is available at the end of the chapter

1. Introduction

The placenta, essential for normal fetal development by providing adequate nutrients to allow appropriate growth and maturation of the fetus in preparation for birth, is also a 'protective' barrier in the sense that it prevents entry into the fetal circulation of substances that are either toxic, or that drive fetal growth at inappropriate rates. An important aspect of this 'filtering' function of the placenta is limiting the entry of glucocorticoids of maternal origin into the fetal compartment. This is achieved by the presence of enzymes, transporters and receptors collectively termed the 'placental glucocorticoid barrier' [1-4].

Antenatal glucocorticoids are routinely administered to the mother for the treatment of a variety of pregnancy and fetal complications. Asthmatic women often experience an increase in severity of their symptoms during pregnancy leading to increased use of glucocorticoids. The threat of preterm birth results in administration of the synthetic glucocorticoid, betamethasone, to rapidly mature fetal organs (especially, the lungs) to promote survival. Further, stressful events during pregnancy such as natural disasters and famines for example, expose fetuses to higher than normal levels of maternally secreted glucocorticoids.

The effects of exposure to high levels of glucocorticoids during fetal development have now been well described [1, 5-9], and the advantages (e.g., maturation of lung surfactant production and increased hepatic glycogen deposition) are offset by effects that limit fetal growth and induce perturbations of brain growth and perfusion [1, 10-11]. However, while fetal/neonatal effects have been intensively investigated, the consequences of glucocorticoid excess on placental structure and function has received little attention to date. The knowledge that male fetuses are more likely to be affected negatively following events that usually increase fetal glucocorticoid exposure, has alerted researchers to the possibility that such sex-related effects could arise in the placenta. This chapter will describe the differences that exist between a male and female placenta with respect to the glucocorticoid barrier, and summarise current human clinical and experimental animal work that has explored the differential response of the placenta of a male and female fetus to glucocorticoid exposure.

2. The placental glucocorticoid barrier

While glucocorticoids are essential for the development of many organs, during pregnancy, the placenta acts as a barrier to prevent excess entry of maternal glucocorticoids into the fetal compartment [12-14]. This placental barrier to glucocorticoids is achieved predominantly by the presence of 11β-hydroxysteriod dehydrogenase type 2 (11βHSD2), which converts the biologically active glucocorticoid (cortisol in humans, corticosterone in mice and rats) to its physiologically inert form [2]. The placental 'barrier' is not complete, and under normal conditions a proportion (~10-15%) of maternal glucocorticoids reaches the fetal circulation [2]. While 11βHSD2 is the major component of the placental glucocorticoid barrier, other proteins contained within the placenta may also help to limit the transfer of maternal glucocorticoid to the fetus. The multi-drug resistance P-glycoprotein (ABCB1) is a membrane-bound protein, which mediates the efflux of glucocorticoids out of the placenta back into the maternal circulation, thus reducing the amount of glucocorticoids able to diffuse down the concentration gradient into the fetal circulation [15-17].

The response of the placenta itself to glucocorticoids is mediated by the glucocorticoid (GR) and mineralocorticoid receptor [18]. The most prominent isoform of the GR, both in the placenta and throughout the whole body, is GRα. This isoform mediates the biological effects of glucocorticoids, which include cell growth, proliferation and differentiation [19]. The placenta has not generally been considered a mineralocorticoid target tissue, however work by Driver et al [20] has suggested that placental trophoblast cells express a functional mineralocorticoid receptor, which is in part responsible for the transport of sodium across the placenta [20]. Because of the limited data on the role of the mineralocorticoid receptor in the placenta, our discussion will focus primarily on GR mediated effects.

3. Causes of elevated glucocorticoids during pregnancy

There are many circumstances during pregnancy in which the circulating levels of maternal glucocorticoids are elevated, resulting in placental and fetal exposure to excess glucocorticoids. The glucocorticoids within the maternal system can either be endogenous, originating from within the mother; or exogenous, where the glucocorticoid has been administered to the mother as a drug or treatment. Exogenous glucocorticoids are generally synthetic, such as betamethasone, dexamethasone or prednisone. The period of time when maternal, and therefore fetal and placental glucocorticoid levels, are elevated will vary considerably depending on the clinical circumstance, and effects arising from either acute or chronic exposures have been identified. Thus, the type of glucocorticoid, duration of exposure, and time in gestation need to be taken into account when determining the consequences for the fetus and placenta.

3.1. Exposure to natural glucocorticoids

Periods of stress, both physical (illness, excess exercise, famine/under nutrition) or psychological (anxiety) in origin, result in the elevation of endogenous glucocorticoids [21]. While cortisol can cross the placenta, it is a good substrate for 11βHSD2, and is readily catalysed by this enzyme under normal levels. However, when levels of cortisol are elevated, the barrier is overwhelmed and more cortisol is able to cross the placenta into the fetal circulation [4]. Deleterious effects of excess endogenous glucocorticoids on the fetus and newborn have been well documented [3, 6, 22-25]. These effects are greater for male fetuses. For example, males have been shown to have greater instances of *in utero* mortality and also increased likelihood of childhood and adult morbidity and mortality [21, 26]. An epidemiology study that examined women who were pregnant at the time of the 2001 terrorist attacks on the World Trade Centre found that there was a higher incidence of low birth weight babies for women who were residing in New York at the time. The greatest proportion of these low birth weight babies came from women who were in their first or second trimester at the time of the attacks [27]. These studies also revealed an increased incidence of male fetal death in New York after September 2001 [28-29]. High maternal stress and thus fetal exposure of cortisol are thought to be the cause of these poor fetal outcomes.

3.2. Exposure to synthetic glucocorticoids

Antenatal glucocorticoids are routinely administered to the mother for the treatment of a variety of pregnancy and fetal complications. Women who suffer from asthma are required to continue their glucocorticoid medication for the ongoing treatment/prevention of their symptoms, which in 33% of cases worsen during pregnancy [30-31]. Women whose babies are at risk of congenital adrenal hyperplasia are administered antenatal glucocorticoid treatment to return fetal adrenal hormone levels to normal and thus virilisation (the abnormal development of male sexual characteristics in a female) and fertility problems are prevented [32]. Further, pregnant mothers threatening preterm birth (~7-10% of all pregnancies), receive antenatal glucocorticoids, to mature the lungs of the fetus prior to birth to reduce neonatal morbidity and mortality [25]. As for cortisol, synthetic glucocorticoids can be catalysed by 11βHSD2, however they are a poor substrate for the enzyme, and more freely cross the placenta than cortisol [33]. The presence of excess maternal glucocorticoids can have positive effects on fetal development and maternal health and in many situations cannot be avoided. The National Institute of Health recommend treatment of all women at risk of preterm delivery, between 24 and 34 weeks of gestation, with synthetic glucocorticoids to prematurely mature fetal organs, primarily the lung, to improve neonatal survival [8]. Therefore a large proportion of this population of babies, are exposed to single, and sometimes multiple courses of synthetic glucocorticoids in the period leading up to birth [25]. While antenatal glucocorticoids are the most effective treatment for improving preterm birth survival rates, the scientific community continues to question whether the use of glucocorticoids to reduce the morbidity and mortality associated with preterm birth, is worth the risk of the potential negative outcomes on metabolism and neurodevelopment seen within these babies during childhood and into adulthood [9]. While the consensus is currently 'yes', the guidelines for women threatening preterm birth state that only a single, and not multiple doses of glucocorticoids, should be given until more convincing data of the benefits of multiple doses are obtained [34]. Much work is examining the outcomes of antenatal glucocorticoids for the fetus, however the effect of glucocorticoids on the placenta, including the potential sex-specific effects, need to be considered as these may contribute to, or compound, the fetal outcomes.

4. Excess glucocorticoids and the programming of disease

The Barker Hypothesis of Developmental Origins of Health and Disease (DoHaD) states that diseases, such as coronary heart disease, hypertension and diabetes, may be consequences of *in utero* 'programming', whereby a stimulus or insult at a critical, sensitive 'window' of fetal life results in long-term changes in structure, physiology or metabolism, leading to diseases later in life [35]. These stimuli are likely to be mediated via a number of different hormones and immune factors, but glucocorticoids have been singled out as one of the most prevalent factors. Epidemiological and experimental animal studies have revealed that excess glucocorticoids *in utero* can be linked to the development of diseases such as hypertension [36-42], depression [43], cardiovascular disease [44], diabetes [45-46] and attention deficit disorders [23, 47]. Further, the outcomes or the severity of these diseases are worse if the offspring affected are male [37-39, 48-51].

Recently, a role for the placenta in mediating developmental programming of excess glucocorticoids and other *in utero* events has been suggested [44, 47, 52-55]. The size (both absolute and relative to fetal size), shape, and vascular development of the placenta have all been identified as potential predictors of adult onset diseases. For instance, a small baby with a large placenta has a relative risk of adult hypertension 3 times that of a large baby with a normal placental size [44]. Further, the abolition of a gene vital for placental, but not cardiac vascular development (*HOXA13*) has been shown to be embryonic lethal in mice, indicating that placental hemodynamics play an important role in the development of the heart, and alterations may lead to the development of cardiovascular problems later in life [56].

5. Susceptibility of the placenta to negative outcomes from glucocorticoid exposure

There are several reasons for the susceptible of the placenta to adverse outcomes caused by excess glucocorticoid exposure. I.) The placenta is in direct contact with the maternal circulation and thus is directly bathed in circulating maternal glucocorticoids. II.) One of the main roles of the placenta, as described above, is as a barrier to prevent fetal exposure to excess glucocorticoids; therefore the placenta may be directly altered by the glucocorticoid exposure *before* 11βHSD2 is able to convert these to their inactive metabolites [57]. III.) The structural development of the placenta occurs through a series of branching events, particularly the placental vasculature. This branching occurs similarly in other organs, such as the lung and kidney, which are particularly vulnerable to excess glucocorticoid exposure during periods of extensive branching [58-60]. Indeed in the evolution of the placenta, the genetic pathways that regulate branching morphogenesis in these other organs has been utilised by the placenta [61-65]. Hence a similar susceptibility could be expected for the placenta.

6. Sex-specific placental regulation of glucocorticoids

The placental is primarily derived from embryonic tissue and therefore has the same genetic content as the fetus. In recent studies examining both human and animal models, a number of fundamental differences between the placenta of a male and female fetus have been uncovered. Differences in placental proportions [66] and surface area [67] have been noted in placentas of males and females. Specifically, females have been shown to have a greater exchange region of the placenta compared to males [66], and within this exchange region, females have been reported to have a larger surface area [67]. Expression of genes and proteins known to have fundamental roles in controlling placental development [66], nutrient transfer, and other placental functions [68-71] differ between a male and female placenta. Specifically, placentas of male fetuses have been reported to have higher levels of the glucose transporter [66], higher levels of epidermal growth factor binding protein at term [68], but lower levels of activity of the sodium-hydrogen exchanger [70]. Levels of pregnancy hormones, produced by the placenta, differ for a male and female. For example, maternal serum human chorionic gonadotrophin levels are significantly higher in pregnancies carrying a female fetus from as early as 3 weeks of pregnancy [72]. Placental levels of progesterone also differ for a male and female fetus in many species, with a study in the gray seal, for example, showing higher levels in females than males [73]. Because progesterone is primarily of placental origin, these differences provide further evidence of the fundamental differences that exist in the placenta of a male and female fetus. Further, the placenta of a male and female fetus have also been shown to respond differently to adverse *in utero* environments including maternal under-nutrition/famine [74] and *in utero* infection [75]. For example, female placentas demonstrated more striking alterations in gene expression in response to restrictions in maternal diet than male placentas when examined by microarray analysis. Further, placentas of male fetuses exhibited a greater immunologicial reaction (greater expression of TNFa, IL-10, and PTGS2) to simulated *in utero* infection. Whether these responses differ because of the fundamental differences that exist between the sexes remains unknown.

Normal physiological glucocorticoid levels: During pregnancy, the term female placenta has significantly higher expression of the GR [31] and 11βHSD2 activity [76] than placentas of male fetuses. Glucocorticoids are known to negatively regulate GR expression [66, 77], therefore the higher GR expression within placentas of female fetuses may be physiological evidence that the female fetal–placental unit is exposed to less bioactive cortisol at term than the male. A downstream consequence of lower glucocorticoid levels may be an enhanced immune response. The activation of the fetal immune system is associated with the activation of the fetal hypothalamic pituitary adrenal axis, which results in the production of glucocorticoids, which in turn modulate the inflammatory response. Glucocorticoids function in a negative feedback loop with the hypothalamic pituitary adrenal axis, such that high glucocorticoid levels suppressing immune function [78]. It has been suggested that this may contribute to the increased viability of female fetuses exposed to a sub-optimal *in utero* environment, compared to males, who are particularly vulnerable to changes in the maternal environment in which increased levels of glucocorticoids are often seen [79] (see above).

Response to excess glucocorticoids: The adverse effects of glucocorticoids during pregnancy on placental weight in the human have been reported as early as 1977 by Koppe and others [80]. Since then, a number of studies, in both humans and animal models, have demonstrated that excess glucocorticoids during gestation have a wide range of consequences for the placenta, which impact its structure and function, ultimately impacting the fetus [22, 81-91]. Recently, these consequences have been shown to occur in a sex-specific manner.

Human evidence

Evidence is beginning to emerge from studies in the clinical setting demonstrating that human placentas are sexually dimorphic in their regulation of normal glucocorticoid levels and these differences are exacerbated in response to excess maternal glucocorticoids. Much of this clinical evidence is arising from the work of Clifton and colleagues, who focus on identifying the effect of glucocorticoids on fetal and placental development, by studying mothers who suffer from asthma and thus use inhaled glucocorticoid treatments throughout their pregnancy. Asthma affects between 3% and 12% of pregnant women worldwide and the prevalence among pregnant women is rising [92]. It is well recognised that women (and their babies) with asthma are at increased risk of poor pregnancy outcomes [93]. Clifton and colleagues have also examined preterm babies and the consequences of excess glucocorticoid exposure on their placentas.

6.1. Effect of glucocorticoids on placental development and other pathways

Female babies born to asthmatic mothers, who utilised inhaled glucocorticoid treatments to manage their symptoms, were found to be growth-reduced unlike male babies born to asthmatic mothers, who were normally grown, despite similar cord blood cortisol levels [76]. Placentas of male and female babies born to these mothers, had reduced vascularisation within the placental villi, resulting in reduced absolute fetal capillary volume [94], although this was most striking in placentas of male fetuses. Further, placentas of glucocorticoid-exposed males also had a reduced fetal capillary length [94], which was not observed in placentas of female fetuses. The authors speculate that glucocorticoid treatment may adversely affect placental vasculogenesis and/or angiogenesis by causing endothelial cell rounding and capillary regression, an observation made in other tissues after glucocorticoid exposure [95-97]. These effects may be mediated by members of the vascular endothelial growth factor family or inflammatory cytokines, both of which play a key role in placental vasculogenesis and angiogenesis [98]. The observed changes in placental morphometry in male placentas would be expected to affect placental heamodynamics, however the absence of these changes in the female placenta do not adequately explain the reduced fetal growth of the female fetus in this high glucocorticoid environment.

A study by Stark et al [99], examined the placental pro-: anti-oxidant balance in response to antenatal betamethasone in placentas of preterm babies. Glucocorticoids have previously been shown to influence fetal reactive oxygen species production and antioxidant defences [100-101]. These pathways are involved in preparing the fetus for the increase in free oxygen radical generation which is experienced during the fetal to neonatal transition [102]. Stark and colleagues observed that a pro-oxidant state was present in placentas of male fetuses, but not females following glucocorticoid exposure. Specifically, they reported that males had higher levels of the oxidative stress marker, protein carbonyl and a decreased level of the anti-oxidant enzyme, glutathione peroxidase. The authors suggested that these findings could contribute to the patho-physiologic processes underlying oxygen radical diseases of the newborn [99]; conditions known to exhibit a male excess [103].

6.2. Sex-specific effects of excess glucocorticoids on the placental glucocorticoid barrier

As the placental glucocorticoid barrier demonstrates sexually dimorphic regulation under normal conditions, and the placental response to glucocorticoids is crucial in determining fetal growth outcomes, the effect of excess maternal glucocorticoids on this barrier have been investigated. The expression of the GR within the placenta of male and female fetuses is reported to be sexually dimorphic under normal conditions (females having higher expression levels), whereas the response of GR to excess glucocorticoids is similar between the sexes [77].

In preterm babies, whose mothers received antenatal betamethasone, the activity of placental 11βHSD2 (predominant component of the glucocorticoid barrier) was reduced in placentas of male fetuses only [104]. This reduction in 11βHSD2 activity would be expected to compound the already increased exposure of the male fetus to cortisol brought about by the decreased term 11βHSD2 activity within male placentas during a normal pregnancy [76]. This may further compound the reduced immune function in male fetuses, thus increasing their susceptibility to disease. Further, glucocorticoids are important for fetal adrenal development [104]. Male preterm babies exposed to excess glucocorticoids *in utero*, have less adrenal activity than female preterm babies exposed to similar levels of glucocorticoids [104], which may explain the increased risk of morbidity and mortality of preterm male babies. We are unaware of any studies that have investigated the other members of the placental glucocorticoid barrier (MR and ABCB1) and their sexually dimorphic response to excess glucocorticoid exposure.

Animal models of glucocorticoid exposure

The effects of excess maternal glucocorticoid exposure, on placental growth and development, has been investigated using a range of animal models including the sheep [105-106], rat [85], mouse [107] and spiny mouse [66]. Most of these studies have utilised synthetic glucocorticoids (namely dexamethasone or betamethasone) and been designed to mimic the level of exposure experienced by the preterm infant. However, there are also a large number of studies using glucocorticoids at other developmental time points including very early in gestation. When considering the data generated from animal models, it is important to take into consideration not only the timing of glucocorticoid exposure but also the timing of placental and fetal development in the species being used, as there is considerable variation in placental development and overall structure between species. Many of these studies, particularly those in the sheep and rat, have not analysed data according to fetal sex. However a couple of recent studies in the mouse and spiny mouse have demonstrated markedly different outcomes in placental development and gene expression in placentas of males and females suggesting that alterations occurring within the placenta, following glucocorticoid exposure, are dependent upon fetal sex.

Sheep

The sheep placenta is made up of 60-70 individual placentomes called cotyledons, which are cup shaped structures with fetal tissue surrounded by maternal tissue. Administration of dexamethasone for 48 hours between 64-66 days of gestation (term=145-150 days) resulted in generally larger cotyledons with overgrowth of the fetal tissue when the placenta was examined at completion of the infusion [105]. However, this was not observed in other studies using betamethasone later in gestation (around 100 days of gestation) [108]. Unfortunately, neither of these studies separated data according to fetal sex. In another study, pregnant ewes received intramuscular injections of dexamethasone on day 40 and 41 of gestation and the placentas were examined at day 50, 100 or 140 days of gestation. In this case, data was analysed separately for males and females and whilst dexamethasone exposure significantly increased placental *11βHSD2* mRNA levels in males compared with controls at 50 and 140 days, in female placentas, levels were not altered by the dexamethasone exposure [106].

Rat

Dexamethasone exposure during late pregnancy has been shown to significantly reduce placental weight in the rat [91, 109]. This was associated with reduced expression of vascular endothelial growth factors (*VEGF*) and placental vascularisation [91] along with altered insulin like growth factor II expression. Neither of these studies looked at sex-specific effects.

Mouse

Given the extensive use of the mouse for development studies, it is somewhat surprising that there has been little research of the effects of glucocorticoids on the mouse placenta. We have recently shown that dexamethasone exposure for 2 days around mid-gestation (day 12.5-14.5 of gestation, term=20 days) caused decreases in fetal body weight at day 14.5, but placental weight was only reduced in placentas from female fetuses [107]. These changes in placental growth were associated with sex-specific changes in placental gene and protein expression: at day 14.5, the placentas from female fetuses had higher mRNA levels of expression of *11βHSD2* and *VEGF*, whilst protein levels of Mitogen-activated protein kinase were significantly reduced. By day 17.5, some 3, days after cessation of the dexamethasone, fetal and placental weights are restored but levels of 11βHSD2 protein are elevated in the placentas of female fetuses. These sex-specific changes in gene and protein levels were not present for nutrient transporters such as glucose transporter 1 and 3 or the major amino acid transports [107].

Spiny mouse

We have also utilised a precocial rodent, the spiny mouse (*Acomys cahirinus*), in which the natural circulating glucocorticoid is cortisol, not corticosterone like other rodents [110], to explore sex-specific effects of glucocorticoids on the placenta. O'Connell et al [66] examined the immediate and long-term consequences of excess maternal glucocorticoids (dexamethasone) administered for a short time (60h) at mid-gestation (day 20, term is 39 days) on placental structure and gene expression. The immediate consequences of glucocorticoid administration were similar between male and female placentas. However, two-weeks post-treatment (day 37), the transcriptional and structural response of the placenta was dependent on the sex of the fetus. Placentas of male fetuses were found to have an increase in the expression of a gene involved in placental patterning, glial cell missing 1 gene; *GCM1*, but also decreases in the expression of the primary placental glucose transporter (solute carrier family 2 (facilitated glucose transporter), member 1; *SLC2A1*). Placentas of male fetuses also had decreased amounts of maternal blood sinusoids, which are involved in the drawing of nutrient poor blood away from the placenta and back into the maternal circulation. Placentas of female fetuses were observed to have increased glucose transporter expression, and an increased amount of maternal blood sinusoids, in other words, the response of a female placenta to excess glucocorticoids was opposite to that of a male. This study highlights that while the immediate response to excess glucocorticoids may be the same for both sexes in this species, these may persist or evolve within the placenta differently, depending on the sex of the fetus [66].

7. Significance

There is now a growing body of evidence to suggest that the placenta of a male and female differs and that this may underlie the greater vulnerability of males to stressors that occur during pregnancy. Here we provided evidence that the placental response to changes in maternal glucocorticoid status differs depending on the sex of the fetus and raises the important question: are differences in fetal outcomes driven by the fetus itself or the placenta. We suggest that the placenta should become an organ of greater interest to clinical obstetrics and perinatology, particularly with respect to how the placenta may function differently for a male and female fetus during periods of high glucocorticoid exposure.

With respect to the clinical use of glucocorticoids, the different response of a male and female to even a small dose of synthetic glucocorticoids must be followed up in a large clinical based study. At least from experimental data, the question has been raised, "Should the sex of the fetus be taken into consideration when synthetic glucocorticoids are administered during pregnancy"?

Author details

Hayley Dickinson*, Bree A. O'Connell and David W. Walker
The Ritchie Centre, Monash Institute of Medical Research, Monash University, Clayton, Australia

Karen M. Moritz
The University of Queensland, School of Biomedical Sciences, St Lucia, Australia

8. References

[1] Harris A, Seckl J (2011) Glucocorticoids, prenatal stress and the programming of disease. Horm Behav; 59:279-89.

[2] Benediktsson R, Calder AA, Edwards CR, Seckl JR (1997) Placental 11 beta-hydroxysteroid dehydrogenase: a key regulator of fetal glucocorticoid exposure. Clin Endocrinol (Oxf); 46:161-6.

[3] Seckl JR (1997) Glucocorticoids, feto-placental 11 beta-hydroxysteroid dehydrogenase type 2, and the early life origins of adult disease. Steroids; 62:89-94.

[4] Seckl JR, Holmes MC (2007) Mechanisms of disease: glucocorticoids, their placental metabolism and fetal 'programming' of adult pathophysiology. Nat Clin Pract Endocrinol Metab; 3:479-88.

[5] Michael AE, Papageorghiou AT (2008) Potential significance of physiological and pharmacological glucocorticoids in early pregnancy. Hum Reprod Update; 14:497-517.

[6] Ortiz LA, Quan A, Weinberg A, Baum M (2001) Effect of prenatal dexamethasone on rat renal development. Kidney Int; 59:1663-9.

[7] Sawady J, Mercer BM, Wapner RJ, Zhao Y, Sorokin Y, Johnson F, et al. (2007) The National Institute of Child Health and Human Development Maternal-Fetal Medicine Units Network Beneficial Effects of Antenatal Repeated Steroids study: impact of repeated doses of antenatal corticosteroids on placental growth and histologic findings. Am J Obstet Gynecol; 197:281 e1-8.

[8] (1995) Effect of corticosteroids for fetal maturation on perinatal outcomes. NIH Consensus Development Panel on the Effect of Corticosteroids for Fetal Maturation on Perinatal Outcomes. JAMA; 273:413-8.

[9] Vos AA, Bruinse HW (2010) Congenital adrenal hyperplasia: do the benefits of prenatal treatment defeat the risks? Obstet Gynecol Surv; 65:196-205.

[10] Wintour EM, Johnson K, Koukoulas I, Moritz K, Tersteeg M, Dodic M (2003) Programming the cardiovascular system, kidney and the brain--a review. Placenta; 24 Suppl A:S65-71.

[11] Uno H, Eisele S, Sakai A, Shelton S, Baker E, DeJesus O, et al. (1994) Neurotoxicity of glucocorticoids in the primate brain. Horm Behav; 28:336-48.

[12] Yang K (1997) Placental 11 beta-hydroxysteroid dehydrogenase: barrier to maternal glucocorticoids. Rev Reprod; 2:129-32.

---

* Corresponding Author

[13] Pepe GJ, Burch MG, Albrecht ED (1999) Expression of the 11beta-hydroxysteroid dehydrogenase types 1 and 2 proteins in human and baboon placental syncytiotrophoblast. Placenta; 20:575-82.

[14] Burton PJ, Waddell BJ (1999) Dual function of 11beta-hydroxysteroid dehydrogenase in placenta: modulating placental glucocorticoid passage and local steroid action. Biol Reprod; 60:234-40.

[15] Parry S, Zhang J (2007) Multidrug resistance proteins affect drug transmission across the placenta. Am J Obstet Gynecol; 196:476 e1-6.

[16] Mark PJ, Waddell BJ (2006) P-glycoprotein restricts access of cortisol and dexamethasone to the glucocorticoid receptor in placental BeWo cells. Endocrinology; 147:5147-52.

[17] Kalabis GM, Kostaki A, Andrews MH, Petropoulos S, Gibb W, Matthews SG (2005) Multidrug resistance phosphoglycoprotein (ABCB1) in the mouse placenta: fetal protection. Biol Reprod; 73:591-7.

[18] Driver PM, Kilby MD, Bujalska I, Walker EA, Hewison M, Stewart PM (2001) Expression of 11 beta-hydroxysteroid dehydrogenase isozymes and corticosteroid hormone receptors in primary cultures of human trophoblast and placental bed biopsies. Mol Hum Reprod; 7:357-63.

[19] Pujols L, Mullol J, Torrego A, Picado C (2004) Glucocorticoid receptors in human airways. Allergy; 59:1042-52.

[20] Driver PM, Rauz S, Walker EA, Hewison M, Kilby MD, Stewart PM (2003) Characterization of human trophoblast as a mineralocorticoid target tissue. Mol Hum Reprod; 9:793-8.

[21] Dickinson H, Wintour EM (2007) Can Life Before Birth Affect Health Ever After? Current Women's Health Reviews; 3:79-88.

[22] Sun K, Yang K, Challis JR (1998) Glucocorticoid actions and metabolism in pregnancy: implications for placental function and fetal cardiovascular activity. Placenta; 19:353-60.

[23] Kapoor A, Petropoulos S, Matthews SG (2008) Fetal programming of hypothalamic-pituitary-adrenal (HPA) axis function and behavior by synthetic glucocorticoids. Brain Res Rev; 57:586-95.

[24] Davis EP, Waffarn F, Sandman CA (2011) Prenatal treatment with glucocorticoids sensitizes the hpa axis response to stress among full-term infants. Dev Psychobiol; 53:175-83.

[25] Matthews SG, Owen D, Kalabis G, Banjanin S, Setiawan EB, Dunn EA, et al. (2004) Fetal glucocorticoid exposure and hypothalamo-pituitary-adrenal (HPA) function after birth. Endocr Res; 30:827-36.

[26] Moritz KM, Cuffe JS, Wilson LB, Dickinson H, Wlodek ME, Simmons DG, et al. (2010) Review: Sex specific programming: a critical role for the renal renin-angiotensin system. Placenta; 31 Suppl:S40-6.

[27] Eskenazi B, Marks AR, Catalano R, Bruckner T, Toniolo PG (2007) Low birthweight in New York City and upstate New York following the events of September 11th. Hum Reprod; 22:3013-20.

[28] Catalano R, Bruckner T, Gould J, Eskenazi B, Anderson E (2005) Sex ratios in California following the terrorist attacks of September 11, 2001. Hum Reprod; 20:1221-7.

[29] Catalano R, Bruckner T, Marks AR, Eskenazi B (2006) Exogenous shocks to the human sex ratio: the case of September 11, 2001 in New York City. Hum Reprod; 21:3127-31.

[30] Murphy VE, Clifton VL, Gibson PG (2006) Asthma exacerbations during pregnancy: incidence and association with adverse pregnancy outcomes. Thorax; 61:169-76.

[31] Clifton VL, Murphy VE (2004) Maternal asthma as a model for examining fetal sex-specific effects on maternal physiology and placental mechanisms that regulate human fetal growth. Placenta; 25 Suppl A:S45-52.

[32] Forest MG (2004) Recent advances in the diagnosis and management of congenital adrenal hyperplasia due to 21-hydroxylase deficiency. Hum Reprod Update; 10:469-85.

[33] Quinkler M, Oelkers W, Diederich S (2001) Clinical implications of glucocorticoid metabolism by 11beta-hydroxysteroid dehydrogenases in target tissues. Eur J Endocrinol; 144:87-97.

[34] Miracle X, Di Renzo GC, Stark A, Fanaroff A, Carbonell-Estrany X, Saling E (2008) Guideline for the use of antenatal corticosteroids for fetal maturation. J Perinat Med; 36:191-6.

[35] Barker DJ, Clark PM (1997) Fetal undernutrition and disease in later life. Rev Reprod; 2:105-12.

[36] Wintour EM, Moritz KM, Johnson K, Ricardo S, Samuel CS, Dodic M (2003) Reduced nephron number in adult sheep, hypertensive as a result of prenatal glucocorticoid treatment. J Physiol (Lond); 549:929-35.

[37] Bertram C, Khan O, Ohri S, Phillips DI, Matthews SG, Hanson MA (2008) Transgenerational effects of prenatal nutrient restriction on cardiovascular and hypothalamic-pituitary-adrenal function. J Physiol; 586:2217-29.

[38] Bertram C, Trowern AR, Copin N, Jackson AA, Whorwood CB (2001) The maternal diet during pregnancy programs altered expression of the glucocorticoid receptor and type 2 11beta-hydroxysteroid dehydrogenase: potential molecular mechanisms underlying the programming of hypertension in utero. Endocrinology; 142:2841-53.

[39] Woods LL, Ingelfinger JR, Nyengaard JR, Rasch R (2001) Maternal protein restriction suppresses the newborn renin-angiotensin system and programs adult hypertension in rats. Pediatr Res; 49:460-7.

[40] Kwong WY, Wild AE, Roberts P, Willis AC, Fleming TP (2000) Maternal undernutrition during the preimplantation period of rat development causes blastocyst abnormalities and programming of postnatal hypertension. Development; 127:4195-202.

[41] Levitt NS, Lindsay RS, Holmes MC, Seckl JR (1996) Dexamethasone in the last week of pregnancy attenuates hippocampal glucocorticoid receptor gene expression and elevates blood pressure in the adult offspring in the rat. Neuroendocrinology; 64:412-8.

[42] Dodic M, Abouantoun T, O'Connor A, Wintour EM, Moritz KM (2002) Programming effects of short prenatal exposure to dexamethasone in sheep. Hypertension; 40:729-34.

[43] Murgatroyd C, Wu Y, Bockmuhl Y, Spengler D (2010) Genes learn from stress: How infantile trauma programs us for depression. Epigenetics; 5.

[44] Thornburg KL, O'Tierney PF, Louey S (2010) Review: The placenta is a programming agent for cardiovascular disease. Placenta; 31 Suppl:S54-9.

[45] Phillips DI, Barker DJ, Fall CH, Seckl JR, Whorwood CB, Wood PJ, et al. (1998) Elevated plasma cortisol concentrations: a link between low birth weight and the insulin resistance syndrome? J Clin Endocrinol Metab; 83:757-60.

[46] De Blasio MJ, Dodic M, Jefferies AJ, Moritz KM, Wintour EM, Owens JA (2007) Maternal exposure to dexamethasone or cortisol in early pregnancy differentially alters insulin secretion and glucose homeostasis in adult male sheep offspring. Am J Physiol Endocrinol Metabol; 293:E75-82.

[47] O'Donnell K, O'Connor TG, Glover V (2009) Prenatal stress and neurodevelopment of the child: focus on the HPA axis and role of the placenta. Dev Neurosci; 31:285-92.

[48] Shoener JA, Baig R, Page KC (2006) Prenatal exposure to dexamethasone alters hippocampal drive on hypothalamic-pituitary-adrenal axis activity in adult male rats. Am J Physiol Regul Integr Comp Physiol; 290:R1366-73.

[49] Mueller BR, Bale TL (2008) Sex-specific programming of offspring emotionality after stress early in pregnancy. J Neurosci; 28:9055-65.

[50] Woods LL, Ingelfinger JR, Rasch R (2005) Modest maternal protein restriction fails to program adult hypertension in female rats. Am J Physiol Regul Integr Comp Physiol; 289:R1131-6.

[51] Rodriguez JS, Zurcher NR, Keenan KE, Bartlett TQ, Nathanielsz PW, Nijland MJ (2011) Prenatal betamethasone exposure has sex specific effects in reversal learning and attention in juvenile baboons. Am J Obstet Gynecol; 204:545 e1- e10.

[52] Burton GJ, Fowden AL (2012) Review: The placenta and developmental programming: Balancing fetal nutrient demands with maternal resource allocation. Placenta; 33 Suppl:S23-7.

[53] Illsley NP, Caniggia I, Zamudio S (2010) Placental metabolic reprogramming: do changes in the mix of energy-generating substrates modulate fetal growth? Int J Dev Biol; 54:409-19.

[54] Godfrey KM (2002) The role of the placenta in fetal programming-a review. Placenta; 23 Suppl A:S20-7.

[55] Fowden AL, Forhead AJ, Coan PM, Burton GJ (2008) The placenta and intrauterine programming. J Neuroendocrinol; 20:439-50.

[56] Shaut CA, Keene DR, Sorensen LK, Li DY, Stadler HS (2008) HOXA13 Is essential for placental vascular patterning and labyrinth endothelial specification. PLoS Genet; 4:e1000073.

[57] Murphy VE, Fittock RJ, Zarzycki PK, Delahunty MM, Smith R, Clifton VL (2007) Metabolism of synthetic steroids by the human placenta. Placenta; 28:39-46.

[58] Dickinson H, Walker DW, Wintour EM, Moritz K (2007) Maternal dexamethasone treatment at midgestation reduces nephron number and alters renal gene expression in the fetal spiny mouse. Am J Physiol Regul Integr Comp Physiol; 292:R453-61.

[59] Oshika E, Liu S, Ung LP, Singh G, Shinozuka H, Michalopoulos GK, et al. (1998) Glucocorticoid-induced effects on pattern formation and epithelial cell differentiation in early embryonic rat lungs. Pediatr Res; 43:305-14.

[60] Bolkenius U, Hahn D, Gressner AM, Breitkopf K, Dooley S, Wickert L (2004) Glucocorticoids decrease the bioavailability of TGF-beta which leads to a reduced TGF-beta signaling in hepatic stellate cells. Biochem Biophys Res Commun; 325:1264-70.

[61] Cross JC, Baczyk D, Dobric N, Hemberger M, Hughes M, Simmons DG, et al. (2003) Genes, development and evolution of the placenta. Placenta; 24:123-30.

[62] Cross JC (2000) Genetic insights into trophoblast differentiation and placental morphogenesis. Semin Cell Dev Biol; 11:105-13.

[63] Rossant J, Cross JC (2001) Placental development: lessons from mouse mutants. Nat Rev Genet; 2:538-48.

[64] Mess A, Carter AM (2007) Evolution of the placenta during the early radiation of placental mammals. Comparative Biochemistry and Physiology - Part A: Molecular & Integrative Physiology; 148:769-79.

[65] Cross JC, Nakano H, Natale DR, Simmons DG, Watson ED (2006) Branching morphogenesis during development of placental villi. Differentiation; 74:393-401.

[66] O'Connell BA, Moritz KM, Roberts CT, Walker DW, Dickinson H (2011) The placental response to excess maternal glucocorticoid exposure differs between the male and female conceptus in spiny mice. Biol Reprod; 85:1040-7.

[67] Grbesa D, Durst-Zivkovic B (1989) The surface of the syncytiotrophoblast in the human placenta at term in relation to the sex of the neonate. Jugosl Ginekol Perinatol; 29:169-71.

[68] Brown MJ, Cook CL, Henry JL, Schultz GS (1987) Levels of epidermal growth factor binding in third-trimester and term human placentas: elevated binding in term placentas of male fetuses. Am J Obstet Gynecol; 156:716-20.

[69] Cleal JK, Day PL, Hanson MA, Lewis RM (2010) Sex differences in the mRNA levels of housekeeping genes in human placenta. Placenta; 31:556-7.

[70] Speake PF, Glazier JD, Greenwood SL, Sibley CP (2010) Aldosterone and cortisol acutely stimulate Na+/H+ exchanger activity in the syncytiotrophoblast of the human placenta: effect of fetal sex. Placenta; 31:289-94.

[71] Haning RV, Jr., Breault PH, DeSilva MV, Hackett RJ, Pouncey CL (1988) Effects of fetal sex, stage of gestation, dibutyryl cyclic adenosine monophosphate, and gonadotropin releasing hormone on secretion of human chorionic gonadotropin by placental explants in vitro. Am J Obstet Gynecol; 159:1332-7.

[72] Yaron Y, Lehavi O, Orr-Urtreger A, Gull I, Lessing JB, Amit A, et al. (2002) Maternal serum HCG is higher in the presence of a female fetus as early as week 3 post-fertilization. Hum Reprod; 17:485-9.

[73] Boyd I (1990) Mass and Hormone Content of Gray Seal Placentae Related to Fetal Sex. J Mammal; 71:101-3.

[74] Mao J, Zhang X, Sieli PT, Falduto MT, Torres KE, Rosenfeld CS (2010) Contrasting effects of different maternal diets on sexually dimorphic gene expression in the murine placenta. Proc Natl Acad Sci U S A; 107:5557-62.

[75] Yeganegi M, Watson CS, Martins A, Kim SO, Reid G, Challis JR, et al. (2009) Effect of Lactobacillus rhamnosus GR-1 supernatant and fetal sex on lipopolysaccharide-induced cytokine and prostaglandin-regulating enzymes in human placental trophoblast cells: implications for treatment of bacterial vaginosis and prevention of preterm labor. Am J Obstet Gynecol; 200:532 e1-8.

[76] Murphy VE, Gibson PG, Giles WB, Zakar T, Smith R, Bisits AM, et al. (2003) Maternal asthma is associated with reduced female fetal growth. Am J Respir Crit Care Med; 168:1317-23.

[77] Hodyl NA, Wyper H, Osei-Kumah A, Scott N, Murphy VE, Gibson P, et al. (2010) Sex-specific associations between cortisol and birth weight in pregnancies complicated by asthma are not due to differential glucocorticoid receptor expression. Thorax; 65:677-83.

[78] Dhabhar FS, McEwen BS (1997) Acute stress enhances while chronic stress suppresses cell-mediated immunity in vivo: a potential role for leukocyte trafficking. Brain Behav Immun; 11:286-306.

[79] Eriksson JG, Kajantie E, Osmond C, Thornburg K, Barker DJ (2010) Boys live dangerously in the womb. Am J Hum Biol; 22:330-5.

[80] Koppe JG, Smolders-de Haas H, Kloosterman GJ (1977) Effects of glucocorticoids during pregnancy on the outcome of the children directly after birth and in the long run. Eur J Obstet Gynecol Reprod Biol; 7:293-9.

[81] Clifton VL, Wallace EM, Smith R (2002) Short-term effects of glucocorticoids in the human fetal-placental circulation in vitro. J Clin Endocrinol Metab; 87:2838-42.

[82] Paakki P, Kirkinen P, Helin H, Pelkonen O, Raunio H, Pasanen M (2000) Antepartum glucocorticoid therapy suppresses human placental xenobiotic and steroid metabolizing enzymes. Placenta; 21:241-6.

[83] Mandl M, Ghaffari-Tabrizi N, Haas J, Nohammer G, Desoye G (2006) Differential glucocorticoid effects on proliferation and invasion of human trophoblast cell lines. Reproduction; 132:159-67.

[84] Matejevic D, Heilmann P, Schuster C, Schoneshofer M, Graf R (1995) Decidua and placenta in mice after treatment with a synthetic glucocorticoid. Reprod Fertil Dev; 7:1551-5.

[85] Waddell BJ, Hisheh S, Dharmarajan AM, Burton PJ (2000) Apoptosis in rat placenta is zone-dependent and stimulated by glucocorticoids. Biol Reprod; 63:1913-7.

[86] Hahn T, Barth S, Graf R, Engelmann M, Beslagic D, Reul JM, et al. (1999) Placental glucose transporter expression is regulated by glucocorticoids. J Clin Endocrinol Metab; 84:1445-52.

[87] Lee MJ, Ma Y, LaChapelle L, Kadner SS, Guller S (2004) Glucocorticoid enhances transforming growth factor-beta effects on extracellular matrix protein expression in human placental mesenchymal cells. Biol Reprod; 70:1246-52.

[88] Siler-Khodr TM, Kang IS, Koong MK, Grayson M (1997) The effect of dexamethasone on CRH and prostanoid production from human term placenta. Prostaglandins; 54:639-53.

[89] Audette MC, Greenwood SL, Sibley CP, Jones CJ, Challis JR, Matthews SG, et al. (2010) Dexamethasone stimulates placental system A transport and trophoblast differentiation in term villous explants. Placenta; 31:97-105.

[90] Jones SA, Brooks AN, Challis JR (1989) Steroids modulate corticotropin-releasing hormone production in human fetal membranes and placenta. J Clin Endocrinol Metab; 68:825-30.

[91] Hewitt DP, Mark PJ, Waddell BJ (2006) Glucocorticoids prevent the normal increase in placental vascular endothelial growth factor expression and placental vascularity during late pregnancy in the rat. Endocrinology; 147:5568-74.

[92] Kurinczuk JJ, Parsons DE, Dawes V, Burton PR (1999) The relationship between asthma and smoking during pregnancy. Women Health; 29:31-47.

[93] Murphy VE, Gibson PG, Smith R, Clifton VL (2005) Asthma during pregnancy: mechanisms and treatment implications. Eur Respir J; 25:731-50.

[94] Mayhew TM, Jenkins H, Todd B, Clifton VL (2008) Maternal asthma and placental morphometry: effects of severity, treatment and fetal sex. Placenta; 29:366-73.

[95] Jung SP, Siegrist B, Wade MR, Anthony CT, Woltering EA (2001) Inhibition of human angiogenesis with heparin and hydrocortisone. Angiogenesis; 4:175-86.

[96] Ingber DE, Madri JA, Folkman J (1986) A possible mechanism for inhibition of angiogenesis by angiostatic steroids: induction of capillary basement membrane dissolution. Endocrinology; 119:1768-75.

[97] Folkman J, Langer R, Linhardt RJ, Haudenschild C, Taylor S (1983) Angiogenesis inhibition and tumor regression caused by heparin or a heparin fragment in the presence of cortisone. Science; 221:719-25.

[98] Charnock-Jones DS, Kaufmann P, Mayhew TM (2004) Aspects of human fetoplacental vasculogenesis and angiogenesis. I. Molecular regulation. Placenta; 25:103-13.

[99] Stark MJ, Hodyl NA, Wright IM, Clifton VL (2011) Influence of sex and glucocorticoid exposure on preterm placental pro-oxidant-antioxidant balance. Placenta; 32:865-70.

[100] Walther FJ, Jobe AH, Ikegami M (1998) Repetitive prenatal glucocorticoid therapy reduces oxidative stress in the lungs of preterm lambs. J Appl Physiol; 85:273-8.

[101] Vento M, Aguar M, Escobar J, Arduini A, Escrig R, Brugada M, et al. (2009) Antenatal steroids and antioxidant enzyme activity in preterm infants: influence of gender and timing. Antioxid Redox Signal; 11:2945-55.

[102] Comporti M, Signorini C, Leoncini S, Buonocore G, Rossi V, Ciccoli L (2004) Plasma F2-isoprostanes are elevated in newborns and inversely correlated to gestational age. Free Radical Biol Med; 37:724-32.

[103] Binet ME, Bujold E, Lefebvre F, Tremblay Y, Piedboeuf B (2012) Role of Gender in Morbidity and Mortality of Extremely Premature Neonates. Am J Perinatol; 29:159-66.

[104] Stark MJ, Wright IM, Clifton VL (2009) Sex-specific alterations in placental 11beta-hydroxysteroid dehydrogenase 2 activity and early postnatal clinical course following antenatal betamethasone. Am J Physiol Regul Integr Comp Physiol; 297:R510-4.

[105] Wintour EM, Alcorn D, McFarlane A, Moritz K, Potocnik SJ, Tangalakis K (1994) Effect of maternal glucocorticoid treatment on fetal fluids in sheep at 0.4 gestation. Am J Physiol; 266:R1174-81.

[106] Braun T, Li S, Sloboda DM, Li W, Audette MC, Moss TJ, et al. (2009) Effects of maternal dexamethasone treatment in early pregnancy on pituitary-adrenal axis in fetal sheep. Endocrinology; 150:5466-77.

[107] Cuffe JS, Dickinson H, Simmons DG, Moritz KM (2011) Sex specific changes in placental growth and MAPK following short term maternal dexamethasone exposure in the mouse. Placenta; 32:981-9.

[108] Braun T, Li S, Moss TJ, Connor KL, Doherty DA, Nitsos I, et al. (2011) Differential appearance of placentomes and expression of prostaglandin H synthase type 2 in placentome subtypes after betamethasone treatment of sheep late in gestation. Placenta; 32:295-303.

[109] Ain R, Canham LN, Soares MJ (2005) Dexamethasone-induced intrauterine growth restriction impacts the placental prolactin family, insulin-like growth factor-II and the Akt signaling pathway. J Endocrinol; 185:253-63.

[110] Dickinson H, O'Connell BA, Quinn T, Cannata D, Moxham A, Walker DW (2010) The spiny mouse - an ideal species to study perinatal biology. Pediatr Res; 68:175.

Chapter 4

Glucocorticoids: Biochemical Group That Play Key Role in Fetal Programming of Adult Disease

Aml Mohammed Erhuma

Additional information is available at the end of the chapter

1. Introduction

1.1. Glucocorticoids discovery started 160 years ago

Glucocorticoids are subclass from corticosteroids. The other subclass of corticosteroids is mineralocorticoids. Historically, the discovery of glucocorticoids has been commenced during the early of last century. In fact, glucocorticoids have revealed themselves by their absence. In 1849, Thomas Addison, who was a physician at Guy`s Hospital in London, had noticed that certain patients were presenting with a cluster of characteristic clinical picture including anemia, weakness, peculiar dark skin color and eventually death (1). He presented his observation on 11 cases at the South London medical society meeting. In 1855 he published monograph entitled (On the Constitutional and Local Effects of Disease of the Supra-Renal capsules), (2, 3). 100 years later, Dr Philip Hench with a collaborated work with Edward Kendall, Professor of Physiological Chemistry, were both at Mayo Clinic which was first rheumatic disease service, had extracted "substance X" and in 21 September 1948 first injection of substance X was given to 29 years old lady who was suffering from severe, erosive arthropathies and became able to walk out of the hospital after 4 days of treatment. Dr Hench then named substance X Cortisone and shared the Nobel prize with professor Kendall in 1950 (4).

1.2. Glucocorticoids characteristics

Glucocorticoids (GCs) are belonging to the steroid group of the hormones that bind to the glucocorticoid receptor, which is present in almost all cells (5). This is the reason why the GCs play wide range of vital physiological roles in the human and other vertebrate bodies (6, 7). They play pivotal role in modulation and regulation of metabolism (8), immune system reaction (9, 10) and more significantly they are essential for normal development and cognition (11).

1.2.1. Biochemical characteristics

To know how GCs exerts their wide range effects, it is crucial to know about their structure and the synthesis pathway. GCs are one of the steroid hormones group. All steroid hormones are derived from cholesterol. These include: sex hormones (Testosterone, estrone (E1), estradiol (E2), estriol (E3), and progesterone) adrenal cortex hormones (Cortisone, the main glucocorticoid and Aldosterone, the main mineralocorticoid) in addition to vitamin D. It is essential to know that androgens are the synthetic precursors of estrogens which mediated mainly by a specific cytochrome P 450 enzyme named aromatase. Each one of these steroid hormones can be a product and precursor in the same time. This is the reason why any defect in the synthesis of one steroid hormone will lead to derangement in the synthesis of the other hormones. For instance, in congenital adrenal hyperplasia (CAH), an autosomal recessive gene defect of the enzyme 21-hydroxylase, there will be blocked synthesis of aldosterone and cortisol pathways. Subsequently, all precursors will be directed toward androgenic pathway which does not involve 21-hydroxylation and eventually lead to excess production of androgens (Figure 1). Fetus with this congenital disease will be exposed to high levels of androgens as early as 3 months of gestation and hence during a critical window of sexual differentiation. As a result a female fetus will develop an ambiguous genitalia or male external genitalia under the influences of adrenal androgens. However, this is associated with varying degrees of GCs and mineralocorticoids deficiencies. In severe cases there will be salt wasting with low sodium and potassium in serum due to aldosterone deficiency (12). Currently, all neonates in the most of world are screened for CAH by measuring 17-Hydroxyprogesteron (17-OHP) in filter-paper blood samples at week one of life. An elevated 17-OHP indicated affected baby. Recently, there are promising clinical trials in prenatal diagnosis and treatments of such condition by giving the mother dexamethasone injections to prevent increased secretion of Adreno-Cortico-Tropic Hormone (ACTH) and subsequently adrenal androgens(13-17).

1.2.2. Physiological characteristics

GCs are needed mainly for energy where as mineralocorticoids are needed for mineral balance. GCs regulates wide range of cellular, molecular and the physiological processes in human body that are crucial for life such as growth, reproduction, essential metabolism, immune responses and inflammatory reactions, as well as central nervous system and cardiovascular functions (19-22). For all these roles to be achieved, adrenal GCs is considered as a ring which coupled with many other rings to form an integrated chain that acts in coordination, this chain is the hypothalamus-pituitary- adrenal axis.

1.2.2.1. Hypothalamus-pituitary-adrenal axis (HPA axis)

HPA axis serves as a master that controls major body systems and is considered as a main connecting pathway between central nervous system and endocrine system. It regulates majority of physiological function as well as it maintains homeostasis in acute stress. In the later situation, the brain will signal the stress to the paraventricular nucleus (PVN) in the hypothalamus which eventually secretes corticotrophin releasing hormone (CRH). CRH is then transported through hypophyseal portal system to the pituitary gland and induces the conversion of pro-opiomelanocortin into ACTH as well as its secretion from anterior pituitary to the systemic circulation. ACTH is the primary regulator of adrenal cortical steroidogenesis. ACTH will induce the synthesis of adrenal steroids (GCs and androgens) in zonae fasciculate and reticularis of adrenal cortex (Figure 1). The ACTH itself is under the influences of negative feedback inhibition which exerted by the plasma levels of circulating free GCs (Figure 2).

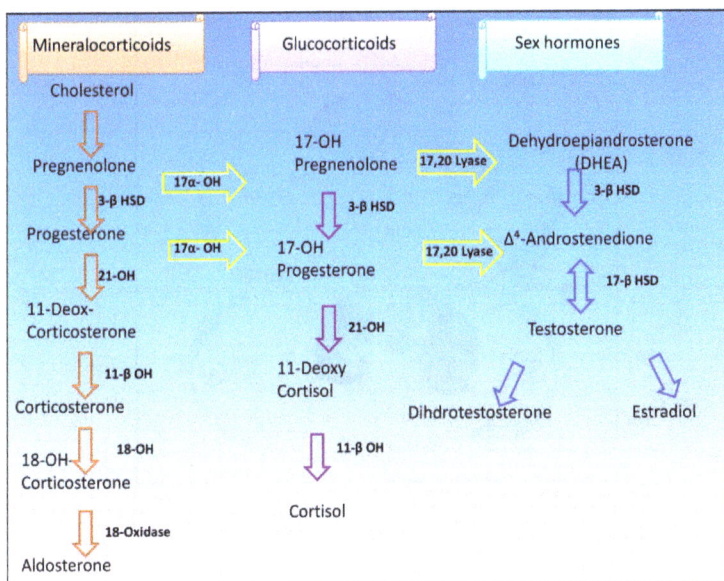

Figure 1. Adrenal gland steroidogenesis. The synthesis of adrenal steroids is started by transfer of cholesterol either from blood or from adrenal gland lipid droplets into mitochondria where it will be converted to pregnenolone. In zona glomerulosa pregnenolone will be hydroxylated to corticosterone and further oxidized to aldosterone where as in zona fasciculate and zona reticularis it will be hydoxylated to cortisol or undergoes cleavage to form the main adrenal androgen (DHEA). HSD: Hydroxysteroid Dehydrogenase, OH: Hydroxylase, (18). Adrenal androgen synthesis is increased about age of 8 years, independent of gonads and puberty, and responsible for pubic and axillary hair growth and termed adrenarche.

1.2.2.2. Molecular mechanisms of GCs action

GCs secretion from zona fasciculata up on ACTH stimulation is not a continuance process but rather in a specific pattern known as circadian rhythm. Once GCs in circulation, 95% of them will be bound to a carrier proteins: 80–90% to corticosteroid binding globulin (CBG) and 10–15% to albumin, leaving only about 5% as active unbound cortisol (23). The free cortisol is the one which mediates the biological effect of GCs since it is able to diffuse through the cell membrane freely. The GCs are metabolized in liver by reduction followed by conjugation rendering them water soluble and ready for renal excretion in urine. Both liver and kidney contain the enzyme 11 β-Hydroxysteroid dehydrogenase (11 β-HSD).There is two isoforms of this enzyme which catalyzes the opposite reactions. 11 β-Hydroxysteroid Dehydrogenase-2 (11 β-HSD 2) will inactivate the cortisol by converting it into cortisone. The 11 β-Hydroxysteroid dehydrogenase-1 (11 β-HSD 1) will convert inactive cortisone into cortisol. The net result will determine the plasma level of active cortisol in the body (24).

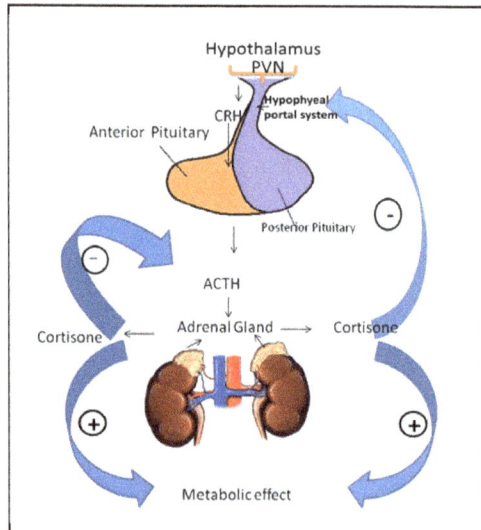

Figure 2. Schematic representation of Hypothalamic-pituitary-adrenal axis. PVN: Paraventricular nucleus, CRH: Corticotrophin releasing hormone, ACTH: Adrenocorticotropic hormone, ⊖: Inhibition, ⊕:Stimulation

Once free GCs defused through the plasma membrane of the target cell they will bind to intra-cytoplasmic receptors called glucocorticoids receptor (GR). GR-GCs complex will be now translocated to the nucleus and bind to glucocorticoids responsive elements (GRE) in the promoter of the target gene (Figure 3).

Human GR is 94 kDa protein which belongs to nuclear receptors known as Steroid/Thyroid/Retinoic acid superfamily and characterizing by being a ligand-dependent transcription factors that induce or suppress target gene expression (25). GCs are also able to alter gene expression of target genes independently to DNA-binding, but through interaction with other transcription factors, such as nuclear factor- κB, activator protein-1, p53 and signal transducers and activators of transcription (25).

Interestingly, there are two isoforms of GR, alpha (α) and beta (β) (26, 27). The GR-α is the one which is able to bind with glucocorticoids and subsequently to the GCs responsive element (GRE) of the DNA promoter region on the target gene. However, GR-β has no such ability to bind to GCs but its main role thought to be inhibitory to GR-α action by competitive interference on the GRE target sites (28). It has been found that the variations in expression of GR-β is responsible for tissue sensitivity and resistance to GCs. Clinically, pathological conditions such as hypertension, rheumatoid arthritis, systemic lupus erythmatosis, ischemic heart disease and nasal carriage of Staphylococcus aureus are all associated with GR-β protein over-expression (29).

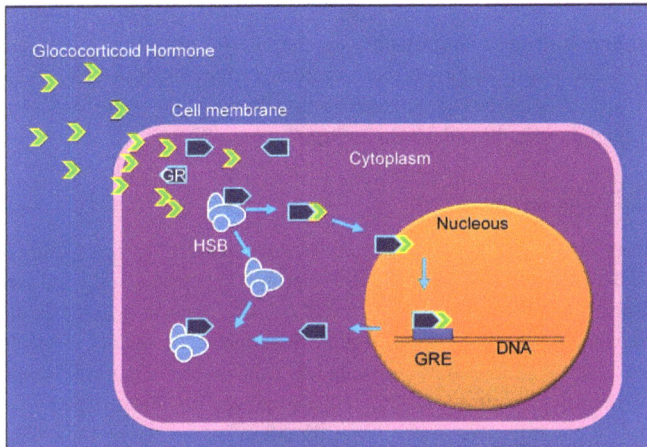

Figure 3. Representation of how glucocorticoid hormone enters to the cell and bind to intracellular glucocorticoids receptors (GR). Up on binding to GR they dissociate from heat shock proteins (HSP). The glucocorticoids-receptor complex enters the nucleus and bind to glucocorticoids responsive element (GRE) in the promoter of the responsive gene (25). Lastly, GR exit nucleus and recycled along with the HSP in the cytoplasm.

2. Tissue responses to glucocorticoids

As mentioned earlier that GR exist in almost every human cell, then we should not get surprised to observe the profound molecular, cellular, metabolic and other known biological events modulation in response to GCs excess or deficiency. Notwithstanding, for more understanding of these complex relationship and the huge difference in the treatment-response equation we categorized the human tissue into adult or mature human tissue and fetal or immature human tissue.

2.1. Adult (mature) tissue response to glucocorticoids

Adult cells and tissue characterized by being fully differentiated and mature. Therefore, influences will mainly affect their function.

2.1.1. Immune system

It is well established that the first medical use of GCs 60 years ago was for inflammation and autoimmune disease (30). GCs have significant influences on both cellular and humeral immunity. They induce plasma cell immunoglobuline production and secretion and hence enhance humeral immunity (31). With regard to cellular immunity, GCs induce T-cell lymphocytosis (32), basophil apoptosis and neutrophilia by increasing bone marrow release of polymorphic neutrophils and decrease their migration to the inflammatory site (33, 34). Moreover, GCs enhances the phagocytosis and hence maximize the tissue clearance ability of the microorganisms and foreign antigens (35). It has been recently revealed that GCs can exert their immune-function manipulation at gene expression level. Galon and colleagues found that GCs significantly suppress the proinflamatory cytokines (IL1b, TNFa, IL-6, IL-8, IL- 12, IL-18) and chemokines gene expression where as the gene expression of anti-inflammatory cytokines (IL-10 and TGFb) are up-regulated (22).

2.1.2. Musculoskeletal system

It is known, from long history of GCs use, that prolonged high doses of GCs results in bone mineralization depletion with subsequent osteoporosis (36). As a result bone formation will be decreased and resorption will be increased (37-41). Bone loss occur in the first few months of treatment and can be improved after cessation of treatment (42-44). Importantly, the GCs induced-osteoporosis can be prevented by calcium and vitamin D supplementation along with GCs treatment course (45). GCs will also cause proximal myopathy which is dose dependent and again improves with discontinuation of treatment (46). GCs treatment increases the risk of femoral head avascular necrosis through a not well established mechanism, although some preliminary evidence pointing to venous endothelial injury (47, 48).

2.1.3. Vascular system

Use of GCs is associated with increased risk of ischemic heart disease and heart failure by increasing the occurrence of hypertension, hyperglycemia, dyslipideamia and obesity (49, 50). Rapid GCs infusion especially in patients with renal and cardiac co-morbidity was associated with sudden death (51).

2.1.4. Serum lipid levels

There are conflicting results from different studies regarding GCs induced hyperlipideamia. Berg and Nilsson-Ehle found that GCs may induce hyperlipideamia through ACTH suppression (52). Whereas others found that GCs may induce favorable lipid profiles in patients aged 60 years or more (53).

2.1.5. Serum glucose levels

GCs are considered diabetogenic hormones. Patients receiving therapeutic doses of GCs will have deranged plasma glucose level and even frank diabetes in glucose intolerant individuals (54, 55). The GCs-induced hyperglycemia is mainly due to reduced glucose peripheral disposal along with increased hepatic gluconeogenesis (56).

2.1.6. Central nervous system

Prolonged use of high doses of GCs is associated with marked behavioral and cognitive deficits. These disorders are more prevalent in those who have risk factors such as pre-existing psychiatric disorders, family history of depression or alcoholism (57). These disturbances are ranging from sleeping disturbances, insomnia, to hypomania, depression and psychosis (58) as well as memory disturbances (59). Recently, more evidences are accumulated to affirm the relationship between exposure to high GCs and impaired cognition. Ioannis and others found that chronic stress, through high endogenous GCs, precipitate cognitive impairment and Alzheimer's like disease (60).

2.1.7. Gastrointestinal system

Gastritis, peptic ulceration, and gastrointestinal hemorrhage all have been found to complicate GCs therapy especially if non-steroidal anti-inflammatory drugs are used concomitantly (61). Although, Chrousos and collegues indicated that GCs therapy could be related to acute pancreatitis in GCs user (62), but more recent studies have proven the opposite that GCs are not an etiological factor (63).

2.2. Fetal (Immature) tissue responses to glucocorticoids

Human intrauterine development is divided mainly into three stages: Zygote, from fertilization to implantation, embryo, from implantation to 8 weeks and fetus, from 8 weeks till term. The embryo and fetal tissues are characterized by rapid division and growth rendering them very susceptible to environmental influences and easily adaptive.

2.2.1. Short term effects of GCs over exposure in fetal life

2.2.1.1. Fetal over exposure to endogenous GCS

Fetal plasma GCs are mainly of maternal adrenal origin (64). This is essentially because of the biochemical, "partial" barrier role played by the placenta. The placenta contains the enzyme 11 β-HSD 2 which is responsible for inactivation of maternal cortisol into cortisone (Section 1.2.2) and hence maintains a normal feto-maternal concentration gradient of the hormone (65). This concentration gradient is species specific where it reaches 180 ng/ml in human; it is only 2 and 15 ng/ml in sheep and pig respectively (66). Therefore, we can assume that fetal exposure to maternal GCs is, at least partly, dependent on the placental activity of this enzyme. This is supported by the finding that in human umbilical cord blood cortisone/cortisol ratio, as a marker of placental 11 β-HSD 2, and the enzyme activity itself and its mRNA expression were lower in human pregnancies which complicated by intrauterine growth restriction (IUGR) (67) and each unit increase in cortisol/cortisone ratio was found to be associated with 1.6 mm Hg higher systolic blood pressure at 3 years of age (68).

GCs are essential for optimal fetal tissue maturation. GR are expressed in brain (69) where it is essential for development of neurons, the building unit in CNS, as well as the formation of synapses by facilitating cortisone-induced axons and dendrites remodeling and neurons myelination (70). Human nervous system development during fetal life is a complex process where extensive proliferation of neurons occurs after initial migration between week 8 and 16 of gestation (71) to reach, at 28 weeks, approximately 40 % higher than total number of neurons in adult (72). These enormous numbers of neurons start to be connected by an extensive network of synapses where between 24 and 34 weeks of gestation more that 10,000 new synapses per second are formed (73). Therefore, exposure to altered plasma level of cortisone during these stages of development and vulnerability is able to alter the basic structure and subsequently the function of the CNS (74). The Maternal and fetal HPA axis are independent (Figure 4) where maternal cortisol is prevented to enter fetal compartment by placental 11 β-HSD 2 until late gestation where placental enzyme drops sharply and allow high levels of maternal free cortisol to enhance fetal lung, CNS and other tissue maturation (75). However, the placenta secretes placental corticotrophin releasing hormone (P-CRH) which is the major, if not the only, mean of cross talk between maternal and fetal HPA axis. As mentioned earlier (Section 1.2.2) that maternal cortisol is exerting negative feedback inhibition on her hypothalamus release of CRH, on contrast, it induces P-CRH secretion as pregnancy advances (76) which in turn will increase maternal and fetal adrenal cortisol secretion (77, 78).

Therefore, maternal either biological stress, like nutritional deprivation, immune reaction, hypertension, or psychological stress will be associated with high maternal cortisol and P-CRH which disrupt fetal nervous system development and affect postnatal cognitive and neuromuscular function. High P-CRH, as a marker of maternal stress, during third trimester associated with weak fetal responsiveness to noval stimuli (79). Postnataly, there is significant reduction in physical and neuromuscular development in neonates who exposed to higher maternal cortisol as well as P-CRH during second and third trimester respectively (80). Those neonates also express prolonged cortisol response to stress, which similar to the effect of synthetic prenatal GCs (81). Interestingly, these behavioral, cognitive and neuromuscular deficiency of offspring exposed to endogenous maternal GCs were accompanied by reduction in the volume of the areas responsible for these functions (82, 83).

Immune system disorder also noted in offspring exposed to maternal prenatal stress with higher incidence of childhood skin, respiratory and other general infections and increased antibiotics use (84). In addition, they have increased body weight which was significantly apparent at age of 10 years (85). More specifically, maternal high CRH during second trimester was found to be associated with offspring adiposity at age of 3 years (86).

2.2.1.2. Antenatal synthetic steroid (dexamethasone and betamethsone) exposure

Maternal administration of synthetic GCs such as dexamethasone and betamethasone, which are poor substrates for 11 β-HSD 2 (87), during pregnancy can cross the placenta (88) in quantities sufficient to induce immediate fetal changes such as reduction in umbilical artery pulsatility index and improved velocity (89) along with transient suppression of fetal breathing and fetal movement resulting in lowering the score of biophysical profile (90). 11 β-HSD 2 is expressed mainly in placental cytotrophoblasts, the progenitors, only upon syncytialization into syncytiotrophoblasts (91). Li and colleagues found that up on syncytialization the expressions of SP1 transcription factor as well as the cAMP pathway are markedly activated (91).

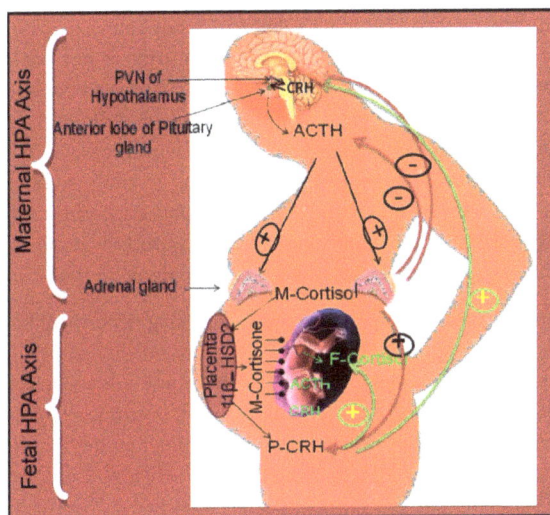

Figure 4. Fetal and maternal HPA axes are two independent systems. The P-CRH stimulates the production of both maternal and fetal cortisol. Maternal cortisol has negative feedback inhibition on her CRH and ACTH but exerts positive feedback stimulation on P-CRH. Placental 11 β-HSD 2 inactivates maternal cortisol into cortisone and hence partially protects the fetus from endogenous maternal GCs over exposure. H: Hypothalamus, P: Pituitary, HPA: Hypothalamo-Pituitary-Adrenal, P-CRH: Placental Corticotrophin Releasing Hormone, ACTH: Adreno-Corticotrophic Hormone, 11 β-HSD 2:11-β-Hydroxysteroid dehydrogenase-2, GCs:Glucocorticoids, M-Cortisol: Maternal cortisol, M-Cortisone: Maternal cortisone, PVN: Paraventricular nucleus, ⊖: Inhibition, ⊕: Stimulation.

GCs are strong inducers of HLA-G gene expression in choriocarcinoma JEG-3 cell lines. The HLA-G molecules play a pivotal role in regulating feto-maternal interface and essential for protecting the allogenic fetus from maternal immune attack (92).

After the finding that surfactant deficiency in premature infants (less than 37 weeks of gestation) is the leading cause of respiratory distress syndrome (RDS) in 1959 (93) and high mortality rate among preterm infants because of this lung immaturity (94, 95) a continuous work was done to prevent such fatal condition. Clinically, GCs has been used to prevent neonatal respiratory distress syndrome successfully (96). Thereafter, many studies found that maternal treatment of GCs will significantly decrease neonatal death due to reduction of intraventricular haemorrhage and necrotising enterocolitis beside reduction in RDS (97, 98). However, randomized controlled trials shown that no differences in the effectiveness of both dexamethasone and betamethasone in reducing the rate of respiratory distress syndrome, need for vasopressor therapy, necrotizing enterocolitis, retinopathy of prematurity, patent ductus arteriosus, neonatal sepsis, and neonatal mortality but reduction in the frequency of intraventricular haemorrhage was more with dexamethasone compared to betamethasone (99).

When synthetic GCs administered during pregnancy they can cross placenta freely since they are not a good substrates to 11 β-HSD 2 (88) and is not bound by CBP (100). Although, the mechanism by which GCs enhance fetal lung maturity is not well established, the administration of antenatal GCs in threatened preterm labour was widely recommended by many institutes. For instance, the National Institutes of Health (NIH) published a Consensus Development Conference Statement in 1994 on the use of antenatal GCs (101) and in 2002, the American College of Obstetricians and Gynecologists' Committee on Obstetric Practice (ACOG) supported the conclusions of the NIH consensus conference (102), whereas, the Royal College of Obstetricians and Gynecologists (RCOG) published guideline in 1996 (103) about antenatal GCs use in preterm labour which then up dated in 1999 and further in 2004.

Recently, there are many evidences that GCs induce fetal lung maturity at both transcriptional and post transcriptional levels (104-106). Pulmonary surfactant is a complex lipoprotein which main action is to reduce surface tension in the alveoli, and subsequently prevent alveolar collapse upon expiration (107). There are four major types of surfactant proteins (SP) A, B, C and D (108). GCs act mainly by increasing the surfactant protein-B (SP-B) mRNA expression at transcription level and its stability at post transcription level (109). Treatment consists of two doses of 12 mg of betamethasone given intramuscularly 24 hours apart or four doses of 6 mg of dexamethasone given intramuscularly 12 hours apart. Optimal benefit begins 24 hours after initiation of therapy and lasts 7 days (101). It has been recently established the use of repeated GCs courses every 14 days for those who still not delivered after the first course. Studies on animal models and also on human showed no additional benefits from repeated courses compared with single GCs course (110-112) and even can be harmful (113-116).

In fact, multiple courses of antenatal GCs have been found to be associated with reduction in ponderal measurements including birth weight, height (116-120) and birth head circumference (117, 119, 121) and higher infant blood pressure and myocardial wall thickness (122, 123) also with maternal infection such as chorioamnionitis and endometritis (116, 121, 124). Rodríguez-Pinilla also reported that antenatal exposure to single steroid course is able to produce similar effects of multiple courses on birth weight and height but not head circumference (117).

With regard to fetal bone metabolism, there were few studies addressing this subject. However, the available data do suggest that both single as well as multiple antenatal steroid courses have no detrimental effects on fetal bone metabolism as evidenced by umbilical cord serum levels of carboxy-terminal propeptide of type I procollagen, a marker for bone formation, and cross-linked carboxy-terminal telopeptide of type I procollagen, a marker of bone resorption (125-127).

The impact of maternal GCs administration antenataly on neonatal hypothalamic-pituitary-adrenal (HPA) axis has been examined extensively but data are controversy. Sandesh Kiran and coworkers found that multiple courses of antenatal dexamethasone causing a significant decrease in RDS without adrenal suppression, decreased growth or impaired neuro-development (128). However, Schäffer and colleagues found that single course of antenatal GCs can lead to absence of stress-induced plasma cortisone and cortisol elevation in neonates at 4 days of life (129). On the other hand, Davis reported that antenatal GCs administration in threatened preterm labour was associated with higher pain-induced plasma cortisol elevation despite no difference in baseline levels than non-treated matched infants at 24 hr after birth (81). Others have assessed the impact of antenatal corticosteroid courses on HPA axis by measuring neonatal 17-OHP in filter-paper blood spots collected between 72 and 96 hr after birth, which usually used for screening the neonates for CAH (Section 1.2.1) (130). These studies revealed a significant reduction of blood 17-OHP in those received multiple courses compared to non-treated matched neonates (130). This fact raise the suspicion in the effectiveness of this screening test in this particular group of neonates as prenatal steroid-induced reduction in 17-OHP could be interpreted falsely as negative test in affected newborns. Ng et al found that at postnatal day 7 and 14 neonatal plasma ACTH and cortisone levels measured after human corticotrophin releasing hormone (hCRH) stimulation test was mildly lower in those exposed to multiple dexamethasone injections antenataly than none treated neonates. Interestingly, there was a negative correlation between plasma cortisone and the number of dexamethasone injections antenataly (131). These finding strongly indicate that antenatal steroid therapy, multiple courses in particular, has impact, which could be transient, on HPA axis harmony and neonatal observation during the first few days is warranted. Animal model of prenatal betamethasone using guinea pigs reported same finding that ACTH and plasma cortisol both suppressed by prenatal betamethasone treatment. This was assosiated with significant reduction in hippocampal mineralococrticoids receptor mRNA and protein expression especially in male offspring with no much difference among GR mRNA and protein expression (132).

It has been found that multiple prenatal steroid courses are not associated with a deleterious effect on auditory neural maturation when assessed at 24 hr after birth (133). However, the use of multiple dexamethasone but not betamethasone are associated with persistent increases in brain parenchymal echogenicity in preterm infants (134) as well as cystic leukomalacia and neurodevelopmental delay at 2 years of age (135). Animal models of prenatal steroid therapy presented some evidence regarding possible mechanism by which antenatal glucocorticoids prevent intraventricular haemorrhage in preterm infants. In mice, prenatal steroid therapy can induce choroid plexus capillary stability and maturation by increasing basement membrane thickness and integrity with subsequent reduction in both peri and intraventricular haemorrhage (136). The frequency and severity of periventricular and intraventricular haemorrhage were even less if vitamin K injection administered antenataly along with steroid course (137).

More recent data comparing the efficacy of single steroid course with multiple courses stated that there were no significant differences in the frequency of respiratory distress syndrome, intraventricular hemorrhage, necrotizing enterocolitis, sepsis and neonatal mortality in neonates receiving either single betamethasone course or multiple courses (138).

According to the same study, the use of multiple courses is not superior to single course. Similar beneficial effect was noted from the use of single and multiple antenatal steroid courses in decreasing the need for postnatal blood pressure support in extreme preterm infants born between 24 to 28 weeks of age (139).

On the same bases, the ACOG Committee on Obstetric Practice (2011) has published its opinion regarding the use of multiple courses. The committee recommended the use of single corticosteroids course to all pregnant women at risk of preterm delivery at 24 to 34 weeks gestation. Another single rescue course of antenatal corticosteroids may be considered if the initial steroid course was given more than 2 weeks earlier (140).

2.2.2. Long term effects of prenatal GCs overexposure

There are accumulating evidence about solid role played by fetal overexposure to both endogenous or synthetic GCs and the risk of developing metabolic and cardiovascular disease in adulthood (141, 142). This remote response to an intrauterine insult has been termed (fetal programming of adult disease).

3. Fetal programming of adult disease

Programming refers to physiological, metabolic, or behavioral adaptation resulting from exposure to or lack of hormones, nutrients, stress, and other agents at critical period during embryonic and fetal development. These insults may encode the function of organs and systems and manifested later as elevated risk for disease in adult life (143, 144). The concept of programming was emerged from many epidemiological studies. For instant, follow up study of a cohort of men who were born during Duch famine in 1944-45 found that exposure to undernutrition during the first half of pregnancy were significantly associated with obesity at adulthood (145). subsequent studies have linked the low birth weight with developing of hypertension, ischaemic heart disease, glucose intolerance, insulin resistance, type 2 diabetes, hyperlipidaemia, hypercortisolaemia, obesity, obstructive pulmonary disease, renal failure and reproductive disorders in the adult (146).

The factors that can programme disease risk in later life are multiple but interact together and include undernutrition (147), stress(148) and endocrine disturbances (149). It has been found that maternal undernutrition leads to decreased placental and fetal birth weight associated with elevated maternal plasma GCs and reduced placental expression of 11 β-Hydroxysteroid Dehydrogenase-2 and subsequently fetal over exposure to maternal corticosterone in rat (150). Maternal low protein diet, for instance, programmed the development of hypertension (151, 152), glucose intolerance (153, 154) and even feeding behavioral abnormalities (155). In human, fetal over exposure to endogenous maternal GCs, such as in maternal psychological stress, programmed the development of metabolic syndrome with higher BMI and body fat percentage, insulin resistance, and atherogenic lipid profile in the offspring at adult life (156). Moreover, adult offspring exposed to prenatal maternal stress, and hence high endogenous GCs, have altered T-helper 1 and 2 balance and abnormal cytokines and ultimately become more prone to develop autoimmune disorders and asthma (157). Similarly, there was impaired cognitive performance as well as memory in the offspring who exposed to maternal stress and higher endogenous GCs. This disturbances in mental function was associated with altered HPA axis in later life where ACTH was increased and plasma cortisol level was decreased (158).

Interestingly, the same programming effect was observed using synthetic GCs such as dexamethasone, which is poor substrate to 11 β-Hydroxysteroid Dehydrogenase-2 (142, 159). Prenatal exposure to synthetic GCs resulted in anxiety and depressive-like behavior in adult offspring. There was altered brain structure with significant increase in volume of the bed nucleus of the stria terminalis and on the other hand decrease amygdala volume due to dendritic atrophy. Dopamin was reduced and dopamin receptor 2 was up regulated in this area (160, 161).

Dexamethasone exposure during late gestation is also able to alter the hepatic and adipose tissue activity and mRNA expression of β-HSD 1 in marmoset monkey with subsequent development of obesity and overt metabolic syndrome (162). It is clear from these data that both fetal exposure to undernutrition, as stress event that lead to fetal over exposure to endogenous maternal GCs, as well as overexposure to synthetic GCs, which are poor substrates to placental 11 β-HSD 2, share common mechanistic pathway in the programming of metabolic syndrome in the offspring at adult life.

3.1. Proposed mechanism of fetal programming of adult disease

The concept of the programming has its roots since 50 years ago (163) and proven by both animal (152, 164) and human studies (119, 149), however, the mechanism that events during intrauterine life are carried in the memory of every molecule, gene, cell, tissue and systems` organs of the body still not completely revealed. Many hypotheses have been proposed with their inherited power and weakness. These include epigenetic modifications of DNA, altered gene expression and regulation, disruption of organ structure by variation in cell number and differentiation and apoptotic remodeling (165, 166). "Hormonal imprinting" where exposure to abnormal levels of a particular hormone during specific window of tissue plasticity is able to exert lifelong abnormal metabolism is another proposed mechanism (167).

3.1.1. Tissue remodeling

In maternal undernutrition model, programming was found to be associated with decreased organ size and total cell mass. Programming of diabetes, in this model, was accompanied by altered pancreatic structure, with predominantly a decrease in β-cell mass (153) due, primarily, to decreased proliferation and increased apoptosis (168). In this model, last week of rat pregnancy was identified as the critical window of programming. Similarly, programming of hypertension was linked to decreased number of nephrons and impaired renal electrolytes and fluid balance (169). GCs, both synthetic one and endogenous, are mediating their programming effects through similar mechanism. As mentioned previously that the observed psychological, behavioral and neuromuscular disturbances were all associated with decreased volume of brain area responsible on that particular function. Moreover, dexamethasone prenatally caused marked reduction in thymus (170). Therefore, antenatal exposure to glucocorticoids above the physiological limit will perturb the growth and ultimate size of the developing fetal organs and eventually their functional capacity which then manifested as disease in adult life.

3.1.2. Epigenetic DNA modification

Epigenetic phenomenon refers to altered heritable genomic function without change in DNA sequence (171). Epigenetic modification involves mainly DNA methylation, histone modification, and miRNA effects (172). DNA methylation has been well explored. In this case there is methylation of cytosine residues within CpG dinucleotides. When this abnormal methylation of CpG islands occur in the promoter region of genes it will result in silencing of genetic information and subsequently to altered biological function (171). Methylation status is a dynamic status and changes are observed since fertilization where both maternal and paternal genomes undergo extensive demethylation followed by selective methylation just prior to implantation (173). This alteration in methylation status has been suggested to play role in cell differentiation and organ development (174). DNA methylation blocks the binding of transcription factors to the promoter of the target gene (Figure 5) and hence prevent gene expression or it promote the binding of the methyl CpG binding protein (MeCP2) which recruits other protein complexes to bind to DNA resulting in a closed chromatin structure and transcriptional silencing (174).

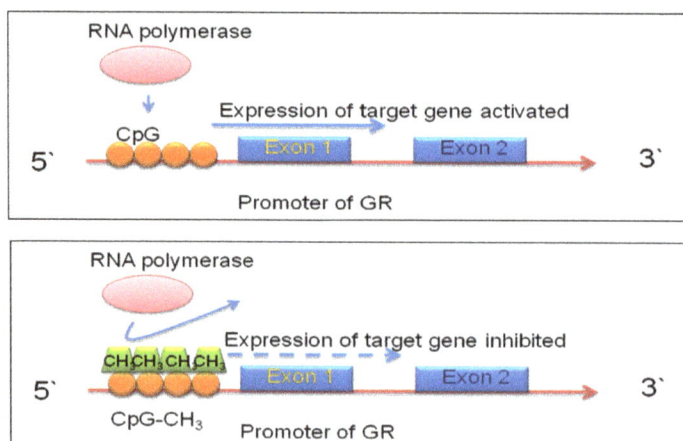

Figure 5. Epigenetic modification of GR promoter by CpG altered methylation.

Maternal low protein diet during pregnancy as experimental model of programming of metabolic syndrome like phenotype has been found to be associated with altered DNA methylation in key genes. For instance, maternal low protein diet resulted in GR over expression and 11 β-HSD 2 decreased expressions in liver, lung, kidney and brain of the offspring (175). GCs induce the hepatic expression and activity of phosphoenolpyruvate carboxykinase (PEPCK) the key enzyme responsible for gluconeogenesis and subsequently produce insulin resistance in this model (176). Interestingly, these changes in expression of target genes were associated with altered methylation status in their promoter area. Namely, GR promoter was found to be hypomethylated in liver tissue of 5 weeks old offspring (177). Some preliminary evidence suggest that hypomethylation of GR occur during early embryogenesis even before cell line differentiation, this was because of finding that GR hypomethylation found in all examined tissue of the offspring in this model (174). GR promoter hypomethylation was associated with histone modification, due to decreased acetylation, in way facilitating transcription (178). Supplementation of maternal low protein diet with glycine or folic acid prevented the development of metabolic syndrome like phenotype as well as GR promoter hypomethylation. Similarly, perinatal stress exposure resulted in altered stress response in the offspring which found to be accompanied with GR promoter hypermethylation at specific CpG dinucleotides in the hippocampus of the offspring. These changes were reversed in adult brain with intra-cranial histone deacetylase inhibitor administration (179). Similarly, in human fetal exposure to maternal stress during second and third trimesters was associated with increased methylation in specific CpG sequence in axon 1F of the GR gene analyzed in cord blood mononuclear cells and at 3 months of offspring age there was significant association between higher CpG methylation in GR gene and higher plasma cortisol response to stress (180). These epigenetic DNA modification seen in antenatal malnutrition or dexamethasone exposure are transmitted to the second generation (181), however, in human it needs to be further explored. It has been suggested that GCs exposure, either endogenous as in maternal psychological stress or in food deprivation or due to antenatal synthetic GCs administration, lead to altered DNA methylation via reduce folic acid availability (182). N5- methyltetrahydrofolate is folic acid derivative and it is considered one of the important methyl donors, therefore, any constrain on folic acid availability will affect methyl donors availability as well.

All these valuable data gave strong evidence that intrauterine life environment has crucial role in human health during adulthood and that the unfavorable conditions will act on the basic unit in the body, that is DNA. Therefore, altered DNA function via epigenetic modification will constrain the functional capacity of key organs when needed to work with their full capacity at adult life and ultimately expressed as disease. The understanding of the mechanism of disease can open the door for discovering early markers for the risk of developing disease and importantly more targeted therapeutic strategies.

3.1.3. Glucocorticoids over exposure

Most of animal models of disease programming and human studies including epidemiological data indicated that glucocorticoids have crucial role in the development of cardio-metabolic and neouro-psychological disease at adulthood. This deleterious effect of glucocorticoids can be exerted directly up on maternal administration of synthetic glucocorticoids and by stress induced endogenous maternal glucocorticoids hypersecretion or indirectly through other types of stress such as food restriction. The development of low birth weight, hypertension, glucose intolerance and insulin resistance in offspring of rat dams fed low protein diet during pregnancy were linked to decreased placental 11 β-HSD 2 expression and activity which resulted in high influx of maternal glucocorticoids to fetal compartment in addition to increased sensitivity of key metabolic organs such as liver, kidney and adipose tissue to glucocorticoids secondary to increased GR expression in these organs (175, 183). The development of metabolic syndrome like phenotype in this animal model has been replicated in human offspring who were exposed to prenatal synthetic glucocorticoids due to threatened preterm delivery to induce lung maturity and also in human offspring who were exposed to high maternal glucocorticoids secondary to maternal stress during pregnancy. Therefore, fetal glucocorticoids over exposure is the main programming pathway despite the variation in the prenatal insult. This hypothesis has many supporting evidence from low protein diet model and other human studies. In rodent, treatment of pregnant dams with placental 11 β-HSD 2 inhibitor, carbenoxolone, resulted in low birth weight and hypertension at adulthood (141). Hypertension in low protein model also was glucocorticoid dependent as maternal adrenalectomy significantly reduced the blood pressure to control levels and corticosterone replacement restored the hypertensive state seen these exposed offspring (151). In human, the placental 11 β-HSD 2 activity correlated with birth weight (184) and reduced in pre-eclampsia (185) and in intrauterine growth restricted fetuses (186). Moreover, 11 β-HSD 2 gene mutation constantly resulted in lower fetal birth weight compared to normal human fetus (187). High maternal GCs associated with decreased placental 11 β-HSD 2, elevated fetal plasma GCs, lower hepatic 11 β-HSD 2 protein expression and enzyme activity which cause over expression and activity of key hepatic gluconeogenesis enzyme, phosphoenolpyruvate kinase (PEPCK), which is linked to insulin resistance and glucose intolerance. In the kidney, the main role of 11 β-HSD 2 is to prevent GCs occupying and activating mineralocorticoid receptor (MR) (188), see figure 6.

GCs-exposed offspring has decreased 11 β-HSD 2 expression and increased GR expression as well as GR promoter hypomethylation in kidney (189). Cortisol will then exert mineralocorticoid activity through MR binding in kidney and resulted in sodium and water retention, hypokalaemia, low plasma renin and aldosterone concentrations, and eventually hypertension in adult life (190). In brain the observed cognitive deficit, altered memory and psychological disturbances in GCs exposed offspring was associated with decreased GR expression in hippocampus (191), which could block the negative feedback regulation of HPA axis by plasma cortisol and hence resulted in abnormal regulation of this crucial nuerohormonal axis. GCs induce the expression of key lipogenic transcription factor, Sterol regulatory element binding protein-1c (SREBP-1c) in liver (192). SREBP-1c transgenic mice, with mRNA and protein over expression of this nuclear factor, developed hyperinsulinaemia, hyperglycaemia, and hepatic steatosis (193, 194).

Interestingly, the metabolic syndrome like phenotype seen in low-protein diet exposed offspring was associated with abnormal expression of SREBP-1c. SREBP-1c mRNA and protein expression were both suppressed from birth until age 9 months in the rat offspring. At 18 months, however, marked over expression seen specially in hepatic tissue with development of non-alcoholic fatty liver, hypercholestreamia, hpertriglycerideamia, hyperglycemia and insulin resistance (147).

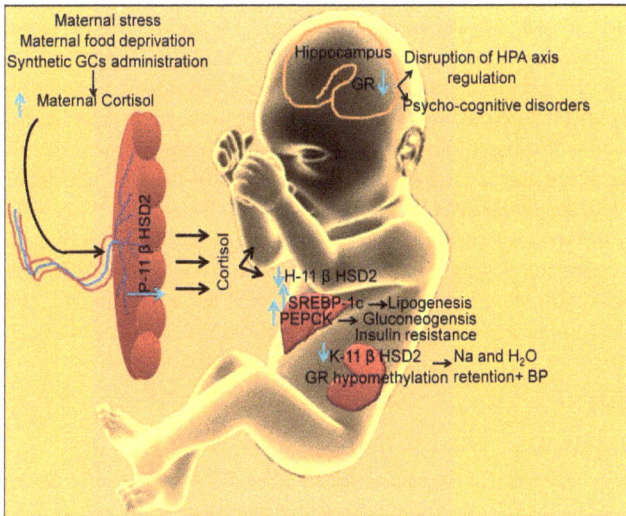

Figure 6. Glucocorticoids central role in the programming of the adult disease. Prenatal exposure to high maternal or synthetic glucocorticoids associated with decreased P-11βHSD2, K-11βHSD2 and H-11βHSD2 expression and activity. In liver this will induce SREBP-1c and lipogenesis and PEPCK and hepatic gluconeogenesis. In kidney, GR hypomethylation and decreased K-11βHSD2 activity associated with more Na and H2O retention and eventually high BP. P-11βHSD2: Placental 11β Hydroxysteroid dehydrogenase 2, K: Kidney, H: Hepatic, SREBP-1c: Sterol Regulatory Element Binding Protein-1c, PEPK: Phosphoenolpyruvate kinase, Na: Sodium, BP: Blood pressure.

4. Conclusions

The understanding of pathogenesis of adult cardio-metabolic and psycho-cognitive disorders is now advanced beyond the idea that such diseases are result of current behavioral and environmental factors. It is well established that adult health originated from wellbeing during fetal life or even at gametes stage. Grandparents' environmental challenges can have impact on human health many generations later. In fact, factors which operate at early life will increase the individual`s susceptibility and vulnerability to adverse environmental events in later life. It is obvious now that different early life environmental events share common programming pathway. The mechanism of programming started to be revealed which include epigenetic DNA modification and promoter methylation status resulting in altered gene expression as well as glucocorticoids over exposure as a primary mechanism where as tissue remodeling and decreased organ and body size as a secondary mechanism. Glucocrticoids over exposure is the main triggering stimulus in this programming, therefore the widely clinical use of prenatal glucocorticoids such as betamethasone and dexamethasone to induce lung maturity in preterm fetus need to be carefully evaluated since they access fetal compartment very easily. Introduction of multiple courses of glucocorticoids as a routine should be discouraged and instead it should be restricted to wisely selected cases. The maximum number of safest courses and lowest therapeutic dose of each subsequent course should be standardized. However, prenatal glucocorticoids have provided the suitable model to study the effects of direct maternal administration of this programming hormone in human candidates. Notwithstanding, these studies still in their neonatal stage and extensive research in this particular area is warranted. The identification of how early life unfavorable environment still able to express pathogenesis at adulthood is crucial to set up pre-disease markers which can be applied clinically in health screening even before the disease itself develops. This will lead to early behavioral and life style interventions which may postponed the onset of disease for many years or even freeze the pathogenesis at its pre-disease stage. Obviously this will lead to decrease financial burden on the health authorities and will markedly cuts the expenses of medical and surgical treatment of the resulted complications.

Author details

Aml Mohammed Erhuma

School of Biomedical Sciences, Nottingham University, Queen`s Medical Centre, Nottingham, UK

Acknowledgement

I would like to express my thanks to Professor Simon Langley-Evans for his valuable advises. My thanks also to my husband and children: Bushra, Tasneem, Lina and Abdul-Rahman for continuance support.

5. References

[1] Addison T. Anemia-disease of supra renal capsule. Med Gazette 1849;43:517-518.

[2] Addison T. On the constitutional and local Effects of Disease of the Supra-Renal Capsules. Samuel Highley, London 1855.

[3] Graner JL. Addison, pernicious anemia and adrenal insufficiency. CMAJ. 1985;133(9):855-7.

[4] Lloyd M. Philip Showalter Hench, 1896-1965. Rheumatology (Oxford) 2002;41(5):582-4.

[5] Nørgaard P, Poulsen H. Glucocorticoid receptors in human malignancies: a review. Ann Oncol. 1991;2(8):541-57.

[6] Chrousos GP, Kino T. Glucocorticoid signaling in the cell. Expanding clinical implications to complex human behavioral and somatic disorders. Ann N Y Acad Sci 2009;1179:153-66.

[7] Zanchi NE, Filho MrAdS, Felitti V, Nicastro H, Lorenzeti FbM, Lancha AH. Glucocorticoids: Extensive physiological actions modulated through multiple mechanisms of gene regulation. Journal of Cellular Physiology 2010;224(2):311-315.

[8]   Dallman MF, Strack AM, Akana SF, Bradbury MJ, Hanson ES, Scribner KA, et al. Feast and Famine: Critical Role of Glucocorticoids with Insulin in Daily Energy Flow. Frontiers in Neuroendocrinology 1993;14(4):303-347.

[9]   Gaillard R. Interaction between the hypothalamo-pituitary-adrenal axis and the immunological system. Ann Endocrinol (Paris). 2001;62(2):155-63.

[10] Da Silva JA. Sex hormones and glucocorticoids: interactions with the immune system. Ann N Y Acad Sci 1999;876:102-17; discussion 117-8.

[11] Giannopoulos G. Early events in the action of glucocorticoids in developing tissues. J Steroid Biochem 1975;6(5):623-31.

[12] Iavazzo C, Myriokefalitaki E, Ntziora F, Bozemberg T, Baskozos I, Papargyriou T, et al. Classic congenital adrenal hyperplasia with virilisation and salt-wasting: from birth to the adult life. Bratisl Lek Listy 2011;112(11):651-2.

[13] Speiser PW, Laforgia N, Kato K, Pareira J, Khan R, Yang SY, et al. First trimester prenatal treatment and molecular genetic diagnosis of congenital adrenal hyperplasia (21-hydroxylase deficiency). J Clin Endocrinol Metab 1990;70(4):838-48.

[14] Forest MG, David M. Antenatal diagnosis and treatment of congenital adrenal hyperplasia due to 21-hydroxylase deficiency. Rev Prat 1991;41(13):1183-7.

[15] Dorr H, Sippell W, Haack D, Bidlingmaier F, Knorr D. Pitfalls of Prenatal treatment of Congenital Adrenal Hyperplasia due to 21-Hydroxylase Deficiency. Program and Abstract. In: 25th Annual meeting of the European Society for Paediatric Endocrinology; 1986; Zurich; 1986.

[16] Evans MI, Chrousos GP, Mann DW, Larsen JW, Jr., Green I, McCluskey J, et al. Pharmacologic suppression of the fetal adrenal gland in utero. Attempted prevention of abnormal external genital masculinization in suspected congenital adrenal hyperplasia. Jama 1985;253(7):1015-20.

[17] Mercado AB, Wilson RC, Cheng KC, Wei JQ, New MI. Prenatal treatment and diagnosis of congenital adrenal hyperplasia owing to steroid 21-hydroxylase deficiency. Journal of Clinical Endocrinology & Metabolism 1995;80(7):2014-20.

[18] Charmandari E, Brook CG, Hindmarsh PC. Why is management of patients with classical congenital adrenal hyperplasia more difficult at puberty? Arch Dis Child 2002;86(4):266-9.

[19] Kino T, Chrousos G. Glucocorticoid effects on gene expression. In: Steckler T KN, Reul JMHM, editor. Handbook of Stress and the Brain. Amsterdam: Elsevier; 2005. p. 295-311.

[20] Chrousos GP. The glucocorticoid receptor gene, longevity, and the complex disorders of Western societies. Am J Med 2004;117(3):204-7.

[21] Chrousos GP, Charmandari E, Kino T. Glucocorticoid action networks--an introduction to systems biology. J Clin Endocrinol Metab 2004;89(2):563-4.

[22] Galon J, Franchimont D, Hiroi N, Frey G, Boettner A, Ehrhart-Bornstein M, et al. Gene profiling reveals unknown enhancing and suppressive actions of glucocorticoids on immune cells. Faseb J 2002;16(1):61-71.

[23] Cameron A, Henley D, Carrell R, Zhou A, Clarke A, Lightman S. Temperature-responsive release of cortisol from its binding globulin: a protein thermocouple. J Clin Endocrinol Metab 2010;95(10):4689-95.

[24] David EG, Armen H, Tashjian J, Ehrin JA, April WA. Pharmacology of the Adrenal Cortex. In: David EG, editor. Principles of pharmacology: the pathophysiologic basis of drug therapy. second ed. USA: Lippincott Williams & Wilkins; 2008. p. 493-508.

[25] Nicolaides NC, Galata Z, Kino T, Chrousos GP, Charmandari E. The human glucocorticoid receptor: molecular basis of biologic function. Steroids 2010;75(1):1-12.

[26] Hollenberg SM, Weinberger C, Ong ES, Cerelli G, Oro A, Lebo R, et al. Primary structure and expression of a functional human glucocorticoid receptor cDNA. Nature 1985;318(6047):635-41.

[27] Duma D, Jewell CM, Cidlowski JA. Multiple glucocorticoid receptor isoforms and mechanisms of post-translational modification. J Steroid Biochem Mol Biol 2006;102(1-5):11-21.

[28] Bamberger CM, Bamberger AM, de Castro M, Chrousos GP. Glucocorticoid receptor beta, a potential endogenous inhibitor of glucocorticoid action in humans. J Clin Invest 1995;95(6):2435-41.

[29] Chung CC, Shimmin L, Natarajan S, Hanis CL, Boerwinkle E, Hixson JE. Glucocorticoid receptor gene variant in the 3' untranslated region is associated with multiple measures of blood pressure. J Clin Endocrinol Metab 2009;94(1):268-76.

[30] Hench P. Effects of cortisone in the rheumatic diseases. Lancet 1950;2(6634):483-4.

[31] Cupps TR, Edgar LC, Thomas CA, Fauci AS. Multiple mechanisms of B cell immunoregulation in man after administration of in vivo corticosteroids. J Immunol 1984;132(1):170-5.

[32] Sbiera S, Dexneit T, Reichardt SD, Michel KD, van den Brandt J, Schmull S, et al. Influence of short-term glucocorticoid therapy on regulatory T cells in vivo. PLoS One 2011;6(9):e24345.

[33] Cox G. Glucocorticoid treatment inhibits apoptosis in human neutrophils. Separation of survival and activation outcomes. J Immunol 1995;154(9):4719-25.

[34] Nakagawa M, Bondy GP, Waisman D, Minshall D, Hogg JC, van Eeden SF. The effect of glucocorticoids on the expression of L-selectin on polymorphonuclear leukocyte. Blood 1999;93(8):2730-7.

[35] van der Goes A, Hoekstra K, van den Berg TK, Dijkstra CD. Dexamethasone promotes phagocytosis and bacterial killing by human monocytes/macrophages in vitro. J Leukoc Biol 2000;67(6):801-7.

[36] Curtiss PH, Jr., Clark WS, Herndon CH. Vertebral fractures resulting from prolonged cortisone and corticotropin therapy. J Am Med Assoc 1954;156(5):467-9.

[37] Lukert BP, Raisz LG. Glucocorticoid-induced osteoporosis: pathogenesis and management. Ann Intern Med 1990;112(5):352-64.

[38] Adler RA, Rosen CJ. Glucocorticoids and osteoporosis. Endocrinol Metab Clin North Am 1994;23(3):641-54.

[39] Canalis E. Clinical review 83: Mechanisms of glucocorticoid action in bone: implications to glucocorticoid-induced osteoporosis. J Clin Endocrinol Metab 1996;81(10):3441-7.

[40] Lane NE, Lukert B. The science and therapy of glucocorticoid-induced bone loss. Endocrinol Metab Clin North Am 1998;27(2):465-83.

[41] Manolagas SC, Weinstein RS. New developments in the pathogenesis and treatment of steroid-induced osteoporosis. J Bone Miner Res 1999;14(7):1061-6.

[42] Pocock NA, Eisman JA, Dunstan CR, Evans RA, Thomas DH, Huq NL. Recovery from steroid-induced osteoporosis. Ann Intern Med 1987;107(3):319-23.

[43] Reid IR, Heap SW. Determinants of vertebral mineral density in patients receiving long-term glucocorticoid therapy. Arch Intern Med 1990;150(12):2545-8.

[44] Reid DM, Hughes RA, Laan RF, Sacco-Gibson NA, Wenderoth DH, Adami S, et al. Efficacy and safety of daily risedronate in the treatment of corticosteroid-induced osteoporosis in men and women: a randomized trial. European Corticosteroid-Induced Osteoporosis Treatment Study. J Bone Miner Res 2000;15(6):1006-13.

[45] Vermaat H, Kirtschig G. Prevention and treatment of glucocorticoid-induced osteoporosis in daily dermatologic practice. Int J Dermatol 2008;47(7):737-42.

[46] Sun L, Trausch-Azar JS, Muglia LJ, Schwartz AL. Glucocorticoids differentially regulate degradation of MyoD and Id1 by N-terminal ubiquitination to promote muscle protein catabolism. Proc Natl Acad Sci U S A 2008;105(9):3339-44.

[47] Nishimura T, Matsumoto T, Nishino M, Tomita K. Histopathologic study of veins in steroid treated rabbits. Clin Orthop Relat Res 1997(334):37-42.

[48] Weinstein RS, Nicholas RW, Manolagas SC. Apoptosis of osteocytes in glucocorticoid-induced osteonecrosis of the hip. J Clin Endocrinol Metab 2000;85(8):2907-12.

[49] Souverein PC, Berard A, Van Staa TP, Cooper C, Egberts AC, Leufkens HG, et al. Use of oral glucocorticoids and risk of cardiovascular and cerebrovascular disease in a population based case-control study. Heart 2004;90(8):859-65.

[50] Wei L, MacDonald TM, Walker BR. Taking glucocorticoids by prescription is associated with subsequent cardiovascular disease. Ann Intern Med 2004;141(10):764-70.

[51] White KP, Driscoll MS, Rothe MJ, Grant-Kels JM. Severe adverse cardiovascular effects of pulse steroid therapy: is continuous cardiac monitoring necessary? J Am Acad Dermatol 1994;30(5 Pt 1):768-73.

[52] Berg AL, Nilsson-Ehle P. ACTH lowers serum lipids in steroid-treated hyperlipemic patients with kidney disease. Kidney Int 1996;50(2):538-42.

[53] Choi HK, Seeger JD. Glucocorticoid use and serum lipid levels in US adults: the Third National Health and Nutrition Examination Survey. Arthritis Rheum 2005;53(4):528-35.

[54] Miller SE, Neilson JM. Clinical Features of the Diabetic Syndrome Appearing after Steroid Therapy. Postgrad Med J 1964;40:660-9.

[55] Gurwitz JH, Bohn RL, Glynn RJ, Monane M, Mogun H, Avorn J. Glucocorticoids and the risk for initiation of hypoglycemic therapy. Arch Intern Med 1994;154(1):97-101.

[56] Olefsky JM, Kimmerling G. Effects of glucocorticoids on carbohydrate metabolism. Am J Med Sci 1976;271(2):202-10.

[57] Minden SL, Orav J, Schildkraut JJ. Hypomanic reactions to ACTH and prednisone treatment for multiple sclerosis. Neurology 1988;38(10):1631-4.

[58] Naber D, Sand P, Heigl B. Psychopathological and neuropsychological effects of 8-days' corticosteroid treatment. A prospective study. Psychoneuroendocrinology 1996;21(1):25-31.

[59] Keenan PA, Jacobson MW, Soleymani RM, Mayes MD, Stress ME, Yaldoo DT. The effect on memory of chronic prednisone treatment in patients with systemic disease. Neurology 1996;47(6):1396-402.

[60] Souza-Talarico JNd, Marin M-F, Sindi S, Lupien SJ. Effects of stress hormones on the brain and cognition Evidence from normal to pathological aging. Dement Neuropsychol 2011;5(1):8-16.

[61] Gabriel SE, Jaakkimainen L, Bombardier C. Risk for serious gastrointestinal complications related to use of nonsteroidal anti-inflammatory drugs. A meta-analysis. Ann Intern Med 1991;115(10):787-96.

[62] Chrousos GA, Kattah JC, Beck RW, Cleary PA. Side effects of glucocorticoid treatment. Experience of the Optic Neuritis Treatment Trial. Jama 1993;269(16):2110-2.

[63] Derk CT, DeHoratius RJ. Systemic lupus erythematosus and acute pancreatitis: a case series. Clin Rheumatol 2004;23(2):147-51.

[64] Mastorakos G, Ilias I. Maternal and fetal hypothalamic-pituitary-adrenal axes during pregnancy and postpartum. Ann N Y Acad Sci 2003;997:136-49.

[65] Seckl JR. Glucocorticoid programming of the fetus; adult phenotypes and molecular mechanisms. Mol Cell Endocrinol 2001;185(1-2):61-71.

[66] Fowden AL, Forhead AJ. Endocrine mechanisms of intrauterine programming. Reproduction 2004;127(5):515-26.

[67] Dy J, Guan H, Sampath-Kumar R, Richardson BS, Yang K. Placental 11beta-hydroxysteroid dehydrogenase type 2 is reduced in pregnancies complicated with idiopathic intrauterine growth Restriction: evidence that this is associated with an attenuated ratio of cortisone to cortisol in the umbilical artery. Placenta 2008;29(2):193-200.

[68] Huh SY, Andrew R, Rich-Edwards JW, Kleinman KP, Seckl JR, Gillman MW. Association between umbilical cord glucocorticoids and blood pressure at age 3 years. BMC Med 2008;6:25.

[69] Sanchez MM, Young LJ, Plotsky PM, Insel TR. Distribution of corticosteroid receptors in the rhesus brain: relative absence of glucocorticoid receptors in the hippocampal formation. J Neurosci 2000;20(12):4657-68.

[70] Raschke C, Schmidt S, Schwab M, Jirikowski G. Effects of betamethasone treatment on central myelination in fetal sheep: an electron microscopical study. Anat Histol Embryol 2008;37(2):95-100.

[71] Kostovic I, Judas M, Rados M, Hrabac P. Laminar organization of the human fetal cerebrum revealed by histochemical markers and magnetic resonance imaging. Cereb Cortex 2002;12(5):536-44.

[72] Huttenlocher PR, Dabholkar AS. Regional differences in synaptogenesis in human cerebral cortex. J Comp Neurol 1997;387(2):167-78.

[73] Levitt P. Structural and functional maturation of the developing primate brain. J Pediatr 2003;143(4 Suppl):S35-45.

[74] Seckl JR, Meaney MJ. Glucocorticoid "programming" and PTSD risk. Ann N Y Acad Sci 2006;1071:351-78.

[75] Murphy VE, Clifton VL. Alterations in human placental 11beta-hydroxysteroid dehydrogenase type 1 and 2 with gestational age and labour. Placenta 2003;24(7):739-44.

[76] Lowry PJ. Corticotropin-releasing factor and its binding protein in human plasma. Ciba Found Symp 1993;172:108-15; discussion 115-28.

[77] Cheng YH, Nicholson RC, King B, Chan EC, Fitter JT, Smith R. Corticotropin-releasing hormone gene expression in primary placental cells is modulated by cyclic adenosine 3',5'-monophosphate. J Clin Endocrinol Metab 2000;85(3):1239-44.

[78] Sandman CA, Davis EP, Buss C, Glynn LM. Prenatal programming of human neurological function. Int J Pept 2011;2011:837596.

[79] Sandman CA, Wadhwa PD, Chicz-DeMet A, Porto M, Garite TJ. Maternal corticotropin-releasing hormone and habituation in the human fetus. Dev Psychobiol 1999;34(3):163-73.

[80] Ellman LM, Schetter CD, Hobel CJ, Chicz-Demet A, Glynn LM, Sandman CA. Timing of fetal exposure to stress hormones: effects on newborn physical and neuromuscular maturation. Dev Psychobiol 2008;50(3):232-41.

[81] Davis EP, Waffarn F, Sandman CA. Prenatal treatment with glucocorticoids sensitizes the hpa axis response to stress among full-term infants. Developmental Psychobiology 2011;53(2):175-183.

[82] Buss C, Davis EP, Muftuler LT, Head K, Sandman CA. High pregnancy anxiety during mid-gestation is associated with decreased gray matter density in 6-9-year-old children. Psychoneuroendocrinology 2010;35(1):141-53.

[83] Connolly JD, Goodale MA, Menon RS, Munoz DP. Human fMRI evidence for the neural correlates of preparatory set. Nat Neurosci 2002;5(12):1345-52.

[84] Beijers R, Jansen J, Riksen-Walraven M, de Weerth C. Maternal prenatal anxiety and stress predict infant illnesses and health complaints. Pediatrics 2010;126(2):e401-9.

[85] Li J, Olsen J, Vestergaard M, Obel C, Baker JL, Sorensen TI. Prenatal stress exposure related to maternal bereavement and risk of childhood overweight. PLoS One 2010;5(7):e11896.

[86] Gillman MW, Rich-Edwards JW, Huh S, Majzoub JA, Oken E, Taveras EM, et al. Maternal corticotropin-releasing hormone levels during pregnancy and offspring adiposity. Obesity (Silver Spring) 2006;14(9):1647-53.

[87] Diederich S, Eigendorff E, Burkhardt P, Quinkler M, Bumke-Vogt C, Rochel M, et al. 11beta-hydroxysteroid dehydrogenase types 1 and 2: an important pharmacokinetic determinant for the activity of synthetic mineralo- and glucocorticoids. J Clin Endocrinol Metab 2002;87(12):5695-701.

[88] Anderson AB, Gennser G, Jeremy JY, Ohrlander S, Sayers L, Turnbull AC. Placental transfer and metabolism of betamethasone in human pregnancy. Obstet Gynecol 1977;49(4):471-4.

[89] Thuring A, Malcus P, Marsal K. Effect of maternal betamethasone on fetal and uteroplacental blood flow velocity waveforms. Ultrasound Obstet Gynecol 2011;37(6):668-72.

[90] Rotmensch S, Liberati M, Celentano C, Efrat Z, Bar-Hava I, Kovo M, et al. The effect of betamethasone on fetal biophysical activities and Doppler velocimetry of umbilical and middle cerebral arteries. Acta Obstet Gynecol Scand 1999;78(9):768-73.

[91] Li JN, Ge YC, Yang Z, Guo CM, Duan T, Myatt L, et al. The Sp1 Transcription Factor Is Crucial for the Expression of 11Î²-Hydroxysteroid Dehydrogenase Type 2 in Human Placental Trophoblasts. Journal of Clinical Endocrinology & Metabolism 2011;96(6):E899-E907.

[92] Akhter A, Das V, Naik S, Faridi RM, Pandey A, Agrawal S. Upregulation of HLA-G in JEG-3 cells by dexamethasone and hydrocortisone. Arch Gynecol Obstet 2012;285(1):7-14.

[93] Avery ME, Mead J. Surface properties in relation to atelectasis and hyaline membrane disease. AMA J Dis Child 1959;97(5, Part 1):517-23.

[94] Dollfus C, Patetta M, Siegel E, Cross AW. Infant mortality: a practical approach to the analysis of the leading causes of death and risk factors. Pediatrics 1990;86(2):176-83.

[95] Wang ML, Dorer DJ, Fleming MP, Catlin EA. Clinical outcomes of near-term infants. Pediatrics 2004;114(2):372-6.

[96] Liggins GC, Howie RN. A controlled trial of antepartum glucocorticoid treatment for prevention of the respiratory distress syndrome in premature infants. Pediatrics 1972;50(4):515-25.

[97] Roberts D, Dalziel S. Antenatal corticosteroids for accelerating fetal lung maturation for women at risk of preterm birth. Cochrane Database Syst Rev 2006;3:CD004454.

[98] Elimian A, Verma U, Canterino J, Shah J, Visintainer P, Tejani N. Effectiveness of antenatal steroids in obstetric subgroups. Obstet Gynecol 1999;93(2):174-9.

[99] Elimian A, Garry D, Figueroa R, Spitzer A, Wiencek V, Quirk JG. Antenatal betamethasone compared with dexamethasone (betacode trial): a randomized controlled trial. Obstet Gynecol 2007;110(1):26-30.

[100] Hughes I, Cutfield W. The adrenal cortex. In: Gluckman P, Heymann M, editors. Pediatrics, perinatology, the scientific basis. London: Arnold; 1996. p. 500- 514.

[101] NIH. ACOG committee opinion. Antenatal corticosteroid therapy for fetal maturation. Number 147--December 1994. Committee on Obstetric Practice. American College of Obstetricians and Gynecologists. Int J Gynaecol Obstet 1995;48(3):340-2.

[102] ACOG. ACOG committee opinion. Antenatal corticosteroid therapy for fetal maturation. American College of Obstetricians and Gynecologists; 2002 Jul.

[103] RCOG. RCOG Guidelines Number 7 ACS to prevent respiratory distress syndrome. London: RCOG; 1996.

[104] Tillis CC, Huang HW, Bi W, Pan S, Bruce SR, Alcorn JL. Glucocorticoid regulation of human pulmonary surfactant protein-B (SP-B) mRNA stability is independent of activated glucocorticocorticoid receptor. American Journal of Physiology - Lung Cellular and Molecular Physiology 2011;300(6):L940-L950.

[105] Whitsett JA, Matsuzaki Y. Transcriptional Regulation of Perinatal Lung Maturation. Pediatric clinics of North America 2006;53(5):873-887.

[106] Venkatesh VC, Iannuzzi DM, Ertsey R, Ballard PL. Differential glucocorticoid regulation of the pulmonary hydrophobic surfactant proteins SP-B and SP-C. Am J Respir Cell Mol Biol 1993;8(2):222-8.

[107] Clements J, King R. Composition of the surface active material. In: RG C, editor. The biochemical basis of pulmonary function. New York: Marcel Dekker; 1976. p. 363-387.

[108] Liley HG, White RT, Warr RG, Benson BJ, Hawgood S, Ballard PL. Regulation of messenger RNAs for the hydrophobic surfactant proteins in human lung. J Clin Invest 1989;83(4):1191-7.

[109] Huang HW, Bi W, Jenkins GN, Alcorn JL. Glucocorticoid regulation of human pulmonary surfactant protein-B mRNA stability involves the 3'-untranslated region. Am J Respir Cell Mol Biol 2008;38(4):473-82.

[110] Smith LM, Qureshi N, Chao CR. Effects of single and multiple courses of antenatal glucocorticoids in preterm newborns less than 30 weeks' gestation. J Matern Fetal Med 2000;9(2):131-5.

[111] Guinn DA, Atkinson MW, Sullivan L, Lee M, MacGregor S, Parilla BV, et al. Single vs weekly courses of antenatal corticosteroids for women at risk of preterm delivery: A randomized controlled trial. Jama 2001;286(13):1581-7.

[112] Wijnberger LD, Mostert JM, van Dam KI, Mol BW, Brouwers H, Visser GH. Comparison of single and repeated antenatal corticosteroid therapy to prevent neonatal death and morbidity in the preterm infant. Early Hum Dev 2002;67(1-2):29-36.

[113] Uno H, Lohmiller L, Thieme C, Kemnitz JW, Engle MJ, Roecker EB, et al. Brain damage induced by prenatal exposure to dexamethasone in fetal rhesus macaques. I. Hippocampus. Brain Res Dev Brain Res 1990;53(2):157-67.

[114] Dunlop SA, Archer MA, Quinlivan JA, Beazley LD, Newnham JP. Repeated prenatal corticosteroids delay myelination in the ovine central nervous system. J Matern Fetal Med 1997;6(6):309-13.

[115] Stewart JD, Gonzalez CL, Christensen HD, Rayburn WF. Impact of multiple antenatal doses of betamethasone on growth and development of mice offspring. Am J Obstet Gynecol 1997;177(5):1138-44.

[116] Ogunyemi D. A comparison of the effectiveness of single-dose vs multi-dose antenatal corticosteroids in pre-term neonates. J Obstet Gynaecol 2005;25(8):756-60.

[117] Rodriguez-Pinilla E, Prieto-Merino D, Dequino G, Mejias C, Fernandez P, Martinez-Frias ML. Antenatal exposure to corticosteroids for fetal lung maturation and its repercussion on weight, length and head circumference in the newborn infant. Med Clin (Barc) 2006;127(10):361-7.

[118] Mazumder P, Dutta S, Kaur J, Narang A. Single versus multiple courses of antenatal betamethasone and neonatal outcome: a randomized controlled trial. Indian Pediatr 2008;45(8):661-7.

[119] Norberg H, Stalnacke J, Heijtz RD, Smedler AC, Nyman M, Forssberg H, et al. Antenatal corticosteroids for preterm birth: dose-dependent reduction in birthweight, length and head circumference. Acta Paediatr 2011;100(3):364-9.

[120] Peltoniemi OM, Kari MA, Hallman M. Repeated antenatal corticosteroid treatment: a systematic review and meta-analysis. Acta Obstet Gynecol Scand 2011;90(7):719-27.

[121] Abbasi S, Hirsch D, Davis J, Tolosa J, Stouffer N, Debbs R, et al. Effect of single versus multiple courses of antenatal corticosteroids on maternal and neonatal outcome. Am J Obstet Gynecol 2000;182(5):1243-9.

[122] Bloomfield F, Knight D, Harding J. Side effects of 2 different dexamethasone courses for preterm infants at risk of chronic lung disease: a randomized trial. J Pediatr. 1998;133(3):395-400.

[123] Mildenhall LF, Battin MR, Morton SM, Bevan C, Kuschel CA, Harding JE. Exposure to repeat doses of antenatal glucocorticoids is associated with altered cardiovascular status after birth. Arch Dis Child Fetal Neonatal Ed 2006;91(1):F56-60.

[124] Mariotti V, Marconi AM, Pardi G. Undesired effects of steroids during pregnancy. J Matern Fetal Neonatal Med 2004;16 Suppl 2:5-7.

[125] Lindahl K, Rubin CJ, Brandstrom H, Karlsson MK, Holmberg A, Ohlsson C, et al. Heterozygosity for a coding SNP in COL1A2 confers a lower BMD and an increased stroke risk. Biochem Biophys Res Commun 2009;384(4):501-5.

[126] Saarela T, Risteli J, Kauppila A, Koivisto M. Effect of short-term antenatal dexamethasone administration on type I collagen synthesis and degradation in preterm infants at birth. Acta PÃ diatrica 2001;90(8):921-925.

[127] Korakaki E, Gourgiotis D, Aligizakis A, Manoura A, Hatzidaki E, Giahnakis E, et al. Levels of bone collagen markers in preterm infants: relation to antenatal glucocorticoid treatment. J Bone Miner Metab 2007;25(3):172-8.

[128] Sandesh Kiran PS, Dutta S, Narang A, Bhansali A, Malhi P. Multiple courses of antenatal steroids. Indian J Pediatr 2007;74(5):463-9.

[129] Schaffer L, Luzi F, Burkhardt T, Rauh M, Beinder E. Antenatal betamethasone administration alters stress physiology in healthy neonates. Obstet Gynecol 2009;113(5):1082-8.

[130] Gatelais F, Berthelot J, Beringue F, Descamps P, Bonneau D, Limal JM, et al. Effect of single and multiple courses of prenatal corticosteroids on 17-hydroxyprogesterone levels: implication for neonatal screening of congenital adrenal hyperplasia. Pediatr Res 2004;56(5):701-5.

[131] Ng PC, Wong GW, Lam CW, Lee CH, Fok TF, Wong MY, et al. Effect of multiple courses of antenatal corticosteroids on pituitary-adrenal function in preterm infants. Arch Dis Child Fetal Neonatal Ed 1999;80(3):F213-6.

[132] Owen D, Matthews SG. Glucocorticoids and sex-dependent development of brain glucocorticoid and mineralocorticoid receptors. Endocrinology 2003;144(7):2775-84.

[133] Amin SB, Guillet R. Auditory neural maturation after exposure to multiple courses of antenatal betamethasone in premature infants as evaluated by auditory brainstem response. Pediatrics 2007;119(3):502-8.

[134] Spinillo A, Chiara A, Bergante C, Biancheri D, Fabiana D, Fazzi E. Obstetric risk factors and persistent increases in brain parenchymal echogenicity in preterm infants. Bjog 2004;111(9):913-8.

[135] Spinillo A, Viazzo F, Colleoni R, Chiara A, Maria Cerbo R, Fazzi E. Two-year infant neurodevelopmental outcome after single or multiple antenatal courses of corticosteroids to prevent complications of prematurity. Am J Obstet Gynecol 2004;191(1):217-24.

[136] Liu J, Feng ZC, Yin XJ, Chen H, Lu J, Qiao X. The role of antenatal corticosteroids for improving the maturation of choroid plexus capillaries in fetal mice. Eur J Pediatr 2008;167(10):1209-12.

[137] Liu J, Wang Q, Zhao JH, Chen YH, Qin GL. The combined antenatal corticosteroids and vitamin K therapy for preventing periventricular-intraventricular hemorrhage in premature newborns less than 35 weeks gestation. J Trop Pediatr 2006;52(5):355-9.

[138] Bontis N, Vavilis D, Tsolakidis D, Goulis DG, Tzevelekis P, Kellartzis D, et al. Comparison of single versus multiple courses of antenatal betamethasone in patients with threatened preterm labor. Clin Exp Obstet Gynecol 2011;38(2):165-7.

[139] Nair GV, Omar SA. Blood pressure support in extremely premature infants is affected by different courses of antenatal steroids. Acta Paediatr 2009;98(9):1437-43.

[140] ACOG. ACOG Committee Opinion No. 475: Antenatal corticosteroid therapy for fetal maturation. Obstet Gynecol 2011;117(2 Pt 1):422-4.

[141] Benediktsson R, Lindsay RS, Noble J, Seckl JR, Edwards CR. Glucocorticoid exposure in utero: new model for adult hypertension. Lancet 1993;341(8841):339-41.

[142] Nyirenda MJ, Lindsay RS, Kenyon CJ, Burchell A, Seckl JR. Glucocorticoid exposure in late gestation permanently programs rat hepatic phosphoenolpyruvate carboxykinase and glucocorticoid receptor expression and causes glucose intolerance in adult offspring. J Clin Invest 1998;101(10):2174-81.

[143] Seckl JR. Physiologic programming of the fetus. Clin Perinatol 1998;25(4):939-62, vii.

[144] Barker DJ. In utero programming of chronic disease. Clin Sci (Lond) 1998;95(2):115-28.

[145] Ravelli GP, Stein ZA, Susser MW. Obesity in young men after famine exposure in utero and early infancy. N Engl J Med 1976;295(7):349-53.

[146] Barker D. Mothers, Babies and Disease in Later Life. London: BMJ Publishing.; 1994.

[147] Erhuma A, Salter AM, Sculley DV, Langley-Evans SC, Bennett AJ. Prenatal exposure to a low-protein diet programs disordered regulation of lipid metabolism in the aging rat. Am J Physiol Endocrinol Metab 2007;292(6):E1702-14.

[148] Lazinski MJ, Shea AK, Steiner M. Effects of maternal prenatal stress on offspring development: a commentary. Arch Womens Ment Health 2008;11(5-6):363-75.

[149] Seckl JR. Prenatal glucocorticoids and long-term programming. Eur J Endocrinol 2004;151 Suppl 3:U49-62.

[150] Belkacemi L, Jelks A, Chen CH, Ross MG, Desai M. Altered placental development in undernourished rats: role of maternal glucocorticoids. Reprod Biol Endocrinol 2011;9:105.

[151] Gardner DS, Jackson AA, Langley-Evans SC. Maintenance of maternal diet-induced hypertension in the rat is dependent on glucocorticoids. Hypertension 1997;30(6):1525-30.

[152] Langley-Evans SC. Hypertension induced by foetal exposure to a maternal low-protein diet, in the rat, is prevented by pharmacological blockade of maternal glucocorticoid synthesis. J Hypertens 1997;15(5):537-44.

[153] Dahri S, Snoeck A, Reusens-Billen B, Remacle C, Hoet JJ. Islet function in offspring of mothers on low-protein diet during gestation. Diabetes 1991;40 Suppl 2:115-20.

[154] Pinheiro AR, Salvucci ID, Aguila MB, Mandarim-de-Lacerda CA. Protein restriction during gestation and/or lactation causes adverse transgenerational effects on biometry and glucose metabolism in F1 and F2 progenies of rats. Clin Sci (Lond) 2008;114(5):381-92.

[155] Bellinger L, Langley-Evans SC. Fetal programming of appetite by exposure to a maternal low-protein diet in the rat. Clin Sci (Lond) 2005;109(4):413-20.

[156] Entringer S, Wust S, Kumsta R, Layes IM, Nelson EL, Hellhammer DH, et al. Prenatal psychosocial stress exposure is associated with insulin resistance in young adults. Am J Obstet Gynecol 2008;199(5):498 e1-7.

[157] Entringer S, Kumsta R, Nelson EL, Hellhammer DH, Wadhwa PD, Wust S. Influence of prenatal psychosocial stress on cytokine production in adult women. Dev Psychobiol 2008;50(6):579-87.

[158] Entringer S, Buss C, Kumsta R, Hellhammer DH, Wadhwa PD, Wust S. Prenatal psychosocial stress exposure is associated with subsequent working memory performance in young women. Behav Neurosci 2009;123(4):886-93.

[159] Tang JI, Kenyon CJ, Seckl JR, Nyirenda MJ. Prenatal overexposure to glucocorticoids programs renal 11beta-hydroxysteroid dehydrogenase type 2 expression and salt-sensitive hypertension in the rat. J Hypertens 2011;29(2):282-9.

[160] McArthur S, McHale E, Dalley JW, Buckingham JC, Gillies GE. Altered Mesencephalic Dopaminergic Populations in Adulthood as a Consequence of Brief Perinatal Glucocorticoid Exposure. Journal of Neuroendocrinology 2005;17(8):475-482.

[161] Oliveira Mr, Rodrigues A-Jo, LeÃ£o P, Cardona D, PÃªgo J, Sousa N. The bed nucleus of stria terminalis and the amygdala as targets of antenatal glucocorticoids: implications for fear and anxiety responses. In: Psychopharmacology: Springer Berlin / Heidelberg; 2012. p. 443-453.

[162] Nyirenda MJ, Carter R, Tang JI, de Vries A, Schlumbohm C, Hillier SG, et al. Prenatal programming of metabolic syndrome in the common marmoset is associated with increased expression of 11beta-hydroxysteroid dehydrogenase type 1. Diabetes 2009;58(12):2873-9.

[163] Neel JV. Diabetes mellitus: a "thrifty" genotype rendered detrimental by "progress"? Am J Hum Genet 1962;14:353-62.

[164] Erhuma A, Bellinger L, Langley-Evans SC, Bennett AJ. Prenatal exposure to undernutrition and programming of responses to high-fat feeding in the rat. Br J Nutr 2007;98(3):517-24.

[165] Waterland RA, Garza C. Potential mechanisms of metabolic imprinting that lead to chronic disease. Am J Clin Nutr 1999;69(2):179-97.

[166] Waterland RA, Jirtle RL. Early nutrition, epigenetic changes at transposons and imprinted genes, and enhanced susceptibility to adult chronic diseases. Nutrition 2004;20(1):63-8.

[167] Csaba G. Phylogeny and ontogeny of hormone receptors: the selection theory of receptor formation and hormonal imprinting. Biol Rev Camb Philos Soc 1980;55(1):47-63.

[168] Berney DM, Desai M, Palmer DJ, Greenwald S, Brown A, Hales CN, et al. The effects of maternal protein deprivation on the fetal rat pancreas: major structural changes and their recuperation. The Journal of Pathology 1997;183(1):109-115.

[169] Langley-Evans SC, Welham SJ, Jackson AA. Fetal exposure to a maternal low protein diet impairs nephrogenesis and promotes hypertension in the rat. Life Sciences 1999;64(11):965-974.

[170] Dietert RR, Lee JE, Olsen J, Fitch K, Marsh JA. Developmental immunotoxicity of dexamethasone: comparison of fetal versus adult exposures. Toxicology 2003;194(1-2):163-76.

[171] Lorenzen JM, Martino F, Thum T. Epigenetic modifications in cardiovascular disease. Basic Res Cardiol 2012;107(2):1-10.

[172] Hussain N. Epigenetic Influences That Modulate Infant Growth, Development, and Disease. Antioxid Redox Signal 2012.

[173] Bird A. DNA methylation patterns and epigenetic memory. Genes Dev 2002;16(1):6-21.

[174] Burdge GC, Hanson MA, Slater-Jefferies JL, Lillycrop KA. Epigenetic regulation of transcription: a mechanism for inducing variations in phenotype (fetal programming) by differences in nutrition during early life? Br J Nutr 2007;97(6):1036-46.

[175] Bertram C, Trowern AR, Copin N, Jackson AA, Whorwood CB. The maternal diet during pregnancy programs altered expression of the glucocorticoid receptor and type 2 11beta-hydroxysteroid dehydrogenase: potential molecular mechanisms underlying the programming of hypertension in utero. Endocrinology 2001;142(7):2841-53.

[176] Burns SP, Desai M, Cohen RD, Hales CN, Iles RA, Germain JP, et al. Gluconeogenesis, glucose handling, and structural changes in livers of the adult offspring of rats partially deprived of protein during pregnancy and lactation. J Clin Invest 1997;100(7):1768-74.

[177] Lillycrop KA, Phillips ES, Jackson AA, Hanson MA, Burdge GC. Dietary protein restriction of pregnant rats induces and folic acid supplementation prevents epigenetic modification of hepatic gene expression in the offspring. J Nutr 2005;135(6):1382-6.

[178] Lillycrop KA, Slater-Jefferies JL, Hanson MA, Godfrey KM, Jackson AA, Burdge GC. Induction of altered epigenetic regulation of the hepatic glucocorticoid receptor in the offspring of rats fed a protein-restricted diet during pregnancy suggests that reduced DNA methyltransferase-1 expression is involved in impaired DNA methylation and changes in histone modifications. Br J Nutr 2007;97(6):1064-73.

[179] Weaver IC, Meaney MJ, Szyf M. Maternal care effects on the hippocampal transcriptome and anxiety-mediated behaviors in the offspring that are reversible in adulthood. Proc Natl Acad Sci U S A 2006;103(9):3480-5.

[180] Oberlander TF, Weinberg J, Papsdorf M, Grunau R, Misri S, Devlin AM. Prenatal exposure to maternal depression, neonatal methylation of human glucocorticoid receptor gene (NR3C1) and infant cortisol stress responses. Epigenetics 2008;3(2):97-106.

[181] Drake AJ, Walker BR, Seckl JR. Intergenerational consequences of fetal programming by in utero exposure to glucocorticoids in rats. Am J Physiol Regul Integr Comp Physiol 2005;288(1):R34-8.

[182] Terzolo M, Allasino B, Bosio S, Brusa E, Daffara F, Ventura M, et al. Hyperhomocysteinemia in patients with Cushing's syndrome. J Clin Endocrinol Metab 2004;89(8):3745-51.

[183] Langley-Evans SC, Phillips GJ, Benediktsson R, Gardner DS, Edwards CR, Jackson AA, et al. Protein intake in pregnancy, placental glucocorticoid metabolism and the programming of hypertension in the rat. Placenta 1996;17(2-3):169-72.

[184] Stewart PM, Rogerson FM, Mason JI. Type 2 11 beta-hydroxysteroid dehydrogenase messenger ribonucleic acid and activity in human placenta and fetal membranes: its relationship to birth weight and putative role in fetal adrenal steroidogenesis. Journal of Clinical Endocrinology & Metabolism 1995;80(3):885-90.

[185] McCalla CO, Nacharaju VL, Muneyyirci-Delale O, Glasgow S, Feldman JG. Placental 11 beta-hydroxysteroid dehydrogenase activity in normotensive and pre-eclamptic pregnancies. Steroids 1998;63(10):511-5.

[186] McTernan CL, Draper N, Nicholson H, Chalder SM, Driver P, Hewison M, et al. Reduced Placental 11 Beta-Hydroxysteroid Dehydrogenase Type 2 mRNA Levels in Human Pregnancies Complicated by Intrauterine Growth Restriction: An Analysis of Possible Mechanisms. Journal of Clinical Endocrinology & Metabolism 2001;86(10):4979-4983.

[187] Kitanaka S, Tanae A, Hibi I. Apparent mineralocorticoid excess due to 11 beta-hydroxysteroid dehydrogenase deficiency: a possible cause of intrauterine growth retardation. Clin Endocrinol (Oxf) 1996;44(3):353-9.

[188] Martinerie L, Pussard E, Meduri G, Delezoide AL, Boileau P, Lombes M. Lack of renal 11 Beta-hydroxysteroid dehydrogenase type 2 at birth, a targeted temporal window for neonatal glucocorticoid action in human and mice. PLoS One 2012;7(2):e31949.

[189] Wyrwoll CS, Mark PJ, Waddell BJ. Developmental programming of renal glucocorticoid sensitivity and the renin-angiotensin system. Hypertension 2007;50(3):579-84.

[190] Ferrari P, Lovati E, Frey FJ. The role of the 11beta-hydroxysteroid dehydrogenase type 2 in human hypertension. J Hypertens 2000;18(3):241-8.

[191] Basta-Kaim A, Budziszewska B, Leskiewicz M, Fijal K, Regulska M, Kubera M, et al. Hyperactivity of the hypothalamus-pituitary-adrenal axis in lipopolysaccharide-induced neurodevelopmental model of schizophrenia in rats: effects of antipsychotic drugs. Eur J Pharmacol 2011;650(2-3):586-95.

[192] Erhuma A, McMullen S, Langley-Evans SC, Bennett AJ. Feeding pregnant rats a low-protein diet alters the hepatic expression of SREBP-1c in their offspring via a glucocorticoid-related mechanism. Endocrine 2009;36(2):333-8.

[193] Shimomura I, Hammer RE, Richardson JA, Ikemoto S, Bashmakov Y, Goldstein JL, et al. Insulin resistance and diabetes mellitus in transgenic mice expressing nuclear SREBP-1c in adipose tissue: model for congenital generalized lipodystrophy. Genes & Development 1998;12(20):3182-3194.

[194] Horton JD, Shimomura I, Ikemoto S, Bashmakov Y, Hammer RE. Overexpression of sterol regulatory element-binding protein-1a in mouse adipose tissue produces adipocyte hypertrophy, increased fatty acid secretion, and fatty liver. J Biol Chem 2003;278(38):36652-60.

The Role of Glucocorticoids in Pregnancy: Four Decades Experience with Use of Betamethasone in the Prevention of Pregnancy Loss

Fortunato Vesce, Emilio Giugliano, Elisa Cagnazzo,
Stefania Bignardi, Elena Mossuto, Tarcisio Servello and Roberto Marci

Additional information is available at the end of the chapter

1. Introduction

'Pregnancy loss' can be defined as the failure by the gestational processes to result in the birth of a viable neonate. Miscarriage is defined as the end of pregnancy before the fetus reaches viability, a condition in turn depending on other variables, among which gestational age, birth weight and maturity, as well as the quality of assistance. Therefore to set, as it is done, at 24 weeks the term before which any birth should be classified as abortion is inadequate, because around this time some fetuses survive. On the other hand, preterm birth, that is strictly related with adverse infant outcome in terms of survival and quality of life, is defined as birth at less than 37 weeks. However it will be recognized that while up to the half of the second trimester no foetus at the moment can survive outside the maternal environment, during the third trimester, rather than from gestational age by itself, pregnancy loss will mainly depend on the pathologic condition leading to premature delivery. Recurrent miscarriage refers to the occurrence of three or even two (von Eye Corleta, 2010) consecutive pregnancy losses. The attempt to distinguish sporadic from repeated abortion stems from the believe that they may have different causes. Nevertheless, although it may be difficult to establish the pathogenic mechanism in single cases, in general it is much better understood today, and it is basically always the same: therefore it appears that separating sporadic from recurrent abortion is no longer needed. Indeed, pregnancy loss can occur at any time throughout gestation and labour as a consequence of a number of pathologic conditions widely recognizing two background pathways, namely the impairment of the blood supply to the foetus and the stimulation of uterine contractions. In the majority of the cases, such complications are triggered by an either pre-existent or acquired inflammatory mechanism. For instance, maternal rheumatic diseases represent a well known condition leading to poor pregnancy outcome (Spinillo et al., 2012), although, as it will be explained ahead, abortion can also represent the only pathologic expression of functional changes resembling inflammation confined at the uterine mucosa level. At this regard, one basic need in approaching the role of glucocorticoids (GCs) in medicine is represented by a reappraisal to the concept itself of inflammation. This, indeed, based on our background medical education, is characterized by classical signs and symptoms (rubor, calor, tumor, dolor and functio laesa) as well as by several hemato-chemical and histological features. However, the cytokines and prostanoids that trigger inflammation are also involved in the regulation of important physiologic functions, among which social behaviour of cells (Biondi et al., 2006), angiogenesis (Suffee et al., 2011), haemostasis (Salgado et al., 1994) and smooth muscle contraction (Shynlova et al., 2009). In obstetrics, processes such as implantation and labour are under the control of these mediators, the **imbalance** of which is able to **deviate a physiological function** towards an inflammatory disease, leading to a wide number of gestational complications, from abortion (Saini et al, 2011) to foetal malformation (Sljivic et al., 2006), intra-uterine growth restriction (Eastabrook et al., 2008), abruptio placentae (Nath et al., 2007), premature delivery (Romero et al., 2002), as well as hyaline membrane disease (Cheah et al., 2005), necrotizing entero-colitis (Xu et al., 2011) and hypoxic ischemic encephalopathy of the newborn (Liu et al., 2010). Such a cytokine and prostanoid **imbalance** may therefore represent the **early change for an eventual, future inflammation**. Surprisingly, instead, implantation and labour themselves are often named as a sort of inflammatory process, thus implying that a pathologic event may be beneficial to human health: such a pointless unsafe concept should be better avoided. Indeed, besides its intrinsic contradiction, it represents an obstacle to the liberal use of some anti-inflammatory drugs, among which GCs, aimed at re-balancing the above mentioned mediators for preventing harmful complications. There is a further point of primary significance to be considered before entering into the specific field of pregnancy regulators, and it deals with the causal relationship between inflammation and infection. At this regard, it is generally accepted that it is the latter to trigger the first, while, based on a number of considerations, at least in some cases the opposite is true. Indeed, most bacteria responsible for infection belong to the saprophytic flora, thus suggesting that their shift to pathogen may be a consequence of an environmental alteration, possibly linked with a cytokine-prostanoid imbalance that leads to the inflammatory response. Such a view is strongly supported in obstetrics, thanks to the fundamental work of professor Romero showing that premature delivery, an ominous condition of pregnancy often complicated by infection, is preceded by an inflammation of gestational tissues: 'the foetal inflammatory response syndrome', that will be explained in a more detailed manner ahead. Being, to the best of our knowledge, the Romero's syndrome the first clinical demonstration of a reversed causal relationship between infection and inflammation, it represents a milestone suggesting to search for similar pathogenic mechanisms in other fields of medicine. In the meantime, it opens to debate upon the role and priority of the drugs currently used in the management of such disease, namely GCs, antibiotics and non steroidal anti-inflammatory compounds.

2. Mediators of physiological pregnancy

Based on the above considerations, we proceed now to analyze the pro- as well as the anti-inflammatory mediators of physiological pregnancy. Cytokines found at the maternal-foetal interface include interferons (IFNs), interleukins (ILs), leukaemia inhibitory factor (LIF), tumour necrosis factors (TNFs), transforming growth factors (TGFs), colony stimulating factors (CSFs), vascular endothelial growth factors (VEGFs) and many others (Chaouat et al., 2007). Although a prevalence of pro-inflammatory cytokines are found during the early stages of pregnancy, the action of the anti-inflammatory is needed as well. For instance, LIF and IL-6 are required for a successful implantation in mice (Robb et al., 1998), but the lack of activity of IL-11 results in reduced fertility (White et al.,2004).

With the aim to shed light upon the complex network of reciprocal influences between cytokines and prostanoids from one side and their trophoblastic target form the other, we provide a more detailed description as regards the macrophage migration inhibitory factor (MIF) system, the interleukin-1 system (IL-1), the Toll-like receptors (TLRs) and the chemicals known as "endocrine disruptors" (EDs). (Figure 1).

2.1. MIF

The need for a balanced action of cytokines, whether or not of the inflammatory type, is confirmed looking at the macrophage migration inhibitory factor (MIF) system. MIF stimulates the production of a large panel of pro-inflammatory molecules, such as TNFα, IFNγ, IL-1β, IL-2, IL-6, IL-8 (Calandra et al., 1995) as well as nitric oxide (NO) (Cunha et al., 1993), matrix metalloproteinases (MMPs) and products of the arachidonic acid pathway (Calandra et al., 2003). MIF protein and mRNA are expressed by first trimester human villous and extra-villous trophoblast, the protein being also found in term placenta, amniotic fluid and maternal serum (Ietta et al. 2002). Their levels are higher at the beginning of first trimester to decline later on. Moreover, they are up-regulated by low oxygen tension, comparable to the values occurring at the very early stage of pregnancy (Ietta et al., 2007). Trophoblast MIF **reduces** the cytotoxicity of decidual natural killer (NK) cells (Arcuri et al., 2006), and intraperitoneal injection of rMIF to pregnant mice induces an increase of endometrial alpha(v),beta-3-integrin subunits and VEGF expression, that are markers of uterine receptivity (Bondza et al., 2008). Accordingly, pregnant MIF-treated mice show an enhanced rate of implanted embryos with respect to controls (Bondza et al., 2008), although fertility is not impaired in MIF knock-out mice (Fingerle-Rowson et al., 2003).

2.2. IL-1

The IL-1 system represents a further regulator of uterine receptivity and embryo implantation At the implantation site, immunoreactive IL-1β was detected in the villous and extravillous trophoblast as well as in the maternal decidual cells (Paulesu et al. 2010). Moreover, interleukin-1 receptor type 1 (IL-1R tI) is expressed by the syncytiotrophoblast, supporting the stimulatory effect of IL-1β on human chorionic gonadotropin (hCG) release (Masuhiro et al., 1991). IL-1 has been reported to stimulate different cytokines in the endometrium, including IL-6, IL-8, LIF and TNF-α, as well as the expression of prostaglandins (PGs)-2 and -2α and their receptor EP1 (Minas et al., 2005). The presence of IL-1α and IL-1β in the embryo culture medium has been correlated with successful implantation after in vitro fertilization (Karagouni et al., 1998). Later studies of endometrial secretions from women before embryo transfer showed the association of lower levels of IL-1β with clinical pregnancy (Boomsma et al., 2009). Since IL-1β and TNFα are significantly related to clinical pregnancy and not embryo implantation, it was suggested that these two cytokines are not associated with the initial apposition and adhesion of the embryo (Boomsma et al., 2009). An inappropriate ratio of IL-1β to IL-α and higher IL-1R tI are involved in the establishment of ectopic pregnancy in the oviduct (Huang et al., 2005). IL-1β mediates the paracrine effect of PG synthesis by inducing COX-2 (Pellicer et al., 2002), and IL-1α induces the production of MMP-1 in stromal fibroblast and raises the activity of MMP-9 in trophoblast (Pellicer et al., 2002). Moreover, it has been shown that trophoblast reduces the secretion of pro-inflammatory cytokines IL-1β, IL-6 and TNFα elicited by low (0.1 µg/mL), but not high, doses lipopolysaccharide (LPS)-activated monocytes (Fest et al., 2007). As the female genital tract is opened to the external environment, cytokine release by gestational tissue can be influenced by external factors. For instance, exposure to seminal plasma factors including TGFβ1 stimulates cytokine production by uterine epithelial cells, with consequent recruitment and activation of macrophages, granulocytes and dendritic cells in the underlying stroma (Gopichandran et al., 2006).

2.3. TLRs

Cytokine release by gestational tissue is further regulated through the action of specific receptors for pathogen-associated molecular patterns, named Toll-like receptors (TLRs). These are present in the epithelial lining as well as in the underlying connective stroma of the human female reproductive tract (Hirata et al., 2007). TLR2 and TLR4 have been detected in villous and extra-villous, but not in syncytial first trimester trophoblast, TLR6, instead, is absent in the first but present in the third trimester trophoblast (Mitsunari et al., 2006). Binding of TLRs with microbial antigens activates the release of pro-inflammatory cytokines, possibly interfering with their physiological gestational balance (Schaefer et al., 2005). In addition to the above mentioned factors, also stress, nutrition, metabolic status, drugs and environmental chemicals (Arck et al., 2008), as well as genetic conditions are known to influence gestational cytokine and prostanoids.

2.4. EDs

Some chemicals defined as "endocrine disruptors" (EDs) are able to act like natural estrogens, interfering with reproductive processes. For instance, it has been recently shown that the ED para-nonylphenol (p-NP) affects trophoblast cytokine secretion as well as cell differentiation and apoptosis (Bechi et al., 2010). In addition to cytokines and prostanoids, also the cellular components of the immune system are involved in the regulation of physiological pregnancy. Among these, NK cells, that are large granular lymphocytes constituting 10-15% of their total circulating number. Even though their main activity is citotoxicity of target cells, in normal pregnancy they provide benefit by secreting cytokines, chemokines and angiogenetic factors which are needed for pregnancy success (Santoni et al., 2008). There is a further class of NK at the decidual level, named uterine NK (uNK), which are provided with phenotypic markers different from peripheral (pNK). uNK cells seem to be necessary for pregnancy success by producing factors that modulate trophoblast invasion and placental vascularization (Saito et al., 1993).

All above evidences outline the concept that there is no single substance, or mediator, or cell type that can be specifically identified as either detrimental or protective towards physiological pregnancy, but rather that it is their imbalance which can lead to an unfavourable outcome.

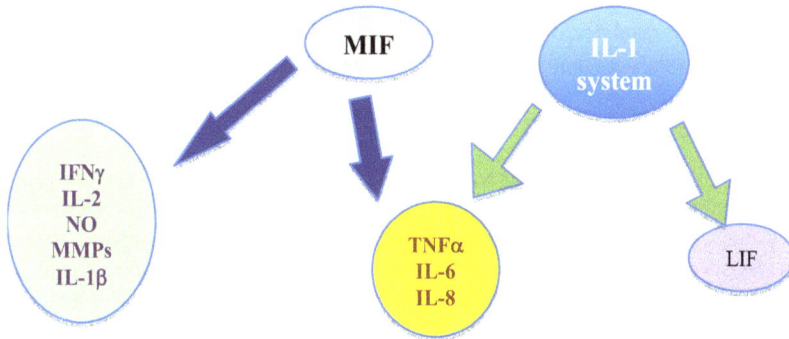

Figure 1. Influences of MIF and IL-1 systems on cytokine network in physiologic pregnancy

3. Hormone regulation of gestational cytokines and prostanoids

Pregnancy can be defined as a vascular phenomenon under the control of steroid hormones. Indeed nearly all above mentioned mediators are directly or indirectly able to interfere with the maternal uterine arteries changes aimed at increasing the foetal blood supply, and they are largely influenced by steroids. Therefore we will look now at the experimental results supporting the specific role of estrogen, progesterone and glucocorticoids in the control of the mediators of gestational functions. In particular, as progesterone and glucocorticoids actions are higly impaired by the abortive drug named mifepristone, we will compare influence of such compounds upon some gestational regulators and functions. Such a comparison should better address to understand the nature of both hormonal protection and drug impairment of pregnancy, provided that their action mechanisms lead to opposite regulatory consequences.

3.1. Estrogen and progesterone

Estradiol and progesterone exert an important role in the regulation of a number of the factors involved in gestational processes thus avoiding harmful inflammatory response (Dekel et al., 2010). By doing so, these hormones also modulate epithelial cells ability to respond to pathogenic microbes. Indeed estradiol suppresses the secretion of MIF, TNFα, IL-6 and IL-8 induced by bacteria in the uterine epithelial cells (EEC-1) (Wira et al., 2010).

Moreover the hormone stimulates IL-1β secretion in LPS-activated human uterine monocytes and down-regulates protein-expression of IL-1RtI, thus inhibiting the IL-1β-mediated inflammatory response. In chorionic explants MIF secretion is dose-dependently modulated by 17β-estradiol (E2) (Ietta et al., 2010). As for progesterone, it favours the secretion of IL-3, IL-4, IL-5 and IL-10, that are reported to inhibit the Th1 response (Pioli et al., 2006). Interestingly, however, dydrogesterone induction of a Th1 to Th2 cytokine shift is also expressed by inhibition of IFN-γ and TNF-α but up-regulation of the production of IL-4 and IL-6. It happens therefore that, given a protective action of progesterone against abortion, IL6, that is able to trigger PG release, thus leading to abortion or premature delivery, being up-regulated by the hormone, should be considered protective in the context of early pregnancy! (Raghupathy et al., 2005).

3.2. Mifepristone

The complexity of the relation between cytokine balance and pregnancy outcome is further expressed by comparison of mifepristone (Ru486), betamethasone and progesterone action mechanisms. As for the antiprogestational action of Ru486, the mechanism by which it inactivates the progesterone receptor (PR) is not completely clarified (Leonhardt et al., 2002). However it appears that its abortive action could be in some way related with an influence on cytokines, as repeated administration of the drug significantly enhances the serum production of TNFα and IFNγ while prolonging LPS-induced depressive-like behaviour in rats (Wang et al., 2011), although it does not exert the same effect in mice (Yang et al., 2008). RU486 also stimulates the expression of IL-6 and LIF protein in human villous trophoblast and stroma cells in early pregnancy, thus questioning the supposed IL6 protective role (Pei et al., 2010). Indeed, while opening to debate the action mechanism of progestogens, GCs and their antagonists at the level of gestational tissues, such contradictory observations do not clarify (whether or not inflammatory) the role of IL6 in pregnancy. RU486 counteracts the hyper-polarization of cell membranes as well as the inhibition of gap-junctions responsible for uterine contraction exerted by the hormone (Garfield et al., 1988). It also stimulates the release of PG and impairs the PG-dehydrogenase activity (Norman et al., 1991). As a consequence, the uterine sensibility to PG is significantly enhanced. Accordingly, the capacity of the drug alone to induce abortion is low, while it raises up to 95% when followed by PG administration (Grimes, 1997). Therefore, once again, it appears that early abortion of an otherwise normal pregnancy is mainly obtained by smooth muscle contraction (and therefore by impairment of utero-placental blood perfusion), rather than by a disturbance of the cellular mechanisms of implantation. However, the antiglucocorticoid nature of RU486 is also well characterized. Indeed, it binds to the glucocorticoid receptor (GR), and oral administration of the drug results in a dose-dependent activation of the hypothalamic-pituitary-adrenal (HPA) axis (Gaillard et al., 1984). Despite the compensatory increase in the serum cortisol concentration, in patients undergoing medical termination of a first trimester pregnancy the net effect of this compound is a profound suppression of circulating GC bioactivity (Heikinheimo et al.; 2003). Given the power of the anti-GC activity of RU486, the question arises whether its abortive action is also due to this property.

Furthermore it is interesting to ascertain whether such an action is to be ascribed to the disturbance of intercellular communication at the earliest stage of blastocyst implantation or to impairment of blood perfusion later on. Indeed, among the potentially positive effects of GC in early pregnancy, promotion of trophoblast growth and invasion have been suggested, along with stimulation of hCG secretion and suppression of NK cells (Michael & Papageorghiou; 2008). By modulating extravillous trophoblast proliferation and invasion, in fact GC may directly influence the capacity of chorionic villi to modify the structure of maternal spiral arteries, a change aimed at meeting the needs of embryo oxygenation and growth. The initial process of invasion belongs to the cross-talk between trophoblast and uterine decidua. Blastocyst attachment appears to be regulated by cell surface signalling molecules among which integrins and fibronectin. At physiological concentrations (100 nmol/l), GCs can suppress the expression of trophoblast integrins while their effects on fibronectin expression are tissue-specific (Burrows et al., 1996). For instance, in human pregnancy at term, dexamethasone suppresses fibronectin expression cytotrophoblasts and amnion while it acts in synergy with transforming growth factor-b towards up-regulation in matched samples of chorion and placental mesenchymal cells (Guller et al., 1995). Moreover, trophoblast functions are regulated by gap-junctional intercellular communication (GJIC) (Malassiné & Cronier, 2005). Gap junctions (GJ) are membrane channels which span the intercellular space, providing a pathway for the exchange of signalling molecules such as second messengers and siRNA. Said channels are constituted by the association of two hemi-channels, termed connexons, each composed of six connexin (Cx) subunits. Trophoblast Cx expression is modulated by hCG and estradiol, and GCs have been shown to enhance trophoblast GJIC in human pregnancy at term (Cronier et al., 1998). We have recently demonstrated that betamethasone selectively modifies trophoblast GR and Cx expression, enhancing the GRα isoform without affecting GRβ, and inhibiting Cx40 expression while increasing that of Cx43 and 45. Furthermore, betamethasone exerts an inhibitory action on cell proliferation. This result could be at least partly due to the inhibitory effect of the reduced expression of Cx40, coupled with an upregulation of Cx43. Indeed, it has been reported that Cx40 is involved in trophoblast proliferation (Winterhager et al. 1999; Nishimura et al. 2004), and that Cx43 upregulation is associated with an inhibition of JEG-3 cell proliferation (Kibschull et al. 2008). By modulating extravillous trophoblast proliferation and invasion, GCs may directly influence the capacity of chorionic villi to modify the structure of maternal spiral arteries, a change aimed at meeting the needs of embryo oxygenation and growth.

RU-486, in spite of its anti-GR property, does not contrast this effect of betamethasone. On the contrary, it induces responses similar to those of the hormone. As for progesterone, it shows the same effect as betamethasone on Cx expression, while it does not affect proliferation. RU-486 does not antagonize the progesterone effect as well. These results, by confirming that neither the abortive action of RU486 nor the protective action of GCs are obtained through their influence on trophoblast Cx expression, along with the other above mentioned evidences, do not exclude that the abortive mechanism of the drug may be also linked to its anti-glucocorticoid action at a level other than Cx (Cervellati et al., 2011).

Moreover, as for the nature of the events leading to pregnancy loss, it appears that it is not to be ascribed to the disturbance of intercellular communication at the earliest stage of blastocyst implantation, but rather to the impairment of blood perfusion and triggering of uterine contractions obtained through an intensive prostaglandin administration later on. If the enhanced responsiveness of myometrium to prostaglandins, that represents the main abortive action of mifepristone, derives from the anti-progesterone or anti-GCs effects, or even both or none of them, remains to be ascertained.

3.3. Influence of GCs on TLR and MIF

Further examples of the regulatory actions of GCs are down-regulation of TLR expression, suppression of pro-inflammatory and up-regulation of anti-inflammatory cytokines by dexamethasone in primary isolated murine liver cells (Broering et al., 2011), as well as inhibition of the human pro-IL-1β gene by decreasing DNA binding of transactivators to the signal-responsive enhancer (Waterman et al., 2006). It is interesting to observe that the GR can be influenced even independently from GCs. Indeed the unliganded GR attenuates TNF-α stimulated IL-6 transcription by a mechanism involving selective phosphorylation and recruitment of the unliganded GR and GRIP-1 to the IL-6 promoter. It is suggested that such an autoregulatory mechanism may prevent overproduction of IL-6 in the endocervix, possibly protecting against negative effects of excessive inflammation (Verhoog et al., 2011). However GCs are also reported **to induce**, rather than to inhibit, the secretion of MIF (Calandra et al., 1995), thus counteracting the hormone inhibition of pro-inflammatory cytokine production. Such an influence is an example of particular relevance in understanding the nature of a balanced protective action against pregnancy loss.

3.4. Trans-placental passageand action site of GCs

A further matter of debate is represented by the regulation of GCs passage into the foetal circulation by placental 11β-hydroxy-dehydrogenase type 2 (11β-HSD2), the level of expression and activity of which is determined by a delicate balance between stimulatory and inhibitory influences. Studies of human and other primate placentas or derived trophoblast cells have shown that placental 11β-HSD2 activity is **reduced** by progesterone, estrogen, NO, PGs, proinflammatory cytokines and infections, β-adrenoceptor agonists, hypoxia and peroxisome proliferator-activated receptor δ agonists. Conversely, placental 11β-HSD2 activity is **stimulated** by **GCs**, retinoids and activators of the pathway that includes cyclic AMP and protein kinase A (Seckl et al., 2007). Moreover, the exposure of foetal tissues to cortisol may be determined locally by 11β-HSD isoenzymes **within** the foetus, rather than simply by GC metabolism at the materno-fetal interface (McNeil et al., 2007). In the trophoblast cells, (the most abundant site of 11β-HSD1), cortisol up-regulates enzyme expression inducing promoter activity, and the effect is enhanced by IL-1β. This suggests that more biologically active GCs could be generated in the foetal membranes in the presence of infection, which may consequently feed forward in up-regulation of PG synthesis. Intriguingly, foetal membranes are a major site of PG synthesis during pregnancy

(Li et al., 2006), the production of which has been reported to be increased by GCs (Sun et al., 2003). However, such stimulatory actions of GCs on the biosynthetic pathways of PG, rather than simply suggesting adverse clinical outcomes, sharpen the complexity of the hormonal regulatory influence upon the internal homeostasis of organic functions, as they, as it will be said ahead, adequately administrated, ultimately contribute to shift the complicate network of cytokines and prostanoids towards a beneficial direction. All above evidences indicate nothing more than the regulation of gestational processes to rely upon an extremely high number of mediators under physiological hormonal control, that are influenced by both maternal and foetal conditions (either congenital or acquired), as well as by external factors able to modify utero-placental perfusion and myometrial quiescence. As pregnancy loss can occur at any time during gestation and labour, it follows that the outcome of pregnancy will depend on the grade and time of the regulators derangement. In other words, speaking of pregnancy loss, there is no difference between the pathogenic mechanism of abortion and that of premature delivery, other than the first to happen very early, the second at a time when the foetus may have already reached the capacity to survive.

4. Direct and indirect relationship between inflammation and pregnancy loss

Aetiology of pregnancy loss includes chromosomal, anatomical, hormonal, immunological and endocrinological abnormalities, but in most cases the cause remains unexplained. It is frequently claimed that an inflammatory microenvironment is required for adequate tissue remodelling during implantation and the early phase of pregnancy (Challis et al., 2009). On the contrary, the second trimester is characterized by a prevalence of anti-inflammatory signals. An inflammatory pattern is then required near term of pregnancy to induce labour contractions and cervical dilatation (Paulesu et al., 2010). At this regard, for instance, we have demonstrated the presence on human amnion-derived WISH cells of binding sites for formyl-methionyl-leucyl-phenylalanine (fMLP), the classical chemotactic receptor for N-formyl peptides. fMLP induces a significant increase of PGE2 release by these human amnion-derived cells. Such a response in turn is impaired by COX, phospholipase A2, and phospholipase C inhibitors (Biondi et al., 2001). Furthermore we have shown that labouring amniotic membranes express both high- and low-affinity specific receptors for 3H-fMLP, while only the low-affinity are found in non-labouring tissue, and that the peptide is able to significantly increase PG synthesis in perifused amnion fragments from labouring and non-labouring women. (Buzzi et al., 1999). Nevertheless, abnormal inflammatory events may lead to adverse pregnancy outcomes, such as implantation failure, pregnancy loss, preeclampsia, preterm labour, intrauterine growth restriction (IUGR), and foetal inflammatory syndrome (Kwak-Kim et al., 2010). Disregulation of cell function mediators can simply derive from genetic conditions, with no need for infectious or inflammatory external stimuli. Indeed, it has been reported that polymorphisms in immunoregulatory genes IL10, MBL2, TNFRSF6 and TGFB1 may influence susceptibility to chorioamnionitis (Annells et al., 2005), and common genetic variants in proinflammatory cytokine genes, such as some selected TNF/LTA haplotypes, increase the risk for spontaneous preterm birth (Engel et al., 2005).

4.1. The Th1/Th2 paradigm

It has been suggested that a successful pregnancy may be a Th2 type phenomenon, whereas a Th1-type prevalence could be detrimental (Kwak-Kim et al., 2003). Immune regulation of pregnancy is mediated by TH1, TH2 and macrphages throughout the release of a number of cytokines (Table 1). Women with recurrent pregnancy loss have higher peripheral concentrations of certain Th1 cytokines (IL-2, TNF-α, TNF-β, IFN-γ) and lower concentrations of Th2 (IL-4, -5, -6, -10) when compared with successful pregnancy. Th1 cytokines, especially IFN-γ, may activate endothelial cell procoagulants and cause thrombotic and inflammatory reactions at the utero-placental level (Clark et al 1998). As for the mechanism by which thrombotic changes are induced, it has been reported an increased expression of pro-coagulant Fg12 in trophoblast cells from failing pregnancy (Knackstedt et al., 2001). Fg12 is a glycoprotein able to directly cleave prothrombin to thrombin, leading to fibrin deposition. Th1 cytokines up regulate this procoagulant, with consequent activation of the coagulation system and disruption of vascular supply to the placenta. On the contrary, Th2 system can hamper this process, suppressing Th1 response (Saini et al., 2011). Among proinflammatory cytokines, TNF-α is of particular interest. Indeed, even though a low concentration is required for successful implantation, it also causes trophoblast apoptosis in combination with Th1 cytokines such INF-γ. The cytokine could even be involved in pregnancy loss by impairing utero-placental perfusion. A recent study on mouse (Renaud et al., 2011) reported a causal link between maternal inflammation induced by LPS administration and impaired placental perfusion. LPS administration determined a disseminated intravascular coagulation(DIC)-like condition, with clot formation within uterine vessels, decreased diastolic uterine artery flow velocity and evidence of prominent diastolic notches, resulting in placental and foetal hypoxia. Many biological effects of LPS are mediated by TNF-α. Oppositely, IL-10 administration decreased serum level of TNF-α, preventing pregnancy loss after LPS exposure. Cytokines of the IL-1 system (IL-1α, IL-1β and IL-1 receptor antagonist) are an important regulatory element of the Th1/Th2 balance. They have been implicated in implantation, and trophoblastic cells proliferation and invasion (Wang et al., 2002). On the other hand, it is interesting to note that IL-1 system can also function as a co-stimulator for Th2 response. Therefore, altered decidual IL-1β production may cause a reduction in Th2-type cytokine production, contributing to early pregnancy failure. The Th1/Th2 paradigm has recently been expanded into the Th1/Th2/Th17 and Treg (T regulatory cells) one (Peck et Mellins, 2010). Indeed increased peripheral and decidual levels of Th17 cells and their related factors (IL-17, IL-23 and - retinoid orphan nuclear receptor (RORC) have been reported in women with unexplained recurrent spontaneous abortion (RSA) (Wang et al., 2010). In addition, an inverse relationship between Th17 cells and Treg cells in the peripheral blood and decidua lymphocytes in unexplained RSA has been found. Treg cells are defined by secretion of TGF-β and IL10 and the presence of intracellular transcription factor FoxP3. Studies in

Cells	Cytokine	Actions
TH1	IFNγ IL1 IL2 TNFβ TNFα	• Inflammatory reactions • Thrombotic events through up-regulation of Fgl2 • Trophoblastic apoptosis, inhibition of trophoblast cell growth and metabolic activity • Promotion of syncytium formation and invasive capacity of trophoblast (TNFα)
TH2	IL4 IL5 IL6 IL10 TGFβ	• Anti-inflammatory action • Enhancement of hCG secretion • Stimulation of growth and differentiation of trophoblast
Macrophage	IL1 system (IL1α, IL1β, IL1ra) LIF	• Stimulation of trophoblast differentiation (LIF)

Table 1. Immune regulation of pregnancy.

animal models (Thuere at al., 2007) have shown that Treg cells are essential for maternal tolerance of the conceptus, and that they exert suppressive actions in the peri-implantation phase. In women, inadequate number of Treg cells or their functional deficiency are linked with infertility, miscarriage and pre-eclampsia (Guerin et al., 2009). It is suggested that impaired Treg function could lead to increased Th1 cytokines (Jin et al., 2009). Nevertheless there are conflicting reports regarding the inflammation state in early pregnancy loss, suggesting adequate balance for Th1/Th2 cytokines, although with a slight shift toward Th2 immunity in successful pregnancy (Saini et al., 2011). A recent study (Calleja-Agius et al., 2012) confirmed an inflammatory state (higher pro-inflammatory cytokines) in normal pregnancy compared with the non pregnant state, which may be disrupted during miscarriage. The study revealed in euploid miscarriage a shift toward Th1 immune response (higher TNF-α/IL-6 ratio) at 6-9 weeks, but a lower TNF-α/IL 10 and IFN-γ/IL10 ratios in the late first trimester compared to normal pregnancy. At this regard it must be noted that the classification of IL-6 remains controversial, as some authors consider it as a Th2 mediator due to its anti-inflammatory properties possibly involved in new vessels generation and tissue remodelling associated with placentation (Jauniaux at al., 1996). A further evidence for an influence of inflammatory mediators in pregnancy is represented by the behaviour of maternal serum MIF (Yamada et al., 2002). Indeed, MIF concentrations in recurrent abortion women with subsequent miscarriage and normal foetal karyotype were lower than those in women with history of RSA with subsequent live birth and those in normal pregnant women. Moreover, MIF acts as an immunosuppressive factor by inhibiting NK cell activity. Since women with RPL and unexplained infertility have increased peripheral blood NK cells and increased NK cytotoxic activity (Yamada et al., 2001), low levels of MIF could lead to insufficient inhibition of NK cell activity and altered cytokines production with impairment of trophoblast proliferation, embryo development, and angiogenesis within placenta. One more pathway leading from inflammation to pregnancy loss acts via the complement system that induces recruitment and activation of inflammatory cells. Antiphospholipid (aPL) antibodies are able to trigger complement system response within decidual tissue, thus inducing inflammation and foetal damage (Salmon & Girardi, 2008). Recruitment of inflammatory cells creates a placental proinflammatory amplification loop, eventually leading to thrombosis, hypoxia, and neutrophil infiltration. Accordingly, increased complement activation is associated with recurrent abortion pre-eclampsia and IUGR (Tincani et al., 2009). A pathogenic mechanism has been postulated for recurrent abortion involving NK cells (Laird et al., 2003). Several studies reported a higher concentration of uNK and pNK as well as a higher proportion of activated pNK in women with history of RSA (Radysh & Chernyshov, 2005).

5. Classical treatment and drugs for preventing pregnancy loss

5.1. Progesterone

Progesterone is secreted by the corpus luteum and the placenta and is necessary for successful implantation and eventually the maintenance of pregnancy. Progesterone is prescribed in 13-40% of women with threatened miscarriage, according to published series because it is expected to support a potentially deficient corpus luteum and induce relaxation of a cramping uterus (Rai & Regan, 2006). This benefit of the hormone could be explained by its immmunomodulatory actions in inducing a pregnancy-protective shift from pro-inflammatoryTh-1 cytokine responses to a more favourable anti-inflammatory Th-2 cytokine response (Raghupathy et al., 2009). The first trial using progesterone for such women was published in the BMJ in 1953 (Swyer & Daley, 1953) and was followed over the decades by several small trials. However, uncertainty remains about the evidence. The latest randomized controlled trial (Haas & Ramsey, 2008) to assess progesterone support for pregnancy showed that it did not reduce the sporadic miscarriage rate. However, in a subgroup analysis of trials involving women with recurrent miscarriage, progesterone treatment appeared to offer a statistically significant decrease in miscarriage rate compared with placebo or no treatment (OR 0.38, 95% CI 0.2–0.7). Nevertheless, in order to understand the limited clinical utility of the conclusions derived from some sort of statistical analysis, it is to be noted that this meta-analysis was based on three small controlled studies, none of which detected a significant improvement in pregnancy outcome! A large multicenter study (PROMISE) is currently under way to assess the benefit of progesterone supplementation in women with unexplained recurrent miscarriage. The trial is expected to report in 2013. At present, progesterone administration is not recommended for unexplained recurrent miscarriage (Coomarasamy et al., 2011).

5.2. Aspirin

Aspirin is largely used in pregnancy because it is believed to increase blood flow to the embryo, act on unrecognized thrombophilias and prevent miscarriage. Pregnancy itself is a hyper-coaguable state associated with increased levels of procoagulant factors and decreased levels of naturally occurring anticoagulants such as protein S (Comp et al., 1986). Microthrombi are a common finding in the placental vasculature of women with recurrent miscarriage (Rushton, 1988). PGs appear to be essential for implantation, although and exogenous administration of high doses induces abortion: the maintenance of pregnancy may be dependent on a mechanism that suppresses prostaglandin synthesis. Aspirin, which suppresses COX, has the potential to support this mechanism. Moreover, the maintenance of pregnancy is said to depend on a shift of pro-inflammatory to anti-inflammatory cytokines. At this regard, aspirin and other antiplatelet agents have been shown to play a role in the inhibition of pro-inflammatory cytokines, such as TNFα and IL-8. In stroke (Al-Bahrani et al., 2007), TNFα induces thrombin generation and IL-8 causes polymorph accumulation (Schraufstatter et al., 2003). Polymorphs react with fibrin and damaged tissues to form clots. However, at present, no report in the medical literature confirms a role for aspirin in preventing recurrent pregnancy loss. Furthermore, it doesn't confer a significant benefit in anti-phospholipid (aPL) syndrome (Pattison et al., 2000) even if the live birth rate increases significantly when heparin is added to treatment. The syndrome is assumed to be responsible for pregnancy loss by causing thrombosis in the small blood vessels of the decidua, leading to subsequent foetal demise. In unexplained pregnancy loss, aspirin had no beneficial effect except for in late pregnancy losses, in cases where hereditary thrombophilias were not excluded. Since there is no study of aspirin in this condition, it's suggested that the positive effects in advanced pregnancy may be due to the action of the drug in such patients (Rai et al., 2000). Nevertheless, the lack of the evidence of any efficacy against RSA, coupled with a reported increased risk of miscarriage and foetal gastroschisis, contraindicate prescribing aspirin in early pregnancy (Carp HJ, 2009).

5.3. COX inhibitors

COX inhibitors impair uterine contractility, are easily administered and have fewer maternal side-effects compared to conventional tocolytics. However, they are not devoid of adverse effects on the foetus and newborn. Indeed, increased neonatal complications including oligohydramnios, renal failure, necrotizing enterocolitis, intraventricular haemorrhage, and closure of the patent ductus arteriosus have been reported with the use of the non-selective COX inhibitor indomethacin (Abou-Ghannam et al. 2011). A recent review includes outcome data from 13 trials for a total of 713 women. with use of indomethacin in 10. When compared with placebo, indomethacin alone resulted in a reduction in birth before 37 weeks gestation, with an increase in gestational age and birth weight. Compared to any other tocolytic, COX inhibition resulted also in reduced maternal drug reaction requiring cessation of treatment. A comparison of non-selective COX inhibitors versus any COX-2 inhibitor did not demonstrate any difference in maternal or neonatal outcomes. However, due to small numbers, all estimates are imprecise and need to be interpreted with caution. Overall, until now there is insufficient information about the role of COX inhibition for women in preterm labour (King et al., 2005).

5.4. Antibiotics

As for antibiotics, their role against infection of the chorioamnionic membranes in preterm labour has been extensively investigated. In these cases, the mechanism by which uterine contractions take place is supposed to be the release of microbial products into the amniotic fluid (Gibbs et al., 1992). There seems to be substantial agreement on the efficacy of antibiotic therapy in the prevention of preterm delivery when there is evidence of infection (Kirshbaum T, 1993), but its utility in idiopathic preterm labour is controversial (Cox et al., 1996). Nevertheless, antibiotics can have beneficial influences not only for their antimicrobial properties but also through a direct tocolytic action on tissues. Indeed, as it will be explained ahead, some among them have the capacity to directly inhibit amniotic IL-6 and PGE2 release, thus offering an explanation for a beneficial response in cases of preterm labour even in the absence of bacterial infection. (Vesce et al., 1998;2004).

5.5. Heparin

Successful pregnancy depending on trophoblast invasion into the uterine vasculature, inadequate placentation and damage to the spiral arteries with impaired flow and prothrombotic changes lead to pregnancy complications that become even more dangerous in hyper-coagulable states. Such complications benefit from prophylactic low molecular weight heparin (LMWH) and unfractionated heparin (UFH), in spite of several drawbacks to their use, including the costs, discomfort of daily injections, risks of bleeding, skin reactions, and thrombocytopenia (Howard, 2009). Indeed, there is general agreement that women with recurrent loss and persistent aPL antibodies positivity should receive antepartum prophylaxis with UFH or LMWH in combination with aspirin (Bates et al., 2008), while, at present, it is claimed that antithrombotic therapy should not be advocated for unexplained recurrent miscarriage in women without an underlying thrombophilia. (Clark et al., 2010). However, although a protective effect in women with heritable thrombophilia is not to be excluded, the British Committee for Standards in Haematology has recently recommended against the antithrombotic therapy in pregnant women with a history of loss based on the results of testing for inherited thrombophilia (Baglin et al., 2010). Low-molecular-weight instead of unfractionated heparin is recommended for the prevention and treatment of venous thromboembolism in pregnant women (Guyatt et al., 2012). In acute cases, anticoagulants should be continued for at least 6 weeks postpartum, for a minimum total duration of the therapy of 3 months. For women who fulfil the laboratory and clinical criteria for aPL antibodies syndrome and history of three or more pregnancy losses, is recommended antepartum administration of prophylactic or intermediate-dose UFH, or prophylactic (LMWH), combined with low-dose aspirin (75-100 mg/d) over no treatment. For women with inherited thrombophilia and a history of pregnancy complications, as well as for those with two or more miscarriages, but without aPL antibodies syndrome or thrombophilia, it is recommended against antithrombotic prophylaxis. (Guyatt et al., 2012).

5.6. Immunotherapy

Idiopathic recurrent miscarriage has traditionally been associated with alloimmune factors, in which uterine CD56+/16 NK cells have been implicated (Quenby et al., 1999). In vitro studies suggest that pregnancy may result in uterine T-cell activation along the Th-2 pathway, resulting in blocking antibodies which mask trophoblast antigens (Wegmann et al., 1993). Activation along the Th-1 pathway, instead, results in the production of abortive cytokines (Raghupathy et al., 2000). Maternal HY-restricting HLA class II alleles are associated with a decreased chance of a live birth in women with secondary recurrent miscarriage with a firstborn boy (Nielsen et al., 2009). Although such mechanisms are intriguing, there is a paucity of validated tests to assess the maternal immune response in pregnancy. Despite this, active and passive immunotherapeutic trials for idiopathic recurrent miscarriage have been reported. Paternal mononuclear cell immunization has been proved not to be effective (Scott, 2003). It is believed that passive immunotherapy with intravenous immunoglobulin (IVIG) may offer benefit in idiopathic secondary (at least one prior ongoing pregnancy), but not idiopathic primary (no prior ongoing pregnancy) recurrent miscarriage (Christiansen et al., 2002). However, such conclusions must be taken with caution because of small heterogeneous sample size. Moreover, IVIG is a highly purified and virally inactivated fractionated blood product made from pooled human plasma, which makes it costly to use and not without risk. Overall, the efficacy of IVIG in women with a history of idiopathic secondary recurrent miscarriage remains controversial, as no significant effect of treatment in these patients was found (Stephenson et al., 2010).

6. Influence of glucocorticoids on foetal development

6.1. Prenatal administration of GCs and HPA function

Several studies in animals have shown that prenatal administration of GCs can cause hormonal changes in the foetus. Epidemiologic research in human even suggested that these may have long-term consequences on health in adult life. This concept is termed 'early life programming' (Seckl, 2004). Great importance is given to the influence of GCs on foetal HPA axis. Several studies assessed basal HPA function in the feto-placental unit by measuring markers of its activity in cord blood and amniotic fluid during gestation and at birth. Compared with unexposed healthy foetuses, cortisol concentrations were significantly lower in otherwise healthy foetuses exposed to synthetic GCs, with values decreasing to the 10% of the controls. These results, however, refer to premature foetuses, which receive 24 mg betamethasone within 24 hours before being delivered (Kajantie et al., 2004). In foetuses of asthmatic mothers who refrained from taking synthetic GCs during pregnancy, cortisol concentrations were even higher compared to those of healthy controls (Murphy et al., 2002). As for placental CRH mRNA, it was slightly higher in asthmatic patients not treated with synthetic GCs. However, treated cases exhibit normal levels irrespective of the treatment dose. Similar to cortisol, ACTH, DHEA and DHEA-S (Parker et al., 1996) concentrations were reduced in treated foetuses.

6.2. Metabolic changes induced by prenatal GCs

The alteration of the HPA activity seems to be closely related to the changes in glucose homeostasis and obesity. In rodent models, administration of dexamethasone leads to permanent hyperglycaemia and hyperinsulinaemia in the offspring (Nyirenda et al., 1998) with life-long elevations in the activity of phosphoenolpyruvate carboxykinase (PEPCK), the enzyme involved in gluconeogenesis. This metabolic effect is correlated with the exposure time, and week 3 of gestation appears to be a critical window for inducing long-term metabolic changes. Similar alterations of glucose homeostasis have been reported in both sheep and non-human primates (de Vries et al., 2007). Although the molecular mechanisms underlying these changes in offspring glucose metabolism have not been fully clarified, the alterations in HPA activity are certainly implicated, as the animals have increased levels of circulating corticosterone, decreased GR expression in the hippocampus, the site of central negative feedback, and increased peripheral GR expression in insulin-sensitive target tissues including liver and muscle in the rat (Nyirenda et al., 1998; Cleasby et al., 2003). The increased PEPCK expression is regulated by transcription factors, including members of the HNF (hepatocyte nuclear factor) and GR that bind to the PEPCK gene promoter. The expression of these factors is increased in liver of rats treated with dexamethasone (Nyirenda et al., 1998), suggesting that the observed increase in PEPCK may be a secondary effect. Thus, changes in key transcription factors may underlie permanent changes in glucose metabolism. The influence of prenatal GCs is also expressed in the foetal pancreas. GC signalling is important in pancreatic beta cell development, with potential underlying mechanisms including their interaction with the transcription factors that control proliferation and differentiation of the Langerhans islets cells (Gesina et al., 2006). Among these, IGF (insulin-like growth factor) 2, the IGF receptor, and several IGF binding proteins (Hill et al., 2000) may lead to a decreased insulin secretion, with consequent hyperglycaemia in adult life. Prenatal GC exposure is also associated with alterations in fat distribution and function. Offspring of rats treated with dexamethasone during days 8, 10 and 12 of pregnancy have increased intra-abdominal fat depots, and a parallel increase in circulating leptin levels (Dahlgren et al., 2001). Moreover, treatment of rats with dexamethasone in the last week of pregnancy leads to an increase in GR expression in visceral adipose tissue and alterations in fat metabolism which may contribute to insulin resistance (Cleasby et al., 2003). Recent evidence also shows that the activity of 11β-HSD type 1 may be 'programmed' by prenatal GC therapy. Indeed, a brief antenatal exposure to GCs in pregnant marmosets resulted in up-regulation of 11β-HSD1 mRNA expression and activity in subcutaneous, but not visceral, fat of the offspring (Nyirenda et al., 2009). The increase in 11β-HSD1 occurred before the animals developed obesity or overt features of the metabolic syndrome. This up-regulation of 11β-HSD1 suggests a novel mechanism underlying the foetal origins of obesity.

6.3. The impact of GCs on foetal bone

Another interesting field of research is represented by the influence of prenatal GCs on foetal bone. Indeed, GCs are known to affect skeletal growth and adult bone metabolism, but their impact on foetal bone remains to be elucidated. Some Authors (Swolin-Eide et al.,

2002) reported prenatal dexamethasone exposure to affect skeletal growth in rats. Dexamethasone-exposed male but not female rat offspring showed transient increases in crown–rump length and tibia and femur lengths at 3–6 weeks of age. In contrast, the cortical bone dimensions were altered in 12-week-old female but not male, and the areal bone mineral densities of the long bones and the spine were unchanged in both male and female suggesting a gender specific effect. Following these results, research was addressed to investigate some biochemical markers of bone turnover such as 4,5 carboxy-terminal propeptide of type I procollagen (PICP) and cross-linked carboxy-terminal telopeptide of type I collagen (ICTP). A single course of antenatal corticosteroids reduced umbilical cord levels of PICP without influence on ICTP (Korakaki et al., 2007). Instead, according to other Authors (Fonseca et al., 2009), umbilical cord serum levels of ICTP, the marker for foetal bone resorption, decreased only when the doses were ≥ 4.

6.4. Conclusion

Overall, it appears that, in animals, programming effects of GCs exposure during gestation involve:

- hyperglycaemia throughout a gluconeogenesis enzyme modulation coupled with a decreased growth of pancreatic islets;
- increased deposition of visceral fat related with an increase in circulating levels of leptin and expression of GR in the fat tissue;
- gender-specific manner stimulation of bone growth without influence on mineralization.

However, the results of these experimental studies, performed on a variety of animal species, using high doses and different types of GC, cannot be extended to human pregnancy, that is provided with distinct metabolising capacity at the utero-placental level. Indeed, GCs are largely prescribed for a variety of maternal and foetal conditions during human pregnancy, where none of the above reported complications and side effects have been confirmed. The absolute indications for using these compounds are Addison syndrome and hypopituarism. Furthermore, they are largely utilized for maternal asthma, collagen disease, ulcerative colitis, regional enteritis, and need of immunosuppression. Moreover, there is a number of specific indications to early administration for pregnancy-induced pathology. Among these foetal atrio-ventricular block, congenital adrenal hyperplasia, cystic adenomatoid malformation of the lung, alloimune thrombocytopenia, recurrent pregnancy loss and antiphospholipid antibody syndrome. In addition, clinical conditions that benefit from use of GCs in advanced pregnancy are related with premature delivery, aimed at the prevention of neonatal respiratory distress syndrome, intraventricular haemorrhage and necrotizing enterocolitis (Lunghi et al., 2010). All above conditions provide evidence for substantial advantages in foetal and maternal prognosis of prenatal administration of GCs, compared to feared, but unproved, side effects such as malformation and intrauterine growth restriction. At this regard, it has been reported that triamcinolone acetonide, a synthetic glucocorticoid, induces cleft palate resulting from poor development of palatal shelves in mice (Furukawa et al., 2004). Nevertheless, direct extrapolation to humans of teratogenic effects of GCs in animals is tenuous. Indeed, a prospective controlled cohort study, based on self-reported drug exposure and maternal interview as a source, collected 311 pregnancies receiving systemic use of different GCs in the first trimester. The rate of major congenital anomalies was compared to that of 790 controls that were counselled for non-teratogenic exposure. There was no case of oral cleft and no pattern of anomalies among the GCs exposed group, supporting the opinion that these hormones do not represent a major teratogenic risk in humans (Gur et al.,2004). A survey of the literature concerning 468 pregnant women treated with corticosteroids outside the transplant setting demonstrated an overall malformation rate of 3.5%, thus within the expected incidence in the general population (Danesi & Del Tacca, 2004). Moreover, a study on more than 6600 infants reported that maternal exposure to orally inhaled budesonide during pregnancy is not associated with an increased risk of congenital malformations or other adverse foetal outcomes (Rahimi et al., 2006). As for foetal growth, a systematic review of animal studies examining the association of GCs on birth outcome reported a reduction in birth weight (Aghajafari, 2002). However, it should be considered that animal experiments demonstrating negative effects employed doses equivalent to 20-100 times a 'replacement' dose of steroids for a human patient. Nevertheless studies in human were addressed to assess both the effect of early exposure protracted for a long time and that of late administration for preventing the complications of premature delivery. Interestingly, although a recent study suggests that foetal growth becomes sensitive to GCs when the treatment starts early and is prolonged for a long time (Gur et al., 2004), dexamethasone given from the 10th week throughout pregnancy in the presence of female foetuses affected by 21-hydroxylase deficiency did not influence weight, length and head circumference of the newborns (Carlson et al., 1999). As for advanced pregnancy, randomized controlled studies have shown that treatment for preventing respiratory distress syndrome of the neonate leads to birth weight reduction only after four or more courses, and that these parameters normalized by the time of hospital discharge (Bonanno et al., 2007). Moreover, a meta-analysis of five trials in which 2028 pregnant women were treated with GCs in late pregnancy found no significant effect on birth weight (Crowther et al., 2007). Two main exceptions can be raised towards human clinical studies: first, the time elapsing between administration of the drug and delivery appears to be too short to influence foetal growth; second, obstetrical diseases affecting foetal growth are necessarily included in the study sample, and therefore it is not possible to discriminate their influence from that of the hormone. The only way to avoid such a bias should be to administrate GC to healthy volunteers along the course of physiological pregnancy, something that happened to us in some way to do, in our long experience with low dose betamethasone therapy throughout gestation (see ahead). Based on our results, there is no persuasive evidence for any adverse effect neither of long duration low dose (see ahead), nor of short duration high dose GC on foetal growth.

7. Need and rules for antibiotic and glucocorticoid therapy in advanced pregnancy: The foetal inflammatory response syndrome.

We have previously treated in a more detailed manner the main indications to glucocorticoid therapy in human pregnancy (Lunghi et al., 2010). Nevertheless, for the purposes of the present chapter, it is necessary to stress the concepts dealing with the "Foetal Inflammatory Response Syndrome" (FIRS) (Romero et al., 1998). Indeed, being paradigmatic of the negative effects of inflammation on pregnancy, it offers the chance to clarify the rationale for the appropriate use of GCs and antibiotics for preventing harmful complications. FIRS is defined as a systemic inflammation characterized by an elevation of foetal plasma IL-6. In this syndrome a foetal plasma IL-6 level above 11 pg/ml is a major independent risk factor for the subsequent development of severe neonatal morbidity. Such a condition can be found even in the absence of microbial invasion of the amniotic cavity and any other sign of infection, as a foetal immune reaction characterized by increase in monocyte and neutrophil activation, and without correlation with maternal plasma or amniotic fluid concentration of the cytokine. It has been suggested that the foetus uses the effector limb of the immune response via the secretion of pro-inflammatory cytokines to signal the onset of labour and exit a hostile intrauterine environment (Romero et al., 1998). Whatever its teleological meaning, FIRS, also expressed by increased concentrations of foetal MMP-9, an enzyme involved in the digestion of type IV collagen and in the patho-physiology of preterm premature rupture of the membranes, can progress towards multiple organ dysfunction. (Romero et al., 2002). A further enzyme involved in such inflammatory process is MMP-8. Indeed an elevated MMP-8 concentration (>23 ng/mL), is present in 81% of the cases with cervical insufficiency, while a positive microbial culture is found only in 8%. These results indicate that, regardless of the eventual microbial involvement, inflammation is a risk factor for impending preterm delivery (Lee et al., 2008). Overall, the evidences above speak in favour of a leading role of inflammation in the pathogenesis not only of premature birth, but also of ominous perinatal complications such as respiratory distress syndrome (RDS), cerebral haemorrhage and necrotizing enterocolitis (NEC). Evidently, in this perspective, the causal role of infection appears substantially scaled. Accordingly, there is no evidence for a clear benefit of antibiotic treatment in infectious conditions that are associated with premature delivery, such as bacterial vaginosis and urinary infections (McDonald et al., 2007). In addition, treating women at risk with antibiotics does not reduce the incidence of subsequent of preterm delivery (Simcox et al., 2007), and among women with Group B streptococcal bacteriuria, exposure to additional antibiotics even increases the risk (Anderson et al., 2008). Conflicting reports do not clarify the role of prophylactic antibiotic therapy for inhibiting preterm labour. For instance, one meta-analysis including 11 trials on 7428 women with intact membranes showed a reduction in maternal infection, but failed to demonstrate benefit or harm for the neonatal outcome (King et al., 2002). On the contrary routine antibiotic prophylaxis during the second or third trimester of pregnancy reduces the risk of pre-labour rupture of the membranes, with beneficial effects on birth weight and the risk of postpartum endometritis in high risk women, according to a further meta-analysis (Thinkhamrop et al., 2002). As regards to the conflicting results of clinical studies about the administration of antibiotics in the prevention and cure of preterm delivery, it must be said that their Authors did not take into account the direct anti-inflammatory capacity that some of them are able to exert on gestational tissues. Indeed, we have demonstrated that ampicillin inhibits PGE release from amnion tissue in vitro, either in basal condition or upon addition of arachidonic acid or oxytocin to the medium (Vesce et al., 1998). Furthermore, it strongly reduces IL-6 level in amniotic fluid of patients sampled 4 hours after drug administration (Vesce et al., 2004). Ceftriaxone and gentamycin significantly and reversibly inhibit both basal and arachidonic acid- or oxytocin-stimulated PGE release from amnion, although to a lesser extent compared with ampicillin. On the contrary tetracycline and erythromycin do not influence the PG output. Of key importance from a clinical standpoint, the inhibitory effect of ampicillin is enhanced in an additive manner by ceftriaxone, reduced by gentamycin, and abolished by tetracycline and erythromycin (Vesce F et al., 1999). The above evidences indicate that, at least in pregnancy, the inhibitory action of β-lactamines on amniotic IL-6 and PGE release could be of value independently from their antibacterial action. Conversely, the classes of antibiotics that do not exert any inhibition on PGE release should not be used when preterm labour is not induced through a bacterial mediation. Furthermore, in cases of premature labour of inflammatory origin subsequently complicated by superimposed infection, macrolides addition to β-lactamines may eradicate infection, but it does not counteract the triggering pathogenic mechanism. In other words, in interpreting the efficacy of antibiotics in the management of premature labour, it is mandatory to know whether or not they directly inhibit inflammatory cytokines and prostanoids. It has been claimed that antibiotic therapy of premature labour in the presence of infection leads to the release of microbial products which may exacerbate the cytokine response and worsen the clinical picture. It has been also hypothesized that a similar scenario may occur in patients with microbial invasion of decidua and amniotic cavity. Such an initial worsening of the inflammatory response may accelerate the process of premature parturition and foetal damage. Nevertheless, it has been also suggested that transient down-regulation of the effects of the inflammatory response would permit the time that is required to eradicate the infectious process, without injury to the foetus. Indeed, anti-inflammatory cytokines, antibody to macrophage migration inhibitory factor and antioxidants, may also play a role in preventing delivery, neonatal injury, and long-term perinatal morbidity. Accordingly, a combination of antibiotics and immunomodulators (dexamethasone and indomethacin), in experimental premature labour induced by intra-amniotic inoculation with group B streptococci. in non human pregnant primates, was effective to eradicate infection, suppress the inflammatory response, and prolong gestation (Tsuzuki et al., 2009). One more aspect needs to be clarified before reporting our experience with use of low dose betamethasone for the prevention of pregnancy loss, and it deals with the necessity to discriminate the pathogenic role of prematurity from inflammation and hypoxia. Indeed, prematurity is still reported everywhere as the leading cause of perinatal morbidity and mortality (Mwaniki et al., 2012). Such a concept is obviously provided with some validity, but in the general contest of pregnancy complications it needs to be adequately scaled. Basically, it appears to stem from the link between prematurity and hyaline membrane disease (HMD) of the lung, an ominous disease that is ascribed to the failure of immature type II alveolar cells to produce sufficient surfactant (i. e. lecithin). As betamethasone was historically recognized to be able to prevent HMD, its efficacy was intended as a sort of "maturational promotion". However, there are good reasons to believe that the main pathogenic mechanism is rather of a hypoxic-inflammatory type. Indeed, premature foetuses express RDS of diverse intensity at the same gestational age, in relation with the grade of the pathology causing premature birth. Pregnancy complications leading to premature birth are largely a consequence of an inflammatory mechanism. Accordingly, prematurity is characterized by two other complications, i. e. NEC and encephalopathy, marked by high levels of inflammatory cytokines that also benefit from the action of betamethasone. Finally, the drug efficacy is limited to its timely prenatal administration, as it lacks when the hormone is given after birth, suggesting that it stimulates the production of an extra amount surfactant at a level other than the foetal alveoli that is subsequently delivered to the lung before birth thru gasping efforts a typical feature of foetal hypoxia. As we have demonstrated, the site of lecithin release in the foetal compartment is represented by amnion tissue (Vesce F et al., 1992). Based on these considerations, chronic intrauterine distress appears to play a major role compared to gestational age in the pathogenic mechanism of the 'prematurity' syndrome. Indeed, all above evidences indicates that FIRS proceeds from inflammatory processes endowed themselves with the capacity to lead to all above mentioned dangerous perinatal complications, infection included. Timely addition of GCs addressed to rebalance cytokines and prostanoids regulating the inflammatory response, represents therefore an unavoidable therapeutic approach.

8. Personal experience with low-dose betamethasone administration throughout pregnancy for prevention of pregnancy loss

The clinical observations by the corresponding author of the present chapter regarding pregnancy loss begun during the early seventies, when progesterone therapy was the main choice in cases of either threatened or recurrent abortion at the Department of Obstetrics and Gynaecology of Ferrara University. However, as ultrasounds became available, it clearly appeared to the echographers that, based on the above mentioned theoretical benefits, the drug was given blindly, even to patient with missed abortion as well as to those who never would have needed it. Indeed, there was no practical way (as it still substantially lacks today) to investigate the causes of abortion in single cases, and the explanation given to the patient dealt almost invariably with either corpus luteum deficiency or aneuploidy. Soon after we were informed that corticosteroids had been occasionally used successfully in patients with recurrent abortion when an "immunological basis" for rejection of the conceptus was hypothesized (Professor Denis Hawkins, of London, personal communication). In addition, administration of cortisone 25-75 mg/day up to 64 days during the first trimester for the treatment of hyperemesis had already been reported long before (Wells, 1953). At that stage, after observing many more cases of recurrent abortion, all treated with various regimens of progesterone, we concluded that there was no reason for further giving this drug to such women. The first case of recurrent abortion occasionally treated with betamethasone was 34 years ago a patient with bronchial asthma that, in spite of progesterone therapy, had experienced three early pregnancy losses. Subsequently she had gone through two years of anovulatory sterility, followed by several attempts to medical induction of ovulation, all ended in ovarian hyperstimulation syndrome. This patient was therefore counselled to assume 0.5 mg betamethasone daily for the next three months for treating asthma, and she started a spontaneous pregnancy one month later. Once adequately informed of a possible protective action of the hormone, she accepted to continue with the same regimen up to the end of pregnancy, when she delivered a normal foetus. Such a successful outcome encouraged us to cautiously adopt over the years low dose betamethasone therapy in all our patients with history of recurrent abortion previously unsuccessfully treated with progesterone. Furthermore, as we became aware of the high efficacy of the hormone, we extended its use to some other cases where protection of the first pregnancy was advisable even in the absence of previous pregnancy loss. These included, for instance, women of advanced age with or without previous sterility. We may say that there are several reasons for such a policy. The first one is represented by the lack of efficacy of progesterone in our experience, coupled with the tenuous and controversial evidence of a protective role in the above reported literature. A further point in favour of preventive GCs administration is that there are women who will not have the chance of a second pregnancy, and therefore they are suitable for prevention of possible inflammatory complications, for the timely diagnosis of which there are no available tests in the clinical practice. Indeed, as it became clear later on, GCs regulate the inflammatory process by modulating cytokine production (IL-6 and $TNF\alpha$) (Thum et al., 2008) and decreasing maternal NK population (Quenby et al., 2005), two among the good reasons to adopt them in the clinical management of these cases. The study of this particular mechanism of GC in early pregnancy has been enhanced in the last years the focus being directed on prednisolone, the role of which in the prevention of recurrent pregnancy loss is currently under trial (Thang et al., 2009). However, its pharmacokinetic characteristics require a high dose to obtain the therapeutic effect. For instance, in the case reported by Quenby et al. (2003), a patient with history of 14 consecutive abortions between the 8th and 10th week of gestation, first received 5 mg/day pre-conceptual prednisolone, leading to 5 further abortions. Only when the dose was raised up to 20 mg/day she became able to deliver a preterm viable baby. Indeed, as it has been explained above, the trans-placental passage of the drug is highly impaired by 11-β-HSD isoenzymes. By contrast, compared to prednisolone, betamethasone is little metabolized by the placenta and it is ten times more effective (Burton & Waddell, 1999). Therefore, we decided to focus on betamethasone that is extensively used in advanced pregnancy for prevention of neonatal respiratory distress syndrome (Sotiriadis et al., 2009) but it is not adopted in early pregnancy, due to all above mentioned possible negative influences in animals, although they have not been confirmed in humans. Taking into account all these evidences, we choose to administer a low dose betamethasone, in order to obtain a better protective effect on pregnancy, avoiding at the same time significant maternal dose-dependent side effects. In our experience this therapeutic approach proved to be coupled with great efficacy and lack of significant complications. We treated over 200 cases until today, as other pregnancies are going on at the moment, the main indication being a history of recurrent pregnancy loss. There were cases in which the usual dose of 0.5 mg/day was ineffective to prevent abortion, and it was doubled during the subsequent pregnancy, to be increased up to 2 mg/day month by month, due to heavy bleeding around the time of the expected menstrual flow. These cases, not included in the sample below, ultimately ended with the birth of healthy babies around term. As expected, there were cases of pregnancy complications, such as premature delivery, IUGR, preeclampsia, abruptio placentae, gestational diabetes, that were handled with the standard obstetric care. Indeed, betamethasone does not represent the panacea for every adverse gestational condition. Overall, besides the high effectiveness of the therapy in preventing pregnancy loss, we can testify that neither foetal malformations nor significant maternal or foetal adverse effect of betamethasone were observed. No chance of a prospective randomized case-control study was offered at our Institution, in order to statistically prove the greater efficacy of betamethasone compared to other therapies. However we were able to analyze retrospectively a total of 101 treated patients as regards to some foetal biometric parameters and birth weight. Furthermore we performed two prospective studies aimed at verify two relevant end-points provided with physio-pathologic and clinical implications:

-   the possible positive correlation of foetal growth restriction with maternal **peripheral** NK cells concentration;
-   the possible efficacy of low-dose betamethasone therapy in decreasing the   maternal **peripheral** NK cells concentration.

Our retrospective analysis includes 166 patients admitted to the Section of Obstetrics and Gynaecology of Ferrara University from the late seventies to 2010. The population was divided into three groups:

-   (Group A): 80 patients treated by low dose betamethasone (0, 5 mg/daily) throughout pregnancy for previous history of recurrent miscarriage;
-   (Group B): 65 patients with physiological pregnancy;
-   (Group C): 21 patients affected by rheumatologic disease treated by prednisone (4-16 mg/daily).

Foetal growth was assessed by measuring the weight, head circumference and length at the birth. First data evaluation revealed neonatal weight and length significantly lower in the treated groups (2843,5 g and 48,14 cm in group A; 3262,92 g and 49,93 cm in group B; 2901,90 g and 49,67 in group C (Figure 2). Instead the head circumference was not statistically different among three groups (respectively 33.6 cm, 34.03 cm and 34.3 cm).

However in evaluating biometric parameters of the newborns, the pathological conditions of pregnancy that may lead to foetal growth restriction must be considered (Grivell et al., 2009). Among these, premature delivery, pre-eclampsia, gestational diabetes, hypothyroidism and bronchial asthma (Murphy & Gibson, 2011; Mitanchez, 2010; Krassas et al., 2010). Therefore, to get a more accurate evidence of the effect of betamethasone alone on foetal growth, we normalized the study population by excluding 26 patients suffering from the above mentioned diseases. By doing so, as expected, the differences among the neonatal biometric parameters were no more significant in the three groups (3144 g, 3262 g and 3171 g respectively for the birth weight; 49.73 cm, 49.3 cm and 49.63 cm for the neonatal length; 34.25 cm, 34.03 cm and 34.53 cm for the head circumference) (Figure 3).

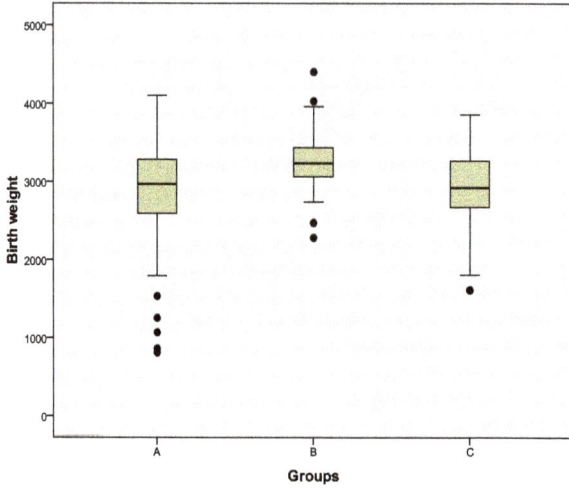

Figure 2. Distribution of birth weight in three groups. Group A (treated by betamethasone): 2843,5 g; Group B (physiologic pregnancy): 3262,92 g; Group C (rheumatologic diseases): 2901,90 g.

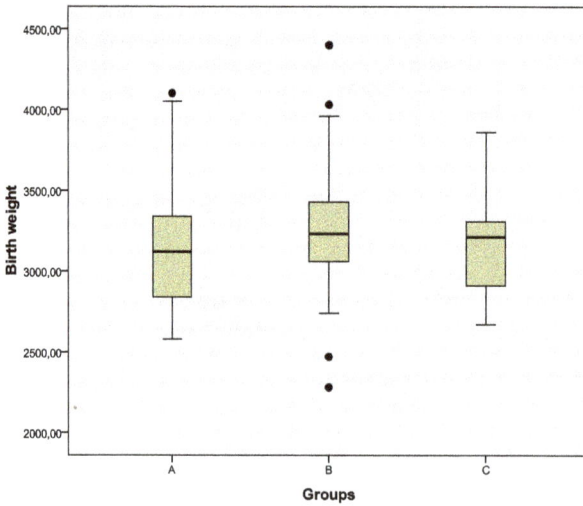

Figure 3. Distribution of birth weight in three groups after normalization of the study population. Group A (treated by betamethasone): 3144 g; Group B (physiologic pregnancy) 3262 g; Group C (rheumatologic diseases): 3171 g.

Moreover, by analyzing the distribution of birth weight values, we observed that one third of the newborns reached a weight higher than the fiftieth percentile in the treated group. Being all the patients upon the same betamethasone regimen, such an observation confirms that the cause of decreased neonatal weight should be ascribed to factors other than the hormone. The result of our attempt to homogenize the study sample highlights the need to take with caution the conclusions of other reports where different classes of patients were accidentally mixed up. As a matter of fact, most cases of GCs administration reported in the literature belong to pathologic conditions leading by themselves to foetal growth restriction (Davis et al., 2009; Kumar & Seshadri, et al., 2005). Coming to our first prospective study, we must recall that impairment of foetal oxygenation and growth, besides being linked with the above mentioned influences of unbalanced cytokines on utero-placental perfusion, is also reflected in the correlation between high values of uNK and IUGR (Williams et al., 2009). Therefore we decided to analyze the circulating lymphocyte subsets, mainly to search for a correlation between **peripheral** maternal NK concentration and foetal growth restriction. Such a possible link, to our knowledge never investigated before, could open the way to a practical test for the early diagnosis of a harmful complication. We selected ten pregnant women with a history of a successful pregnancy as a control group (group 1), plus ten with a diagnosis of IUGR, i.e. with foetal ultrasound biometric parameters below the 10th percentile (group 2). The course of pregnancy was normal in both groups, ending in spontaneous or elective caesarean delivery at term. Fresh blood samples drawn during the third trimester were analyzed at the Laboratory of the Haematological Unit of Ferrara University. Our study demonstrates that the number of peripheral leukocytes, the number of lymphocytes and their percentage were constant ($p<0,75$; $p<0,93$; $p<0,49$) while significant changes are observed for the NK cells. In particular:

- Significantly higher NK percentage (% $CD56^+$ cells) in group 2 (20,9) compared to group 1 (15,1) ($p<0,01$) (Figure 4);
- No significant increase in NK total number ($CD56^+$ U/µl cells) (419,6) in group 2 compared to group 1 (341,4) ($p< 0,10$);
- Significantly higher percentage NK subset ($CD2^+CD56^+$ cells) in group 2 (18,8) compared to group 1 (13,4) ($p<0.02$) (Figure 5).

By analyzing the other lymphocyte subsets, we observed a non significant $CD4^+$ T decrease along with a $CD8^+$ T increase, with a consequent decrease of their ratio. Moreover, there were no differences in the absolute count and percentage of the following lymphocyte subsets: T($CD3^+$) lymphocytes, T activated lymphocytes ($CD3^+$ HLA-DR$^+$), CD45 leukocytes, HLA-DR cells and B lymphocytes ($CD19^+$ e $CD19^+CD5^+$).

Therefore, increased peripheral NK percentage was the only significant feature of lymphocyte subset linked with IUGR in our study sample. Subsequently, with the aim to contribute to a better knowledge of the basic mechanisms of GCs protection, we evaluated the influence of betamethasone on the percentage of maternal pNK and other components of the lymphocyte subset in women with history of RSA. The patients with known anatomical, hormonal, genetic, infectious, autoimmune causes of abortion, as well as those with psychiatric disease were excluded from the study. Ten pregnant women with history of RSA

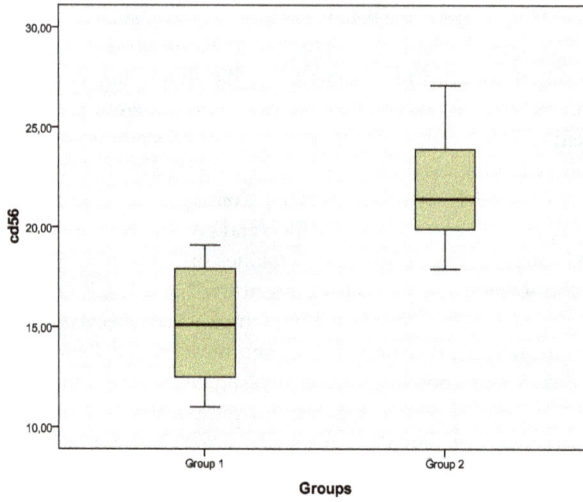

Figure 4. Comparison of pNK percentage (% CD56 +) between patients with adequate foetal growth (Group 1) and those with growth restriction (Group 2)

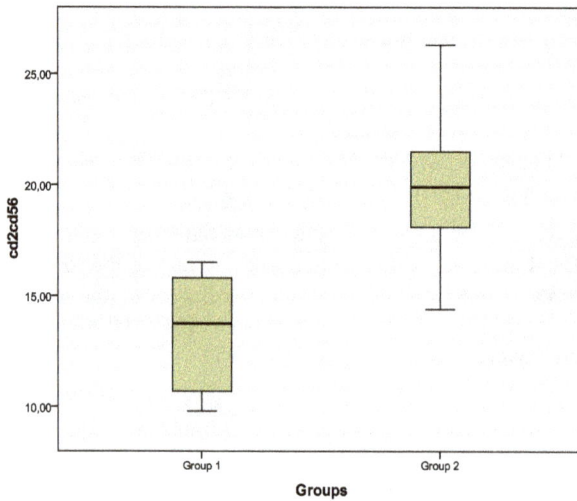

Figure 5. Comparison of the mean value of the CD2 + CD56 + subset percentage between patients with adequate foetal growth (Group 1) and those with growth restriction (Group 2).

were consecutively recruited (group 1). They were given oral betamethasone 0.5mg/daily from the fifth week of pregnancy until delivery. Ten normal pregnant women with previous history of successful pregnancies served as a control group (group 2). Blood samples were drawn at each one of the three trimesters (t1-first trimester, t2-second, t3-third). Fresh samples were analyzed at the Laboratory of the Haematology Unit of Ferrara University. The comparison between the two groups showed that lymphocytes percentage was significantly lower upon betamethasone therapy only in the third trimester (p-value =0,035). The percentage of T CD4+ cells in the third trimester was higher in treated women (46,4%) compared with controls (42,2%) (p-value =0,031), while that of T CD8+ cells was significantly lower in RSA in the second and in the third trimester. Comparison of CD2+, CD3+, CD5+, CD19+, CD45+, CD3+HLA-DR+ and CD19+CD5+ cells percentage between groups revealed no difference. As for NK, during the first trimester their percentage in RSA did not differ from that of the controls (gr1=15,0%, gr2=15,3%). However in the second trimester it became significantly lower (gr1=15,2%, gr2=17,6%, p-value=0,045). In the third trimester, despite a drop of their percentage (reaching 12,0%), only the absolute NK count decrease reached statistical significance. The percentage of NK subset CD2+CD56+ in the second and third trimester was significantly lower in group 1 (Figure 6). Our data on controls show the absence of significant changes in leukocyte and NK count and percentage throughout pregnancy. Coming to leukocyte subsets, we registered a lymphocytes decrease in the second trimester and a subsequent raise in the third, and a T CD4+ lymphocytes decrease with a T CD8+ increase throughout pregnancy. All together, these results substantially agree with the previous studies on physiologic pregnancy (Radysh et al., 2005).

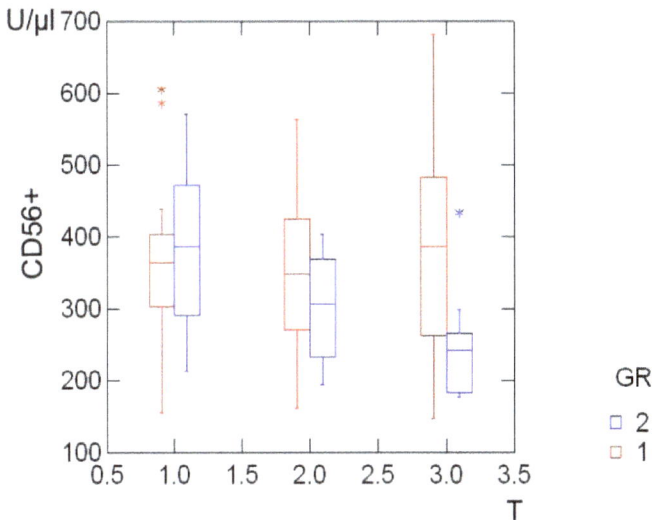

Figure 6. Trend of CD56 + cells U / l in group 1 and group 2 in the three trimesters. Time = 1.0 1^ trimester, 2.0 = 2^ trimester, 3.0 = 3^ trimester. Gr1 = normal pregnancy, Gr.2 = pregnancy with history of RSA treated with betamethasone

In the present study, moreover, we found that chronic low dose betamethasone administration leads to a significant decrease of leukocyte total number. Such behaviour is opposite to the well known leukocyte increase that follows 24 mg betamethasone administration during the third trimester for the prevention of hyaline membrane disease of the newborn. In addition, the lymphocytes percentage decrease caused by betamethasone reached statistical significance compared with controls in the third trimester. Such a result is likely to be related to the reduction of pNK. In treated cases NK percentage and number during the second and third trimester respectively reached lower values compared to controls. However, their values during the first trimester did not differ. Since it has been reported that women with history of RSA have a higher peripheral NK percentage, the absence of a difference between treated cases and physiological pregnancies during the first trimester in our data can be interpreted as an effect of betamethasone administration. In other words, betamethasone in RSA was able to decrease NK to values equal to (first trimester) and lower than (second and third) those in physiological pregnancy. With regard to the other lymphocyte subsets, it had been reported that women with RSA have a higher T cytotoxic CD8+ and T activated cells (CD3+HLA-DR+) percentage as compared to physiological pregnancy. Our work showed that betamethasone is able to decrease T CD8+ percentage to the same or even lower values compared to physiological pregnancy. In addition, we found no differences for T activated cells, between physiological pregnancy and treated RSA group, probably due to a suppressive action of the hormone. Previous studies demonstrated a CD19+CD5+ decrease in normal pregnancy. These are B lymphocytes producing auto-antibodies, and their percentage typically raises in RSA and in ANA positive women. Indeed, their percentage is reported to fall from 4,17% in the first trimester to 1,92% in the third. In contrast, we did not find any difference in CD19+CD5+ percentage between the 2 groups. In conclusion, our research shows that 0.5 mg/day betamethasone therapy throughout pregnancy in RSA women reduces pNK cells, CD19+CD5+ and CD3+HLA-DR+ lymphocytes. Such a finding, based on the above reported data in the literature, suggests that, besides the possible rebalancing effect of the drug upon the inflammatory cytokines at the implantation site, successful outcome probably derives also from an action on the cellular components of the immune system. It is noteworthy that the clinical result is obtained with use of a low dose that proved to be harmless for the foetus and devoid of maternal side effects.

9. Conclusive remarks

We have reported in the present chapter the regulation of the gestational processes as it appears from the data in the literature. Pregnancy can be essentially interpreted as a vascular phenomenon resulting from a balanced activation and release of a great number of mediators upon hormonal control. Corpus luteum progesterone is required before conception in order to adapt the uterine decidua to the subsequent early phase of implantation. However it was shown long ago that from the seventh week onward the corpus luteum is no more needed, as at this stage castration becomes unable to interrupt pregnancy. In spite of such evidence, the hormone is extensively used for prevention of abortion, and it keeps on being advocated even later on (Lucovnik et al., 2011), mainly based on its immuno-modulatory and myometrial relaxing effects. Recent research shed light on a more relevant cause of pregnancy loss than progesterone deficiency that is represented by inflammation at any stage of the gestational process. It can be triggered along a number of pathways, infection included. Nevertheless, infection, although accounting for ominous complications, has been found in some cases to represent a consequence rather than the cause of gestational inflammation. Inflammatory changes appear quite often to derive from a derangement of cytokines and prostanoids involved in the regulation of gestational physiological processes. A great number of cell function mediators has been found to be linked either with favourable outcome or with pregnancy loss, depending on the experimental model as well as on the gestational stage, but none can be identified alone as the keystone, successful pregnancy appearing the result of a balanced action of all mediators together. On the contrary, their imbalance leads to the activation of blood coagulation and stimulation of uterine contraction, the basic mechanisms for any pregnancy loss, aneuploid included (Vesce et al., 1996; Vesce et al., 2001; Vesce 2002). Myometrial activity is triggered by the release of prostanoids, mainly PGs of the E type, upon the action of many unbalanced cytokines. During the first trimester such abnormalities are confined to the feto-placental unit, while from late second to the third they can involve the maternal organism as well, leading to the variable clinical signs of preeclampsia. Outcome of pregnancy depends on the time of onset, the grade and the duration of cytokine imbalance. Moreover it must be considered that the maternal vascular adaptation is induced by the foetus itself, through the action of mediators released by trophoblastic cells on the uterine spiral arteries, and that even apparently late complications, such as preeclampsia, derive their origin from early foetal inadequacy (Vesce et al., 1997) Derangement of such mediators largely recognizing an inflammatory pathogenic mechanism, and low dose betamethasone being devoid of significant foetal side effects, there is no reason for administrating the glucocorticoids whose transfer to the foetus is highly impaired by 11β-HSD iso-enzymes. Indeed two possible scenarios can be identified:

- the trophoblast is able to modify the uterine vessels, but the unfavourable decidual environment impairs such a potential capacity;
- the maternal environment is favourable, but the trophoblast is unable to correctly operate.

In either one of the cases, there are several possible treatments that, like in any other disease, can be classified as symptomatic or etiological: the first are addressed to counteract uterine contractions and blood clotting, the second aimed at rebalancing maternal, as well as foetal, cytokine derangement that leads to abnormal prostanoids release. However, none of the available therapeutic options is able to reverse endothelial damage, once it is already established. Moreover, only etiological therapies are provided with the capacity to prevent the clinical pictures of pregnancy loss in high risk cases. Therefore, once the risk identified, etiological prevention and cure must start as early as possible, in some cases even before conception, and last enough to ensure foetal survival. In our opinion, GCs are the best preventive choice, as they represent the natural controller of the cross-talk that trophoblast entertains with maternal cells, throughout their entangled cytokine network. In this perspective, their efficacy is not to be intended simply as the result of a mere anti-inflammatory action, but rather as a complex direct and indirect regulatory influence on the mediators of cell functions. For instance, betamethasone, from one hand directly down-regulates the synthesis of inflammatory cytokines, while from the other it indirectly does the opposite by stimulating the MIF system. Unfortunately, in spite of the clinical evidence of the lack of significant maternal and foetal side effects of appropriate doses extensively reported in the literature, coupled with the great therapeutic benefits in life-threatening pregnancy complications, the concern for a negative impact on foetal morphogenesis and growth, mainly derived from experiments in animals with use of high doses, still impairs the correct adoption of GCs in the prevention of gestational risk. In the present chapter we reported some data from our long term use of low dose betamethasone throughout gestation for the prevention of pregnancy loss. Basically it is justified by the concept that pregnancy loss is the results of a cytokine imbalance possibly leading to inflammation, a derangement for which the use of progesterone is clinically proved to be either unsuitable or ineffective. In our experience, low dose betamethasone therapy is provided with great efficacy and devoid of significant foetal and maternal side effects. It will keep on representing the first choice therapy for protection of pregnancy in our practice.

Author details

Fortunato Vesce, Emilio Giugliano, Elisa Cagnazzo,
Stefania Bignardi, Elena Mossuto, Tarcisio Servello and Roberto Marci
Department of Biomedical Sciences and Advanced Therapy,
Section of Obstetrics and Gynecology, University of Ferrara, Italy

10. References

Abou-Ghannam G, Usta IM, Nassar AH (2011) Indomethacin in Pregnancy: Applications and Safety Am J Perinatol In press

Aghajafari F (2002) Repeated doses of antenatal corticosteroids in animals: a systematic review. American Journal of Obstetrics and Gynecology 186:843

Al-Bahrani A, Taha S, Shaath H & Bakhiet M (2007) TNF-alpha and IL-8 in acute stroke and the modulation of these cytokines by antiplatelet agents. Curr Neurovasc Res 4:31-7

Anderson BL, Simhan HN, Simons K & Wiesenfeld HC (2008) Additional antibiotic use and preterm birth among bacteriuric and nonbacteriuric pregnant women. Int J Gynaecol Obstet 102:141-5

Annells MF, Hart PH, Mullighan CG, Heatley SL, Robinson JS & McDonald HM (2005) Polymorphisms in immunoregulatory genes and the risk of histologic chorioamnionitis in Caucasoid women: a case control study. BMC Pregnancy Childbirth.5:4

Arck PC, Gilhar A, Bienenstock J & Paus R (2008) The alchemy of immune privilege explored from a neuroimmunological perspective. Curr Opin Pharmacol 8: 480-9.

Arcuri, F., Ricci, C., Ietta, F., Cintorino, M., Tripodi, S.A., Cetin, I., Garzia, E., Schatz, F., Klemi, P., Santopietro, R. et al. (2001) Macrophage migration inhibitory factor in the human endometrium: expression and localization during the menstrual cycle and early pregnancy. Biol. Reprod., 64, 1200–1205.

Arcuri F, Cintorino M, Carducci A, Papa S, Riparbelli MG, Mangioni S, Di Blasio AM, Tosi P & Viganò P (2006) Human decidual natural killer cells as a source and target of macrophage migration inhibitory factor. Reproduction. 131:175-82.

Baglin T, Gray E, Greaves M, Hunt BJ, Keeling D, Machin S, Mackie I, Makris M, Nokes T, Perry D, Tait RC, Walker I & Watson H (2010) Clinical guidelines for testing for heritable thrombophilia. Br J Haematol 149: 209–220

Bates SM, Greer AI, Pabinger I, Sofaer S & Hirsh J (2008) Venous thromboembolism, thrombophilia, antithrombotic therapy, and pregnancy: American College of Chest Physicians Evidence- Based Clinical Practice Guidelines (8th edition). Chest. 133: 844S-88

Bechi N, Ietta F, Romagnoli R, Jantra S, Cencini M, Galassi G,Serchi T, Corsi I, Focardi S & Paulesu L (2010) Environmental levels of para-nonylphenol are able to affect cytokine secretion in human placenta. Environ Health Perspect 118: 427-31

Biondi C, Pavan B, Ferretti ME, Corradini FG, Neri LM & Vesce F (2001) Formyl-methionyl-leucyl-phenylalanine induces prostaglandin E2 release from human amnion-derived WISH cells by phospholipase C-mediated [Ca+]i rise. Biol Reprod. 64:865-70.

Biondi C, Ferretti ME, Pavan B, Lunghi L, Gravina B, Nicoloso MS, Vesce F & Baldassarre G (2006) Prostaglandin E2 inhibits proliferation and migration of HTR-8/SVneo cells, a human trophoblast-derived cell line. Placenta 27:592-601.

Bonanno C, Fuchs K & Wapner RJ (2007) Single versus repeat courses of antenatal steroids to improve neonatal outcomes: risks and benefits. Obstet Gynecol Surv 62:261-71

Bondza PK, Metz CN & Akoum A (2008) Postgestational effects of macrophage migration inhibitory factor on embryonic implantation in mice. Fertil Steril.90:1433-43

Boomsma CM, Kavelaars A, Eijkemans MJ, Lentjes EG, Fauser BC, Heijnen CJ & Macklon NS (2009) Endometrial secretion analysis identifies a cytokine profile predictive of pregnancy in IVF. Hum Reprod. 24:1427-35.

Broering R, Montag M, Jiang M, Lu M, Sowa JP, Kleinehr K, Gerken G & Schlaak JF (2011) Corticosteroids shift the Toll-like receptor response pattern of primary-isolated murine liver cells from an inflammatory to an anti-inflammatory state.Int Immunol 23:537-44

Burrows TD, King A & Loke YW (1996) Trophoblast migration during human placental implantation. Hum Reprod Update 2:307-21.

Burton PJ & Waddell BJ (1999) Dual function of 11beta-hydroxysteroid dehydrogenase in placenta: modulating placental glucocorticoid passage and local steroid action. Biol Reprod. 60:234-40

Buzzi M, Vesce F, Ferretti ME, Fabbri E & Biondi C (1999) Does formyl-methionyl-leucyl-phenylalanine exert a physiological role in labor in women? Biol Reprod. 60:1211-6.

Calandra T, Bernhagen J, Metz CN, Spiegel LA, Bacher M, Donnelly T, Cerami A & Bucala R (1995) MIF as a glucocorticoid-induced modulator of cytokine production. Nature 377: 68-71.

Calandra T & Roger T (2003) Macrophage migration inhibitory factor: a regulator of innate immunity. Nat Rev Immunol 3: 791-800

Calleja-Agius J, Jauniaux E, Pizzey AR & Muttukrishna S (2012) Investigation of systemic inflammatory response in first trimester pregnancy failure. Hum Reprod. 27:349-57.

Cardaropoli S, Paulesu L, Romagnoli R, Ietta F, Marzioni D, Castellucci M, Rolfo A, Vasario E, Piccoli E, Todros T. Macrophage migration inhibitory factor in fetoplacental tissues from preeclamptic pregnancies with or without fetal growth restriction. Clin Dev Immunol. 2012;2012:639342.

Carlson AD, Obeid JS, Kanellopoulou N, Wilson RC & New MI (1999) Congenital adrenal hyperplasia: update on prenatal diagnosis and treatment. J Steroid Biochem Mol Biol. 69:19-29.

Carp HJ (2009) Aspirin in Recurrent Miscarriage: Is There an Indication? Isr Med Assoc J 11:178-82

Cervellati F, Pavan B, Lunghi L, Manni E, Fabbri E, Mascoli C, Biondi C, Patella A & Vesce F (2011) Betamethasone, progesterone and RU-486 exert similar effects on connexin expression in trophoblast-derived HTR-8/SVneo cells. Reprod Fertil Dev. 23:319-28

Challis JR, Lockwood CJ, Myatt L, Norman JE, Strauss JF 3rd, Petraglia F. Inflammation and pregnancy. Reprod Sci. 16:206-15

Chaouat G, Dubanchet S & Ledée N (2007) Cytokines: important for implantation? J Assist Reprod Genet 24: 491-505

Cheah FC, Winterbourn CC, Darlow BA, Mocatta TJ & Vissers MC (2005) Nuclear factor kappaB activation in pulmonary leukocytes from infants with hyaline membrane disease: associations with chorioamnionitis and Ureaplasma urealyticum colonization. Pediatr Res. 57:616-23.

Christiansen OB, Pedersen B, Rosgaard A & Husth M (2002) A randomized, double-blind, placebo-controlled trial of intravenous immunoglobulin in the prevention of recurrent miscarriage: evidence for a therapeutic effect in women with secondary recurrent miscarriage. Hum Reprod 17:809–816

Clark DA, Chaouat G, Arck PC, Mittruecker HW & Levy GA (1998) Cytokine-dependent abortion in CBA x DBA/2 mice is mediated by the procoagulant fgl2 prothrombinase. J Immunol. 160:545-9.

Clark P, Walker ID, Langhorne P,Crichton L, Thomson A, Greaves M, Whyte S & Greer IA (2010) The Scottish Pregnancy Intervention Study: a multicenter randomized controlled trial of low molecular weight heparin and low dose aspirin in women with recurrent miscarriage. Blood 115:4162–4167

Cleasby ME, Kelly PA, Walker BR & Seckl JR (2003) Programming of rat muscle and fat metabolism by in utero overexposure to glucocorticoids, Endocrinology 144:999–1007

Comp PC, Thurnau GR, Welsh J & Esmon CT (1986) Functional and immunologic protein S levels are decreased during pregnancy. Blood 68: 881-5

Coomarasamy A, Truchanowicz EG & Rai R (2011) Does first trimester progesterone prophylaxis increase the live birth rate in women with unexplained recurrent miscarriages? BMJ. 342:d1914.

Cox SM,Bohman VR,Sherman ML & Leveno KJ (1996) Randomized investigation of antimicrobials for the prevention of preterm birth. Am J Obstet Gynecol 174: 296-10

Cowchock S & Reece EA (1997) Do low-risk pregnant women with antiphospholipid antibodies need to be treated? Organizing Group of the Antiphospholipid Antibody Treatment Trial. Am J Obstet Gynecol 176: 1099-100

Cronier L, Alsat E, Harve' JC, De'le'ze J & Malassine' A (1998) Dexamethasone stimulates gap-junctional communication, peptide hormone production and differentiation in human term trophoblast. Placenta 19(Suppl. 1), 35–49

Crowther CA & Harding JE (2007) Repeat doses of prenatal corticosteroids for women at risk of preterm birth for preventing neonatal respiratory disease. Cochrane Database Syst Rev 3:CD003935

Cunha FQ, Weiser WY, David JR, Moss DW, Moncada S & Liew FY (1993) Recombinant migration inhibitory factor induces nitric oxide synthase in murine macrophages. J Immunol 150: 1908-12.

Dahlgren J, Nilsson C, Jennische E, Ho HP, Eriksson E, Niklasson A, Björntorp P, Albertsson Wikland K & Holmäng A. (2001) Prenatal cytokine exposure results in obesity and gender-specific programming, Am. J. Physiol. Endocrinol. Metab. 281:E326–E334

Danesi R & Del Tacca M (2004) Teratogenesis and immunosuppressive treatment. Transplant Proc 36:705-7

Davis EP, Waffarn F, Uy C, Hobel CJ, Glynn LM & Sandman CA (2009) Effect of prenatal glucocorticoid treatment on size at birth among infants born at term gestation. J Perinatol 29:731-7

de Vries A, Holmes MC, Heijnis A, Seier JV, Heerden J, Louw J, Wolfe-Coote S, Meaney MJ, Levitt NS & Seckl JR (2007) Prenatal dexamethasone exposure induces changes in nonhuman primate offspring cardiometabolic and hypothalamic–pituitary–adrenal axis function. J. Clin. Invest. 117:1058–1067

Dekel N, Gnainsky Y, Granot I & Mor G (2010) Inflammation and implantation. Am J Reprod Immunol 63: 17-21

Eastabrook G, Hu Y & von Dadelszen P (2008) The role of decidual natural killer cells in normal placentation and in the pathogenesis of preeclampsia. J Obstet Gynaecol Can. 30:467-76.

Engel SA, Erichsen HC, Savitz DA, Thorp J, Chanock SJ & Olshan AF (2005) Risk of spontaneous preterm birth is associated with common proinflammatory cytokine polymorphisms. Epidemiology 16:469-77.

Fest S, Aldo PB, Abrahams VM, Visintin I, Alvero A, Chen R, Chavez SL, Romero R & Mor G (2007) Trophoblast-macrophage interactions: a regulatory network for the protection of pregnancy. Am J Reprod Immunol.57:55-66.

Fingerle-Rowson G, Petrenko O, Metz CN, Forsthuber TG, Mitchell R, Huss R, Moll U, Müller W & Bucala R (2003) The p53-dependent effects of macrophage migration inhibitory factor revealed by gene targeting. Proc Natl Acad Sci U S A. 100:9354-9

Fonseca L, Ramin SM, Mele L, Wapner RJ, Johnson F, Peaceman AM, Sorokin Y, Dudley DJ, Spong CY, Leveno KJ, Caritis SN, Miodovnik M, Mercer B, Thorp JM, O'sullivan MJ, Carpenter MW, Rouse DJ & Sibai B; Eunice Kennedy Shriver National Institute of Child

Health and Human Development (NICHD) Maternal Fetal Medicine Units Network (MFMU) (2009) Bone metabolism in fetuses of pregnant women exposed to single and multiple courses of corticosteroids. Obstet Gynecol. 114:38-44

Furukawa S, Usuda K, Abe M & Ogawa I (2004) Histopathological findings of cleft palate in rat embryos induced by triamcinolone acetonide. J Vet Med Sci 66:397-402

Gaillard R, Riondel A, Muller A, Herrmann W & Baulieu EE (1984) RU 486: A steroid with antiglucocorticosteroid activity that only disinhibits the human pituitary-adrenal system at a specific time of day. Proc Natl Acad Sci USA 81:3879–3882

Garfield RE, Blennerhasset MG & Miller SM (1988) Control of myometrial contractility: role and regulation of gap-junctions. Oxf Rev Reprod Biol 10:436-90

Gesina E, Blondeau B, Milet A, Le Nin I, Duchene B, Czernichow P, Scharfmann R, Tronche F & Breant B (2006) Glucocorticoid signalling affects pancreatic development through both direct and indirect effects, Diabetologia 49:2939–2947

Gibbs RS, Romero R, Hiller SL, Eschenbach DA, Sweet RL (1992) A review of premature birth and subclinical infection. Am J obstet Gynecol 166. 1515-28

Gopichandran N, Ekbote UV, Walker JJ, Brooke D & Orsi NM (2006) Multiplex determination of murine seminal fluid cytokine profiles. Reproduction 131: 613-21

Grimes DA (1997) Medical abortion in early pregnancy: a review of the evidence. Obstet Gynecol 89:790-6

Grivell R, Dodd J & Robinson J (2009) The prevention and treatment of intrauterine growth restriction. Best Pract Res Clin Obstet Gynaecol. 2009 23:795-807

Guerin LR, Prins JR & Robertson SA (2009) Regulatory T-cells and immune tolerance in pregnancy: a new target for infertility treatment? Hum Reprod Update 15:517-35.

Guller S, Kong L, Wozniak R & Lockwood CJ (1995) Reduction of extracellular matrix protein expression in human amnion epithelial cells by glucocorticoids: a potential role in preterm rupture of the fetal membranes. J Clin Endocrinol Metab. 80:2244-50.

Gur C, Diav-Citrin O, Shechtman S, Arnon J & Ornoy A (2004) Pregnancy outcome after first trimester exposure to corticosteroids: a prospective controlled study. Reprod Toxicol 18: 93-101

Guyatt GH, Akl EA, Crowther M, Gutterman DD & Schuünemann HJ; American College of Chest Physicians Antithrombotic Therapy and Prevention of Thrombosis Panel. (2012) Executive summary: Antithrombotic Therapy and Prevention of Thrombosis, 9th ed: American College of Chest Physicians Evidence-Based Clinical Practice Guidelines. Chest 141(2 Suppl):7S-47S

Haas DM & Ramsey PS (2008) Progestogen for preventing miscarriage. Cochrane Database Syst Rev (2):CD003511

Heikinheimo O, Raivio T, Honkanen H, Ranta S & Jänne OA.Termination of pregnancy with mifepristone and prostaglandin suppresses transiently circulating glucocorticoid bioactivity. J Clin Endocrinol Metab. 88:323-6

Hill DJ & Duvillie B (2000) Pancreatic development and adult diabetes. Pediatr. Res.48:269–274

Hirata T, Osuga Y, Hamasaki K, Hirota Y, Nose E, Morimoto C, Harada M, Takemura Y, Koga K, Yoshino O, Tajima T, Hasegawa A, Yano T & Taketani Y (2007) Expression of toll-like receptors 2, 3, 4, and 9 genes in the human endometrium during the menstrual cycle. J Reprod Immunol. 74: 53-60

Huang HY, Chan SH, Wu CH, Wang CW, Lai CH & Soong YK (2005) Interleukin-1 system messenger ribonucleic acid and protein expression in human fallopian tube may be associated with ectopic pregnancy. Fertil Steril.84:1484-92.

Ietta F, Todros T, Ticconi C, Piccoli E, Zicari A, Piccione E & Paulesu L (2002) Macrophage migration inhibitory factor in human pregnancy and labor. Am J Reprod Immunol. 48:404-9.

Ietta F, Wu Y, Romagnoli R, Soleymanlou N, Orsini B, Zamudio S, Paulesu L & Caniggia I (2007) Oxygen regulation of macrophage migration inhibitory factor in human placenta. Am J Physiol Endocrinol Metab. 292:E272-80.

Ietta F, Bechi N, Romagnoli R, Bhattacharjee J, Realacci M, Di Vito M, Ferretti C & Paulesu L (2010) 17β-Estradiol modulates the macrophage migration inhibitory factor secretory pathway by regulating ABCA1 expression in human first-trimester placenta.Am J Physiol Endocrinol Metab. 298:E411-8

Jauniaux E, Gulbis B, Schandene L, Collette J & Hustin J (1996) Distribution of interleukin-6 in maternal and embryonic tissues during the first trimester. Mol Hum Reprod 2:239-43.

Jin LP, Chen QY, Zhang T, Guo PF, Li DJ. The CD4+CD25 bright regulatory T cells and CTLA-4 expression in peripheral and decidual lymphocytes are down-regulated in human miscarriage. Clin Immunol. 2009 Dec;133(3):402-10.

Kajantie E, Raivio T, Janne OA, Hovi P, Dunkel L & Andersson S (2004) Circulating glucocorticoid bioactivity in the preterm newborn after antenatal betamethasone treatment. J Clin Endocrinol Metab 89:3999–4003

Karagouni EE, Chryssikopoulos A, Mantzavinos T, Kanakas N & Dotsika EN (1998) Interleukin-1beta and interleukin-1alpha may affect the implantation rate of patients undergoing in vitro fertilization-embryo transfer. Fertil Steril. 70:553-9.

Kibschull M, Gellhaus A & Winterhager E. (2008). Analogous and unique functions of connexins in mouse and human placental development. Placenta 29, 848–854. doi:10.1016/J.PLACENTA.2008.07.013

King J & Flenady V (2002) Prophylactic antibiotics for inhibiting preterm labour with intact membranes. Cochrane Database Syst Rev 4:CD000246

King J, Flenady V, Cole S, Thornton S (2005) Cyclo-oxygenase (COX) inhibitors for treating preterm labour. Cochrane Database Syst Rev (2):CD001992.

Kirshbaum T (1993)Antibiotics in the treatment of preterm labor. Am J Obstet Gynecol 16 1239-46

Knackstedt M, Ding JW, Arck PC, Hertwig K, Coulam CB, August C, Lea R, Dudenhausen JW, Gorczynski RM, Levy GA & Clark DA (2001) Activation of the novel prothrombinase, fg12, as a basis for the pregnancy complications spontaneous abortion and pre-eclampsia. Am J Reprod Immunol. 46:196-210.

Korakaki E, Gourgiotis D, Aligizakis A, Manoura A, Hatzidaki E, Giahnakis E, Marmarinos A, Kalmanti M & Giannakopoulou C (2007) Levels of bone collagen markers in preterm infants: relation to antenatal glucocorticoid treatment. J Bone Miner Metab 25:172–178

Krassas GE, Poppe K & Glinoer D (2010) Thyroid function and human reproductive health.Endocr Rev 31:702-55

Kumar P & Seshadri R. Neonatal morbidity and growth in very low birth-weight infants after multiple courses of antenatal steroids. J Perinatol 25:698–702.

Kwak-Kim JY, Chung-Bang HS, Ng SC, Ntrivalas EI, Mangubat CP, Beaman KD, Beer AE & Gilman-Sachs A (2003) Increased T helper 1 cytokine responses by circulating T cells are present in women with recurrent pregnancy losses and in infertile women with multiple implantation failures after IVF. Hum Reprod.18:767-73.

Kwak-Kim J, Park JC, Ahn HK, Kim JW & Gilman-Sachs A (2010) Immunological modes of pregnancy loss. Am J Reprod Immunol. 63:611-23.

Laird SM, Tuckerman EM, Cork BA, Linjawi S, Blakemore AI & Li TC (2003) A review of immune cells and molecules in women with recurrent miscarriage. Hum Reprod Update 9:163-74

Lee SE, Romero R, Park CW, Jun JK & Yoon BH (2008) The frequency and significance of intraamniotic inflammation in patients with cervical insufficiency. Am J Obstet Gynecol 198:633.e1-8

Leonhardt SA & Edwards DP (2002) Mechanism of action of progesterone antagonists. Exp Biol Med 227:969-80

Li W, Gao L, Wang Y, Duan T, Myatt L & Sun K (2006) Enhancement of cortisol-induced 11beta-hydroxysteroid dehydrogenase type 1 expression by interleukin 1beta in cultured human chorionic trophoblast cells. Endocrinology 147: 2490-5.

Liu J & Feng ZC (2010) Increased umbilical cord plasma interleukin-1 beta levels was correlated with adverse outcomes of neonatal hypoxic-ischemic encephalopathy. J Trop Pediatr. 56:178-82

Lucovnik M, Kuon RJ, Chambliss LR, Maner WL, Shi SQ, Shi L, Balducci J & Garfield RE (2011) Progestin treatment for the prevention of preterm birth. Acta Obstet Gynecol Scand. 90:1057-69

Lunghi L, Pavan B, Biondi C, Paolillo R, Valerio A, Vesce F & Patella A (2010) Use of glucocorticoids in pregnancy. Curr Pharm Des. 16:3616-37.

Malassine´ A & Cronier L. (2005). Involvement of gap junctions in placental functions and development. Biochim. Biophys. Acta 1719:117–124.

Masuhiro K, Matsuzaki N, Nishino E, Taniguchi T, Kameda T, Li Y, Saji F & Tanizawa O (1991) Trophoblast-derived interleukin-1 (IL-1) stimulates the release of human chorionic gonadotropin by activating IL-6 and IL-6-receptor system in first trimester human trophoblasts. J Clin Endocrinol Metab.72:594-601.

McDonald HM, Brocklehurst P & Gordon A (2007) Antibiotics for treating bacterial vaginosis in pregnancy. Cochrane Database Syst Rev 1:CD000262;

McNeil CJ, Nwagwu MO, Finch AM, Page KR, Thain A, McArdle HJ & Ashworth CJ. (2007) Glucocorticoid exposure and tissue gene expression of 11beta HSD-1, 11beta HSD-2, and glucocorticoid receptor in a porcine model of differential fetal growth. Reproduction 133: 653-61

Michael AE & Papageorghiou AT (2008) Potential significance of physiological and pharmacological glucocorticoids in early pregnancy. Hum Reprod Update 14:497-517

Minas V, Loutradis D & Makrigiannakis A (2005) Factors controlling blastocyst implantation. Reprod Biomed Online. 10:205-16.

Mitanchez D (2010) Fetal and neonatal complications of gestational diabetes: perinatal mortality, congenital malformations, macrosomia, shoulder dystocia, birth injuries, neonatal outcomes. J Gynecol Obstet Biol Reprod (Paris). 39:S189-99

Mitsunari M, Yoshida S, Shoji T, Tsukihara S, Iwabe T, Harada T & Terakawa N (2006) Macrophage-activating lipopeptide-2 induces cyclooxygenase-2 and prostaglandin E(2) via toll-like receptor 2 in human placental trophoblast cells. J Reprod Immunol 72:46-59

Murphy VE, Zakar T, Smith R, Giles WB, Gibson PG & Clifton VL (2002) Reduced 11β-hydroxysteroid dehydrogenase type 2 activity is associated with decreased birth weight centile in pregnancies complicated by asthma. J Clin Endocrinol Metab 87:1660–1668

Murphy VE & Gibson PG (2011) Asthma in pregnancy. Clin Chest Med.32:93-110

Mwaniki MK, Atieno M, Lawn JE & Newton CR (2012) Long-term neurodevelopmental outcomes after intrauterine and neonatal insults: a systematic review. Lancet. 379:445-52

Nath CA, Ananth CV, Smulian JC, Shen-Schwarz S & Kaminsky L (2007) Histologic evidence of inflammation and risk of placental abruption. Am J Obstet Gynecol.197:319.e1-6.

Nielsen HS, Steffensen R, Varming K, Van Halteren AG, Spierings E, Ryder LP, Goulmy E & Christiansen OB (2009) Association of HY-restricting HLA class II alleles with pregnancy outcome in patients with recurrent miscarriage subsequent to a firstborn boy. Hum Mol Genet 18:1684–1691

Nishimura T, Dunk C, Lu Y, Feng X, Gellhaus A, Winterhager E, Rossant J & Lye SJ. (2004). Gap junctions are required for trophoblast proliferation in early human placental development. *Placenta* 25, 595–607. doi:10.1016/J.PLACENTA.2004.01.002

Norman JE, Kelly RW & Baird DT (1991) Uterine activity and decidual prostaglandin production in women in early pregnancy in response to mifepristone with or without indomethacin in vivo. Hum Reprod 6:740-4

Nyirenda MJ, Lindsay RS, Kenyon, Burchell A & Seckl JR (1998) Glucocorticoid exposure in late gestation permanently programs rat hepatic phosphoenolpyruvate carboxykinase and glucocorticoid receptor expression and causes glucose intolerance in adult offspring, J. Clin. Invest. 101:2174–2181

Nyirenda MJ, Carter R, Tang JI, de Vries A, Schlumbohm C, Hillier SG, Streit F, Oellerich M, Armstrong VW, Fuchs E & Seckl JR. (2009) Prenatal programming of metabolic syndrome in the common marmoset is associated with increased expression of 11beta-hydroxysteroid dehydrogenase type 1, Diabetes 58:2873–2879

Parker Jr CR, AtkinsonMW,Owen J & AndrewsWW (1996) Dynamics of the fetal adrenal, cholesterol, and apolipoprotein B responses to antenatal betamethasone therapy. Am J Obstet Gynecol 174:562–565

Pattison NS, Chamley LW, Birdsall M, Zanderigo AM, Liddell HS & McDougall J (2000) Does aspirin have a role in improving pregnancy outcome for women with the antiphospholipid syndrome? A randomized controlled trial. Am J Obstet Gynecol 183: 1008-12

Paulesu L, Bhattacharjee J, Bechi N, Romagnoli R, Jantra S & Ietta F (2010) Pro-inflammatory cytokines in animal and human gestation. Curr Pharm Des. 16:3601-15

Peck A & Mellins ED (2010) Plasticity of T-cell phenotype and function: the T helper type 17 example. Immunology. 129:147-53.

Pei K, Yu C, Shi X & Jia M (2010) The effects of mifepristone on the expressions of osteopontin, interleukin-6 and leukemia inhibitory factor in the villi of early pregnant women. Contraception. 82:379-84

Pellicer A, Dominguez F, Remohi J & Simón C (2002) Molecular basis of implantation. Reprod Biomed Online. 5:44-51. J Reprod Immunol. 72:46-59.

Pioli PA, Weaver LK, Schaefer TM, Wright JA, Wira CR & Guyre PM (2006) Lipopolysaccharide-induced IL-1 beta production by human uterine macrophages up-regulates uterine epithelial cell expression of human beta-defensin 2. J Immunol 176: 6647-55

Quenby S, Bates M, Doig T, Brewster J, Lewis-Jones DI, Johnson PM & Vince G (1999) Pre-implantation endometrial leukocytes in women with recurrent miscarriage. Hum Reprod 14:2386–2391

Quenby S, Farquharson R, Young M & Vince G (2003) Successful pregnancy outcome following 19 consecutive miscarriages: case report. Hum Reprod. 18:2562-4.

Quenby S, Kalumbi C, Bates M, Farquharson R & Vince G (2005) Prednisolone reduces preconceptual endometrial natural killer cells in women with recurrent miscarriage. Fertil Steril. 84:980-4.

Radysh TV & Chernyshov VP (2005) Immunopathophysiologic characteristics of early pregnancy in women with recurrent miscarriage. Fiziol Zh. 51:65-72.

Raghupathy R, Makhseed M, Azizieh F, Omu A, Gupta M & Farhat R (2000) Cytokine production by maternal lymphocytes during normal human pregnancy and in unexplained recurrent spontaneous abortion. Hum Reprod 15:713–718

Raghupathy R, Al Mutawa E, Makhseed M, Azizieh F & Szekeres-Bartho J (2005) Modulation of cytokine production by dydrogesterone in lymphocytes from women with recurrent miscarriage. BJOG. 112:1096-101.

Raghupathy R, Al-Mutawa E, Al-Azemi M, Makhseed M, Azizieh F & Szekeres-Bartho J (2009) Progesterone-induced blocking factor (PIBF) modulates cytokine production by lymphocytes from women with recurrent miscarriage or preterm delivery. JReprod Immunol 80:91–9

Rahimi R, Nikfar S & Abdollahi M (2006) Meta-analysis finds use of inhaled corticosteroids during pregnancy safe: a systematic meta-analysis review. Hum Exp Toxicol. 25:447-52.

Rai R, Backos M, Baxter N, Chilcott I, Regan L. Recurrent miscarriage – an aspirin a day? Hum Reprod 2000; 15: 2220-3

Rai R & Regan L (2006) Recurrent miscarriage. Lancet 368:601-1

Renaud SJ, Cotechini T, Quirt JS, Macdonald-Goodfellow SK, Othman M, Graham CH. Spontaneous pregnancy loss mediated by abnormal maternal inflammation in rats is linked to deficient uteroplacental perfusion. J Immunol. 2011 Feb 1;186(3):1799-808.

Robb L, Li R, Hartley L, Nandurkar HH, Koentgen F & Begley CG (1998) Infertility in female
mice lacking the receptor for interleukin 11 is due to a defective uterine response to
implantation. Nat Med 4: 303-8

Romero R, Gomez R, Ghezzi F, Bo Hyun Yoon, Mazor M, Edwin SS & Berry SM (1998) A
fetal systemic inflammatory response is followed by the spontaneous onset of preterm
parturition. Am J Obstet Gynecol 179:186-93.

Romero R, Chaiworapongsa T, Espinoza J, Gomez R, Yoon BH, Edwin S, Mazor M,
Maymon E & Berry S (2002) Fetal plasma MMP-9 concentrations are elevated in
preterm premature rupture of the membranes. Am J Obstet Gynecol 187:1125-30

Ryu JS, Majeska RJ, Ma Y, LaChapelle L & Guller S (1999) Steroid regulation of human
placental integrins: suppression of alpha2 integrin expression in cytotrophoblasts by
glucocorticoids. Endocrinology. 140:3904-8

Rushton DI (1988) Placental pathology in spontaneous miscarriage. In: Beard RW, Sharp F,
eds. Early Pregnancy Loss: Mechanisms and Treatment. London: Royal College of
Obstetricians and Gynaecologists : 149-58

Saini V, Arora S, Yadav A & Bhattacharjee J (2011) Cytokines in recurrent pregnancy loss.
Clin Chim Acta.412:702-8

Saito S, Nishikawa K, Morii T, Enomoto M, Narita N, Motoyoshi K & Ichijo M (1993)
Cytokine production by CD16-CD56bright natural killer cells in the human early
pregnancy decidua. Int Immunol. 5:559-63

Salgado A, Bóveda JL, Monasterio J, Segura RM, Mourelle M, Gómez-Jiménez J & Peracaula
R (1994) Inflammatory mediators and their influence on haemostasis. Haemostasis
24:132-8

Salmon JE & Girardi G (2008) Antiphospholipid antibodies and pregnancy loss: a disorder
of inflammation. J Reprod Immunol. 77:51-6.

Santoni A, Carlino C & Gismondi A (2008) Uterine NK cell development, migration and
function. Reprod Biomed Online 16:202-10

Schaefer TM, Fahey JV, Wright JA & Wira CR (2005) Innate immunity in the human female
reproductive tract: antiviral response of uterine epithelial cells to the TLR3 agonist poly
(I:C). J Immunol 174: 992-1002

Schraufstatter IU, Trieu K, Zhao M, Rose DM, Terkeltaub RA & Burger M (2003) IL- 8-
mediated cell migration in endothelial cells depends on cathepsin B activity and
transactivation of the epidermal growth factor receptor. J Immunol 171: 6714-22

Scott JR (2003) Immunotherapy for recurrent miscarriage. Cochrane Database Syst Rev
1:CD000112

Seckl JR (2004) Prenatal glucocorticoids and long-term programming, Eur. J. Endocrinol
151:49–62

Seckl JR & Holmes MC (2007)Mechanisms of Disease: glucocorticoids, their placental
metabolism and fetal 'programming' of adult pathophysiology.   Nature Clinical
Practice Endocrinology & Metabolism 3:479-88.

Shynlova O, Tsui P, Jaffer S & Lye SJ (2009) Integration of endocrine and mechanical signals
in the regulation of myometrial functions during pregnancy and labour. Eur J Obstet
Gynecol Reprod Biol 144 Suppl 1:S2-10

Simcox R, Sin WT, Seed PT, Briley A & Shennan AH (2007) Prophylactic antibiotics for the prevention of preterm birth in women at risk: a meta-analysis. Aust N Z J Obstet Gynaecol 47:368-77.

Sljivic S, Kamenov B, Maglajlic S, Djordjevic V, Stojkovic-Eferica I, Stojanovic M, Stefanovic M, Mihailovic D, Mrkaic L & Tasic G (2006) Possible interactions of genetic and immuno-neuro-endocrine regulatory mechanisms in pathogenesis of congenital anomalies. Med Hypotheses. 67:57-64.

Sotiriadis A, Makrydimas G, Papatheodorou S & Ioannidis JP (2009) Corticosteroids for preventing neonatal respiratory morbidity after elective caesarean section at term. Cochrane Database Syst Rev. CD006614

Spinillo A, Beneventi F, Ramoni V, Caporali R, Locatelli E, Simonetta M, Cavagnoli C, Alpini C, Albonico G, Prisco E & Montecucco C. (2012) Prevalence and significance of previously undiagnosed rheumatic diseases in pregnancy. Ann Rheum Dis. In press

Stephenson MD, Kutte WH, Purkiss S, Librach C, Schultz P, Houlihan E & Liao C (2010) Intravenous immunoglobulin and idiopathic secondary recurrent miscarriage: a multicentered randomized placebo-controlled trial, Human Reproduction 25:2203–2209

Suffee N, Richard B, Hlawaty H, Oudar O, Charnaux N & Sutton A (2011) Angiogenic properties of the chemokine RANTES/CCL5. Biochem Soc Trans 39:1649-53.

Sun K, Ma R, Cui X, Campos B, Webster R, Brockman D & Myatt L (2003) Glucocorticoids induce cytosolic phospholipase A2 and prostaglandin H synthase type 2 but not microsomal and cytosolic prostaglandin E synthase (PGES) expression in cultured primary human amnion cells. J Clin Endocrinol Metab 88: 5564–71.

Swolin-Eide D, Dahlgren J, Nilsson C, Albertsson Wikland K, Holmäng A & Ohlsson C. Affected skeletal growth but normal bone mineralization in rat offspring after prenatal dexamethasone exposure. J Endocrinol. 174:411-8.

Swyer GI, Daley D. Progesterone implantation in habitual abortion. BMJ 1953;1:1073-7

Tang AW, Alfirevic Z, Turner MA, Drury J & Quenby S. (2009) Prednisolone Trial: Study protocol for a randomised controlled trial of prednisolone for women with idiopathic recurrent miscarriage and raised levels of uterine natural killer (uNK) cells in the endometrium. Trials. 10;10:102

Thinkhamrop J, Hofmeyr GJ, Adetoro O & Lumbiganon P (2002) Prophylactic antibiotic administration in pregnancy to prevent infectious morbidity and mortality. Cochrane Database Syst Rev 4:CD002250

Thuere C, Zenclussen ML, Schumacher A, Langwisch S, Schulte-Wrede U, Teles A, Paeschke S, Volk HD & Zenclussen AC (2007) Kinetics of regulatory T cells during murine pregnancy. Am J Reprod Immunol. 58:514-23

Thum MY, Bhaskaran S, Abdalla HI, Ford B, Sumar N & Bansa (2008) Prednisolone suppresses NK cell cytotoxicity in vitro in women with a history of infertility and elevated NK cell cytotoxicity. l A.Am J Reprod Immunol. 59:259-65

Tincani A, Cavazzana I, Ziglioli T, Lojacono A, De Angelis V & Meroni P (2010) Complement activation and pregnancy failure. Clin Rev Allergy Immunol. 39:153-9

Tsuzuki Y, Takeba Y, Kumai T, Matsumoto N, Mizuno M, Murano K, Asoh K, Takagi
    M, Yamamoto H & Kobayashi S (2009) Antenatal glucocorticoid therapy increase
    cardiac alpha-enolase levels in fetus and neonate rats. Life Sci 85:609-16.
Verhoog NJ, Du Toit A, Avenant C & Hapgood JP (2011) Glucocorticoid-independent
    repression of tumor necrosis factor (TNF) alpha-stimulated interleukin (IL)-6 expression
    by the glucocorticoid receptor: a potential mechanism for protection against an
    excessive inflammatory response. J Biol Chem 286:19297-310.
Vesce F, Pareschi MC, Travagli S, Tarabbia C, Pansini F, Salvatorelli G, Gulinati AM, Grandi
    E & Biondi C (1992) Betamethasone-induced lecithin release in vitro from the fetal
    membranes. Gynecol Obstet Invest. 33:134-7
Vesce F, Farina A, Jorizzo G, Tarabbia C, Calabrese O, Pelizzola D & Giovannini G, Piffanelli
    A (1996) Raised level of amniotic endothelin in pregnancies with fetal aneuploidy. Fetal
    Diagn Ther. 11:94-8.
Vesce F, Farina A, Giorgetti M, Jorizzo G, Bianciotto A, Calabrese O & Mollica G (1997)
    Increased incidence of preeclampsia in pregnancies complicated by fetal malformation.
    Gynecol Obstet Invest. 44:107-11.
Vesce F, Buzzi M, Ferretti ME, Pavan B, Bianciotto A, Jorizzo G & Biondi C (1998) Inhibition
    of amniotic prostaglandin E release by ampicillin. Am J Obstet Gynecol 178: 759-64
Vesce F, Pavan B, Buzzi M, Pareschi MC, Bianciotto A, Iorizzo G & Biondi C (1999) Effect of
    different classes of antibiotics on amniotic prostaglandin E release. Prostaglandins
    Other Lipid Mediat. 57:207-18
Vesce F, Scapoli C, Giovannini G, Piffanelli A, Geurts-Moespot A & Sweep FC (2001)
    Plasminogen activator system in serum and amniotic fluid of euploid and aneuploid
    pregnancies. Obstet Gynecol. 97:404-8.
Vesce F, Scapoli C, Giovannini G, Tralli L, Gotti G, Valerio A & Piffanelli A (2002) Cytokine
    imbalance in pregnancies with fetal chromosomal abnormalities. Hum Reprod. 17:803-8
Vesce F, Pavan B, Lunghi L, Giovannini G, Scapoli C, Piffanelli A &Biondi C (2004)
    Inhibition of amniotic Interleukin-6 and Prostaglandin E2 release by ampicillin Obstet
    Gynecol 103: 108-113
von Eye Corleta H (2010) It is time to respect the American Society for Reproductive
    Medicine definition of recurrent pregnancy loss. Fertil Steril 94(4):e61
Wang ZC, Yunis EJ, De los Santos MJ, Xiao L, Anderson DJ & Hill JA (2002) T helper 1-type
    immunity to trophoblast antigens in women with a history of recurrent pregnancy loss
    is associated with polymorphism of the IL1B promoter region. Genes Immun. 3:38-42
Wang WJ, Hao CF, Yi-Lin, Yin GJ, Bao SH, Qiu LH & Lin QD (2010) Increased prevalence of
    T helper 17 (Th17) cells in peripheral blood and decidua in unexplained recurrent
    spontaneous abortion patients. J Reprod Immunol. 84:164-70.
Wang D, Lin W, Pan Y, Kuang X, Qi X & Sun H (2011) Chronic blockade of glucocorticoid
    receptors by RU486 enhances lipopolysaccharide-induced depressive-like behaviour
    and cytokine production in rats. Brain Behav Immun. 25:706-14
Waterman WR, Xu LL, Tetradis S, Motyckova G, Tsukada J, Saito K, Webb AC, Robinson
    DR & Auron PE (2006) Glucocorticoid inhibits the human pro-interleukin lbeta gene

(ILIB) by decreasing DNA binding of transactivators to the signal-responsive enhancer. Mol Immunol 43:773-82

Wegmann TG, Lin H, Guilbert L & Mosmann TR (1993) Bidirectional cytokine interactions in the maternal-fetal relationship: is successful pregnancy a TH2 phenomenon? Immunol Today 14:353–356

Wells C N (1953) Treatment of hyperemesis gravidarum with cortisone. Am J Obstet Gynecol 66:598-601

White CA, Robb L & Salamonsen LA (2004) Uterine extracellular matrix components are altered during defective decidualization in interleukin-11 receptor alpha deficient mice. Reprod Biol Endocrinol 2: 76

Williams PJ, Bulmer JN, Searle RF, Innes BA & Robson SC (2009) Altered decidual leucocyte populations in the placental bed in pre-eclampsia and foetal growth restriction: a comparison with late normal pregnancy. Reproduction. 138:177-84

Wira CR, Fahey JV, Ghosh M, Patel MV, Hickey DK & Ochiel DO (2010) Sex hormone regulation of innate immunity in the female reproductive tract: the role of epithelial cells in balancing reproductive potential with protection against sexually transmitted pathogens. Am J Reprod Immunol 63: 544-65

Winterhager E, Von Ostau C, Gerke M, Gruemmer R, Traub O & Kaufmann P. (1999). Connexin expression patterns in human trophoblast cells during placental development. *Placenta* 20, 627–638. doi:10.1053/PLAC.1999.0434

Xu J, Treem WR, Roman C, Anderson V, Rubenstein R & Schwarz SM (2011) Ileal immune dysregulation in necrotizing enterocolitis: role of CD40/CD40L in the pathogenesis of disease. J Pediatr Gastroenterol Nutr. 52:140-6.

Yamada H, Kato EH, Kobashi G, Ebina Y, Shimada S, Morikawa M, Sakuragi N & Fujimoto S (2001) High NK cell activity in early pregnancy correlates with subsequent abortion with normal chromosomes in women with recurrent abortion. Am J Reprod Immunol. 46:132-6.

Yamada H, Kato EH, Morikawa M, Shimada S, Saito H, Watari M, Minakami H & Nishihira J (2003) Decreased serum levels of macrophage migration inhibition factor in miscarriages with normal chromosome karyotype. Hum Reprod. 18:616-20.

Yang B, Trump RP, Shen Y, McNulty JA, Clifton LG, Stimpson SA, Lin P & Pahel GL (2008) RU486 did not exacerbate cytokine release in mice challenged with LPS nor in db/db mice. BMC Pharmacol.8:7

Glucocorticoids in Modern Clinical Therapy

Chapter 6

The Use of Glucocorticoids in the Treatment of Acute Asthma Exacerbations

Abdullah A. Alangari

Additional information is available at the end of the chapter

1. Introduction

1.1. Pathophysiology of asthma and acute asthma exacerbations: Brief overview

Asthma is a chronic respiratory disease that is prevalent worldwide. It is considered as a major cause of morbidity and a main contributor to the high health care expenditure especially in developed countries (Subbarao et al, 2009). There are two major pathological features in asthmatics' airways, inflammation and hyperresponsiveness. These features are interrelated but not totally dependent on each other. Airway inflammatory changes include increased airway mucus secretions, airway wall edema, inflammatory cellular infiltrates, epithelial cell damage, smooth muscle hypertrophy, and submucosal fibrosis (Bergeron et al, 2009). The cellular infiltrates are mainly composed of eosinophils, neutrophils, mast cells, lymphocytes, basophils and macrophages. The ratio of these cells may widely vary between patients pointing to asthma heterogeneity (Holgate, 2008). Overall, asthma can be divided into eosinophilic, neutrophilic, and pauci-granulocytic phenotypes. The eosinophilic phenotype is characterized by predominant eosinophilic infiltration of the airways. Patients tend to be allergic, have asthma triggered by exposure to allergens and tend to respond well to glucocorticoids. The neutrophilic phenotype is characterized by predominant neutrophil infiltration of the airways. Patients tend to have severe, more aggressive, poorly controlled asthma, or acute asthma triggered by viral infection. They usually do not respond to glucocorticoids as good as the eosinophilic type. In the pauci-granulocytic phenotype neutrophils and eosinophils are almost absent (Holgate, 2008).

Triggers of acute asthma exacerbation include allergens like pollens, animal dander, dust mites and mold; viral respiratory tract infections; irritants like smoke and dust; cold air and exercise. When pollens, for instance, are inhaled by an allergic individual, the allergenic protein is taken up by antigen presenting cells (dendritic cells) in the airway. It is then presented to naïve T-helper (Th) cells that develop into Th2 cell phenotype. These cells respond by secreting Th2 cytokines like IL-4 and IL-13 that cause allergen specific B-cells to switch from IgM producing to IgE producing cells. These cytokines could also contribute to epithelial cell damage, increased mucus secretion and airway hyperresponsiveness. Th2 cells also secrete IL-5 that stimulates eosinophil development, release from the bone marrow and their recruitment to the site of inflammation. IgE antibodies bind to their receptors on the surface of mast cells. Cross linking of adjacent IgE molecules leads to degranulation and release of mediators like histamine and tryptase that are key to features of immediate hypersensitivity reaction. Activation of mast cells and eosinophils will also stimulate the synthesis and release of lipid derived mediators like prostaglandins and cysteinyl leukotrienes that are very potent bronchoconstrictors. Moreover, activation of eosinophils leads to the release of mediators like eosinophil cataionic protein and major basic protein, which can cause airway epithelial cell damage and submucosal fibrosis. New evidence suggests that Th1 cells contribute to chronic changes in the airways including epithelial cells damage and smooth muscle cells activation. Regulatory T cells (Treg) inhibit Th2 cells by secreting IL-10 and tansforming growth factor β (TGFβ). Also, antigen specific Th17 cells were found to play an important role in neutrophilic airway inflammation and the process of airway remodeling (fixed changes to the airway) through the secretion of IL-17A and IL-17F (figure 1). This is a very quick overview, but many other changes take place during this process that are beyond the scope of this chapter.

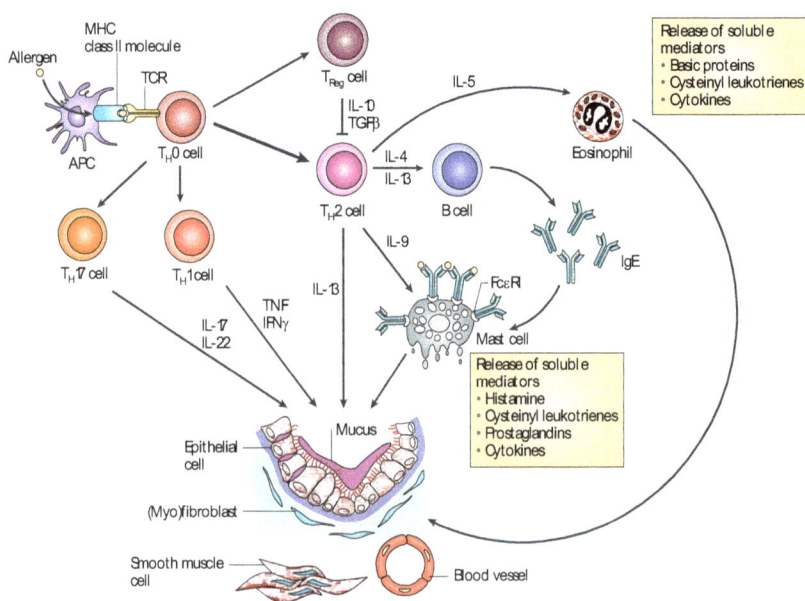

Figure 1. Major immunopahtologic processes that take place in the bronchial airways of patients with asthma. Please see the text for detailed description. FcεRI, high-affinity receptor for IgE; IFNγ, interferon-γ; TCR, T-cell receptor; TNF, tumour-necrosis factor. Reprinted by permission from Macmillan Publishers Ltd: Nature Reviews Immunology. Stephen T. Holgate and Riccardo Polosa. Treatment strategies for allergy and asthma. Vol. 8(3):Page 220, Copyright 2008.

The most common cause of acute asthma exacerbation in both adults and children, but more in children, is viral respiratory tract infections. Viruses may be responsible for up to 80% of wheezing episodes in children and 50-75% of episodes in adults (Jackson et al, 2011b). Many viruses can cause exacerbation of asthma symptoms, the most important and most common is rhinovirus (Khetsuriani et al, 2007). Respiratory syncycial virus and influenza virus also cause significant proportion of exacerbations. The pathology of virally induced asthma exacerbation is more related to the airway epithelial cells which, in response to infection secret chemokines like IL-8 and CCL-5 that can attract inflammatory cells including neutrophils and lymphocytes and augment allergic inflammation (Gern & Busse, 2002). This finding is supported by epidemiological observations that allergen sensitization and respiratory viral infections can synergize to cause asthma exacerbation (Green et al, 2002). Children who are atopic are more likely to have virally induced wheezing and respiratory distress than non-atopic children (Jackson et al, 2011a).

1.2. Treatment of acute asthma exacerbation: general overview

Acute asthma exacerbations are defined as "episodes of progressive increase in shortness of breath, cough, wheezing, or chest tightness, or some combination of these symptoms" (EPR3, 2007; GINA, 2011). Most recently an expert group formed by the NIH agreed to define acute asthma as "a worsening of asthma requiring the use of systemic corticosteroids to prevent a serious outcome" (Fuhlbrigge et al, 2012). Acute exacerbation of asthma symptoms is a common complication of the disease. The frequency in which exacerbations happen vary widely depending on the severity of disease (Moore et al, 2007), the degree of control with prophylactic medications (Peters et al, 2007), and exposure to triggers. In a multicenter study from the US (Pollack et al, 2002) the admission rate of all comers to the ER with acute asthma was 23%. On the other hand, a European study showed that only about 7% of all patients with acute asthma exacerbation required hospitalization (Rabe et al, 2000). We have a similar experience in Saudi Arabia where about 8% of all asthmatics with acute exacerbation are hospitalized, but if we look at only the severe group the rate goes up to 40% (unpublished data). These epidemiological data underscores the importance of effective treatment of asthma exacerbations and their prevention.

Patients with acute asthma exacerbation usually present with increasing cough, and dyspnea. On examination patients may have increased respiratory rate, retractions (accessory respiratory muscle use), wheezing, oxygen desaturation on pulse oxymetry and, in more severe cases, inability to speak, silent chest, with reduced respiratory lung volumes, cyanosis and change in mental status. Asthma exacerbations can be classified as mild, moderate, or severe based on the level of severity of the signs and symptoms as illustrated in Table 1. (Adams et al, 2011)

Different asthma scoring systems have been developed to assess the severity of asthma exacerbations more objectively, which is more useful for research purposes. An example is shown in table 2. (Qureshi et al, 1998). This scoring system is becoming more widely used because of its high reliability and objectivity.

Severity	Mild	Moderate	Severe
PEFR*	≥ 70%	40-69%	<40%
Speech	Sentences	Phrases	Words
Mental Status	Anxious	Agitated	Distressed
Accessory muscle use	No	Sometimes	Commonly
Oxygen saturation	≥ 95%	90-95%	<90%

Table 1. General classification of asthma severity. * PEFR: Peak Expiratory Flow Rate

Other frequently used scoring systems in the literature include; the Pulmonary Index Score (Scarfone et al, 1993) (table 3), and to a lesser degree the Preschool Respiratory Assessment Measure (PRAM) (Ducharme et al, 2008)(table 4), and the Pediatrics Asthma Severity Score (PASS) (Gorelick et al, 2004) (table 5).

Variable	Asthma score		
	1 point	2 points	3 points
Respiratory rate (breaths/min)			
2-3 years	≤ 34	35 - 39	≥ 40
4-5 years	≤ 30	31 - 35	≥ 36
6-12 years	≤ 26	27 - 30	≥ 31
>12 years	≤ 23	24 - 27	≥ 28
Oxygen saturation (%)	> 95 with room air	90 - 95 with room air	<90 with room air or supplemental oxygen
Auscultation	Normal breathing or end-expiratory wheezing	Expiratory wheezing	Inspiratory and expiratory wheezing, diminished breath sounds, or both
Retractions	None or intercostal	Intercostal and substernal	Intercostal, substernal, and supraclavicular
Dyspnea	Speaks in sentences or coos and babbles	Speaks in partial sentences or utters short cries	Speaks in single words or short phrases or grunts

Table 2. Asthma severity score (Qureshi et al). Score interpretation: Mild asthma 5-7, Moderate 8-11, Severe 12-15

In patients with mild asthma exacerbation, inhaled β2-agonists like albuterol (salbutamol) is usually sufficient to resolve symptoms. The dose can be repeated 3 times every 15-20 minutes. Levalbuterol, the (R)-enantiomer of albuterol is the effective form of the drug, but clinical trials did not show any advantage of using it over albuterol in terms of efficacy or side effects (Kelly, 2007). Most patients with mild asthma exacerbation will not require systemic glucocoricoids. However, it is recommended that patients who take them regularly or patients who fail initial treatment with albuterol should be given systemic glucocorticoids.

Score	0	1	2	3
Respiratory Rate* (breaths/min)	< 30	31-45	46-60	> 60
Wheezing	None	End expiration	Entire expiration	Inspiration and expiration without stethoscope
Inspiratory / Expiratory Ratio	5/2	5/3 - 5/4	1/1	<1/1
Accessory Muscle Use	0	+	++	+++

Table 3. Pulmonary Index Score. * For patients aged 6 years or older: <20 = 0; 21-35 = 1; 36-50 = 2; >50 = 3

Signs	0	1	2	3
Suprasternal retractions	Absent		Present	
Scalene muscle contraction	Absent		Present	
Air entry*	Normal	Decreased at bases	Widespread decrease	Absent/minimal
Wheezing*	Absent	Expiration only	Inspiratory and expiratory	Audible without stethoscope/silent chest with minimal air entry
O$_2$ saturation	≥95%	92%-94%	<92%	

Table 4. The Preschool Respiratory Assessment Measure (PRAM). *If asymmetric findings between right and left lungs, the most severe side is rated.

Current guidelines recommend that patients with mild-moderate or moderate exacerbation should receive 3 doses of inhaled or nebulized β2-agonist every 15-20 minutes in the first hour (Camargo et al, 2003). Additional doses may be repeated in the next 2-3 hours every 30-60 minutes. All those patients should be treated with systemic glucocorticoids at a dose of 2mg/kg or a maximum dose of 80 mg early in the course of management as it takes at least 4 hours to start working (Rowe et al, 2004). Doses more than 80 mg will not confer any additional benefit. Systemic glucocorticoids were found to speed resolution of symptoms, decrease the rate of admission and decrease the rate of relapse if administered for 3-5 days after the acute exacerbation. More detailed discussion about the use of systemic glucocoricoids in the treatment of acute asthma can be found below in section 2.1.

Clinical Finding	Definition	0	1	2
Wheezing	High-pitched expiratory sound heard by auscultation	None or mild	Moderate	Severe wheezing due to poor air exchange
Air entry	Intensity of inspiratory sounds by auscultation	Normal or mildly diminished	Moderately diminished	Severely diminished
Work of breathing	Observed use of accessory muscles, retractions, or in-breathing	None or mild	Moderate	Severe
Prolongation of expiration	Ratio of duration of expiration to inspiration	Normal or mildly prolonged	Moderately prolonged	Severely prolonged
Tachypnea	Respiratory rate above normal for age	Absent	Present	
Mental status	Observation of the child's state of alertness	Normal	Depressed	

Table 5. The Pediatrics Asthma Severity Score (PASS)

Patients with severe asthma exacerbation should obviously be treated more aggressively. High dose inhaled (8-12 puffs) or nebulized β2-agonist should be given every 15-20 minutes at least in the first hour, which could be repeated for up to 4 hours then as required. The data are conflicting whether continuous nebulization using β2-agonist is superior to intermittent nebulaization or not (Camargo et al, 2003; Rodrigo & Rodrigo, 2002). Practically, continuous high dose nebulization could be used for the first hour and then intermittent nebulization thereafter as required. Ipratropium bromide has been shown to decrease the rate of hospitalization and shorten the stay in the emergency room in patients with severe or moderate to severe asthma exacerbation in many clinical trials (Qureshi et al, 1998; Rodrigo & Castro-Rodriguez, 2005; Zorc et al, 1999). Therefore, it is recommended to add it to each treatment of β2-agonist at least in the first hour of therapy. Its use in patients after admission to the hospital was not shown to make a difference. Systemic steroids should be used as mentioned in patients with moderate exacerbation. Other treatment modalities may be considered like magnesium sulfate and helium oxygen (heliox) therapy in the more severe and non-responsive patients. Subcutaneous or intravenous β2-agonists (Travers et al, 2002), intravenous aminophylline (Parameswaran et al, 2000), intravenous montelukast (Camargo et al, 2010; Morris et al, 2010), or oral montelukast added to standard therapy in the ER (Todi et al, 2010) were not shown to be helpful in the treatment of patients with severe asthma exacerbation and therefore are not recommended. Moreover, oral montelukast given to patients post discharge for 5 days was also shown not to be helpful (Schuh et al, 2009).

β2-agonists can be delivered via a nebulizer or by metered dose inhaled (MDI) with a holding chamber. An MDI dose of 4-8 puffs depending on age is equivalent to a nebulized dose of 2.5-5 mg of albuterol (Cates et al, 2006). Nebulizer is preferable in cases of severe symptoms when patients are unable to use the MDI effectively or if other nebulized medications are needed to be mixed with albuterol at the same time or if the patient is requiring oxygen supplementation. Oxygen therapy should be given to maintain saturation ≥ 90% in adults and ≥95% in pregnant women or children.

Patients who maintain normal oxygen saturation, have no or minimal wheezing on chest auscultation, and have no or mild intercostal retractions can be discharged home after 1 hour of assessment on no additional medications in the emergency room. However, these patients should have a step up in their maintenance medications to prevent relapse. Patients who fail to achieve improvement after 4 hours of treatment should be admitted to the hospital for further aggressive therapy.

1.3. Introduction and evolution of glucocorticoids in the management of asthma: Historical background

Shortly after the discovery of the structure of adrenal steroid hormones, Hench and his colleagues examined using cortisone to treat arthritis in 1949. The effect was remarkable and that work won the Nobel Prize the next year. It also started a series of trials of corticosteroids in various inflammatory conditions. The first use of corticosteroid to treat acute asthma exacerbation occured in 1956 (Subcommittee on clinical trials in asthma, 1956). Development of corticosteroids that have less mineralocorticoid activity, like prednisone, and later those that have no mineralocorticoid activity, like dexamethasone, made glucocorticoids more attractive therapies to use in asthma. In 1972, Clerk et. al. showed for the first time that inhaled beclomethasone was effective in the management of asthma with less adverse effects than systemic steroids (Clark, 1972). Numerous reports came afterwards describing the efficacy of oral prednisone and prednisolone, intravenous methylprednisolone and inhaled glucocorticoids (IGC) like triamcinolone, budesonide, and fluticasone in the management of asthma. Table 3 shows some common systemic glucocorticoids and their relative potency.

Preparation	Potency relative to hydrocortisone	Relative sodium retention potency	Biological half life (h)
Hydrocortisone	1	1	8-12
Prednisone/Prednisolone	4	0.8	12-36
Methylprednisolone	5	0.5	12-36
Dexamethasone	25	0	36-72

Table 6. Common types of systemic glucocorticoids and their relative properties

1.4. Adverse effects of glucocorticoids

There are many adverse effects that may result from the use of oral or IGC in the treatment of asthma especially in high doses. I will summarize here the most pertinent ones.

a. Suppression of the hypothalamic-pituitary-adrenal axis. Soon after the commencement of high dose oral glucocorticoids adrenal suppression may be noticeable. It also occurs with longer use of lower doses. IGC can also be systemically absorbed in their active form through particle deposition in the orophaynx or the lungs (particles deposited in the stomach usually undergo first pass hepatic metabolism where they are deactivated). High doses of IGC, more than 400 mcg of becloemthasone and 200 mcg of fluticasone or budesonide per day, could cause systemic adverse effects especially in children (Gulliver & Eid, 2005). Patients who undergo a stressful situation like major surgery should receive systemic steroid coverage to avoid symptoms of adrenal crises. These symptoms include lethargy, vomiting, change in mental status, and electrolyte disturbances. The hypothalamic-pituitary-adrenal axis can be evaluated by measuring early morning cortisol level.

b. Osteoporosis. A common and serious complication of prolonged oral or high dose IGC therapy. Patients on such treatment, especially women and those with limited physical activity or who are taking medications that increase vitamine D metabolism in the liver, should undergo bone densitometry evaluation because this complication cannot be detected clinically. In one specialized center in the US, 40% of adolescent females admitted with severe asthma had osteopenia (Covar et al, 2000).

c. Growth suppression. Glucocorticiods have been consistently shown to suppress growth in children. This seems to be independent from the growth suppression caused by the disease itself (Covar et al, 2000). The degree of growth suppression may reach 1 cm especially in the first year after starting IGC treatment. However, children eventually reach their expected height as adults (Agertoft & Pedersen, 2000; Sharek & Bergman, 2000).

d. Ophthalmologic adverse effects. Long-term administration of oral glucocorticoids or high doses IGC can lead to the development of posterior capsular cataract (Cumming et al, 1997). Some patients may need lens replacement surgery. Another ophthalmic complication is glaucoma that also may result from prolonged therapy with high dose IGC (Garbe et al, 1997). However, short-term treatment for less than 2 years or the use of moderate doses of IGC was found to be safe (Li et al, 1999; Pelkonen et al, 2008).

e. Local adverse effects: Chronic use of IGC can be associated with the development of oral thrush (candidiasis), which could be minimized by washing the mouth with water after the inhalation. It may also be associated with hoarseness of voice and dysphonia due probably to laryngeal edema. These effects can be managed by changing the mode of inhalation (e.g: from dry powder inhaler to MDI) and the use of a holding chamber.

f. Other adverse effects: These include immune suppression, metabolic changes like hyperglycemia, acne, hirsutism, skin thinning, delayed wound healing, myopathy, psychosis or mood changes.

2. Clinical evidence of the effect of glucocorticoids in acute asthma

2.1. Systemic glucocorticoids

Systemic glucocorticoids given early in the course of treatment of acute asthma exacerbations in the emergency room were overall shown to be effective and are recommended by different asthma guidelines like GINA and EPR3. Littenberg et al. initially showed that they decrease hospital admission rate (Littenberg & Gluck, 1986). Five subsequent studies had, however, conflicting results. Rodrigo & Rodrigo reviewed all these six studies and concluded that there was no improvement in hospital admission rate or lung function (Rodrigo & Rodrigo, 1999). They, however, reported a trend of improvement in lung function only with medium or high doses systemic glucocorticoids. So data in terms of lung function are more encouraging (Fanta et al, 1983; Lin et al, 1999). In terms of effect on exacerbation relapse after discharge from the emergency room, most studies showed less relapse with systemic glucocorticoids (Schneider et al, 1988; Subcommittee on clinical trials in asthma, 1956) although others did not (Rodrigo & Rodrigo, 1994). One important issue with all these studies is the low number of patients recruited. Almost all had subject number less than 100 per study and all were performed in adults. On the other hand, Krishnan et al recently reviewed 9 published studies in the use of systemic glucocorticoids in acute asthma in adults and concluded "systemic corticosteroids provide clinically meaningful benefits in patients presenting with acute asthma" (Krishnan et al, 2009). In children, more limited data showed benefit of systemic steroids used early in the emergency room with decreased rate of admission (Scarfone et al, 1993). A Cochrane database review by Rowe et al showed decrease rate of admission in patients with acute asthma with the use of systemic glucocorticoids in adults and children especially those with severe asthma and those not currently receiving steroids (Rowe et al, 2001).

There is no significant difference in efficacy of systemic glucocorticoids at doses above 60-80 mg/d or 2 mg/kg/d in regards to pulmonary function, rate of admission, or length of stay in the hospital. For example, Marquette et al compared 1 mg/kg/d to 6 mg/kg/d methylprednisolone in 47 adults hospitalized with severe acute asthma and found no benefit of the high dose over the low dose (Marquette et al, 1995). Manser et al performed a systematic review of randomized controlled studies of patients with acute severe asthma comparing different doses of glucocorticoids with a minimum follow up of 24 hours. They divided the different doses used in the trials included into 3 groups as equivalent dose of methylprednisolone in 24 hours; low dose ($\leq$80 mg), medium dose (>80 mg and $\leq$360 mg), and high dose (>360 mg). Nine trials were included with a total of 344 adults. They found no difference between the different doses (Manser et al, 2001).

Studies also showed no difference in efficacy between oral or intravenous administration or in their onset on action. Fifty-two adults with severe acute asthma were treated with either IV hydrocortisone or PO prednisolone. There was no difference in their peak flow measurements 24 hours after admission (Harrison et al, 1986). Ratto et al compared four different doses of methylprednisolone; 160 or 320 mg given orally, or 500 or 1000 mg given IV in four divided doses in adults with acute asthma and found no difference in their FEV_1, days of hospitalization (Ratto et al, 1988). In children oral prednisolone was found equivalent to IV methylprednisolone in regards to patients' length of hospital stay (Becker et al, 1999). In addition, oral treatment was cost saving. GINA and the EPR3 guidelines prefer oral administration because it is less invasive except in patients with absorption problems or those who are not able to take orally due to the severity of their respiratory distress or because they are vomiting.

Prescribing oral glucocorticoids for the treatment of acute asthma exacerbations for longer than 5 days was not found to provide any additional benefit (Hasegawa et al, 2000; Jones et al, 2002). In children, a single dose of dexamethasone 0.6 mg/kg (max. 18 mg) was found to be equivalent to prednisolone 2 mg/kg/d in two divided doses for 5 days in terms of symptoms resolution (Altamimi et al, 2006). There is also no benefit from using a dose taper over fixed-dose regimen (Krishnan et al, 2009). Because of poor compliance on oral prednisone after discharge from the emergency, intramuscular injection of methylprednisolone was studied as an alternative but was not found superior, plus there was an evidence of injection-site adverse reaction (see last reference).

2.2. Inhaled glucocorticoids

IGC were studied in the treatment of acute asthma in 4 contexts: as compared to placebo, as compared to systemic glucocorticoids, as add on therapy to systemic steroids for up to few weeks after discharge from the ER, or as add on therapy to systemic steroids in the ER only.

In the first context, a review that looked at 8 randomized and blinded studies comparing the efficacy of IGC to placebo in acute asthma exacerbation suggested that IGC are superior to placebo especially when given at high doses (> 1mg of budesonide or fluticasone) and to patients with severe exacerbations (Rodrigo, 2006). It is important to note that those studies were quite heterogeneous in terms of the severity of asthma in recruited patients, the dose and frequency of IGC administered, and in the outcome measures that included clinical symptoms, pulmonary function, oxygen saturation, admission rate, or relapse rate. A recent study found that preemptive use of high dose fluticasone (750 mcg BID) at the onset of an upper respiratory tract infection in children with recurrent virus induced wheezing and continuing it for 10 days, reduced the use of rescue oral glucocorticoids (Ducharme et al, 2009).

When IGCs were compared with systemic glucocorticoids in randomized and blinded studies the data were more controversial. Some studies reported superiority of systemic steroids in reducing admission rate (Schuh et al, 2000), some reported equal efficacy in relation to admission rate as well (Lee-Wong et al, 2002; Levy et al, 1996; Scarfone et al, 1995), and some reported clear superiority of IGC (Devidayal et al, 1999; Rodrigo, 2005). A study compared high dose fluticasone in the ER and for 5 days post discharge to systemic glucocorticoids in the same period in patients with mild to moderate asthma found that oral steroids lead to faster improvement in FEV_1 at 4 hours in the ER and less relapse rate at 48 hours post discharge (Schuh et al, 2006). One recent study showed that in patients who were given systemic glucocorticoids plus IGC post discharge from the ER, stopping the systemic glucocorticoids after 1 week resulted in rebound in the level of exhaled NO 2 weeks post discharge despite continuing IGC with no effect on the use of rescue medications or on FEV_1 (Khoo & Lim, 2009). GINA guideline state that "IGC are effective as part of therapy for asthma exacerbations….and can be as effective as oral glucocorticoids at preventing relapses"(GINA, 2011), while the EPR3 guidelines state that "high doses of IGC may be considered in the ER, although current evidence is insufficient to permit conclusions about using IGC rather than oral systemic corticosteroids in the ER"(EPR3, 2007).

When IGC were used as add on therapy to systemic glucocorticoids in the ER and continued after discharge for few weeks, Rowe et al found decrease in relapse rate when 1600 mcg/d budesonide for 21 days was added to a course of 50 mg/d prednisone for 7 days as compared to placebo (Rowe et al, 1999). On the other hand, Brenner et al found no difference in the peak expiratory flow rate between high dose flunisolide used for 24 days added to prednisone 40 mg/d for 5 days as compared to placebo (Brenner et al, 2000). A systematic review of ten trials concluded no benefit of adding inhaled to systemic glucocorticoids in reducing the relapse rate of acute asthma (Edmonds et al, 2000).

There are few randomized and blinded studies examining only the short-term effect of IGC in the ER as add on therapy to systemic glucocorticoids plus other standard acute asthma therapy. One study looked at the addition of high dose beclomethasone versus placebo to methylprednisolone in 60 adults and found no difference in FEV_1 or symptoms between the two groups (Guttman et al, 1997). One study looked at the addition of budesonide nebulizations to methylprednisolone in a population of 26 children with moderate asthma (Nuhoglu et al, 2005) and found no difference in the primary outcome of pulmonary index score but there was an improvement in the PEFR in the budesonide group compared to placebo. However, the patient number included is very small and PEFR is generally not reliable in young children. The two other randomized and blinded studies that were larger and more rigorous examined the effect of adding 2 mg of budesonide nebulization to prednisone in children with moderate to severe asthma (Sung et al, 1998; Upham et al, 2011). In the study by Sung et al, 44 children with moderate to severe asthma were included. Both groups had no difference in the pulmonary index score. In the Upham et al study, 180 children with moderate to severe asthma were included. There was no difference in the asthma score (adopted form (Qureshi et al, 1998)) at 2 hours after intervention or in the admission rate or time to discharge from the ER between the two groups. Collectively, all these studies, although small in subjects number, indicate that the addition of IGC to systemic steroid is not helpful in patients with moderate to severe acute asthma. We are conducting a larger study that will hopefully shed more light on that question, the results of which should be available quite soon.

3. A brief overview of the use of glucocorticoids in asthma prophylaxis

3.1. Inhaled glucocorticoids

IGCs are the main stay of asthma management. They were shown to very consistently change many of the pathologic inflammatory features of asthma in the lung airways. They lead to decrease cellular infiltrates including T-lymphocytes, mast cells, eosinophils, and macrophages. Also, epithelial damage, goblet cell hyperplasia, and vascular blood flow significantly decreases with IGC therapy (Fanta, 2009). Consistent with the histological changes, clinical changes are observed. Compliant use of IGC is associated with decreased airway hyperresponsiveness and improved asthma symptomatology (CAMP, 2000; Haahtela et al, 1991). Most patients will also have improved lung function demonstrated by increased FEV_1. In addition, the risk of patients' hospitalization from asthma exacerbations is decreased by up to 50% (Donahue et al, 1997). Moreover, the risk of death from asthma is decreased, an effect that is dependent on the patients' compliance on IGC and the duration of their use (Suissa et al, 2000).

It is important here to note several points. First, the local anti-inflammatory effect of IGC usually plateaus after reaching low to moderate dosages, except probably for the most severe patients. However, the other systemic effects of IGC increase steeply after exceeding the low to moderate dose (Szefler et al, 2005). Therefore, efforts should be made to maintain patients on the lowest possible dose of IGC and, in cases of inappropriate response, long acting beta-agonists (LABA) or leukotriene receptor antagonists (LTRA) or both should be added before doubling the dose of IGC (Fanta, 2009). Second, there is great heterogeneity among asthmatics in their response to IGC. This variability can be attributed to several factors, most importantly are genetic variations between individuals (Lima et al, 2009). Third, multiple studies have shown that IGC therapy over the years do not change the natural history of the disease or prevent decline in lung function. They may have little effect on some features of remodeling but not all of them. Also, IGC, even when used in high risk infants who are very likely to develop asthma, were not able to prevent its development (Murray, 2008).

3.2. Systemic glucocorticoids

Systemic glucocorticoids are only occasionally used for long-term asthma control. There use is limited to the most severe patients who are difficult to control using other common modalities (EPR3, 2007). This is due to their side effects that can be very serious as stated above. The side effects are dose and duration dependent. Prolonged low dose therapy (<7.5 mg prednisone-equivalent in adults/day) is usually associated with mild adverse effects. Moderate doses (7.5 mg – 30 mg/day) are usually associated with significant adverse effects, and high doses (30 mg – 100 mg) may be associated with serious adverse effects (Stahn & Buttgereit, 2008).

4. Mechanism of action of glucocorticoids in asthma

Discussion of the mechanism of action of glucocorticoids in asthma is beyond the scope of this chapter and was recently reviewed (Alangari, 2010). Glucocorticoids act either by altering the rate of transcription of certain genes at the DNA level or through non-genomic pathways. Some of these effects could lead to the desirable anti-inflammatory action and some may result in adverse reactions.

4.1. Genomic action

The main mechanism whereby glucocorticoids deliver their anti-inflammatory action involves genomic action. This mechanism entails binding of glucocorticoids to their cytoplasmic receptors forming complexes that then translocate to the nucleus, where they either homo-dimerize then bind to their glucocorticoid response elements (GRE) in the DNA, or bind to different transcription factors (protein-protein interaction) as monomers (Ito et al, 2006; Lowenberg et al, 2008). Because of this, the genomic action of glucocorticoids takes at least 4 hours to start showing an effect and the duration of action is also prolonged and may exceed 24 hours.

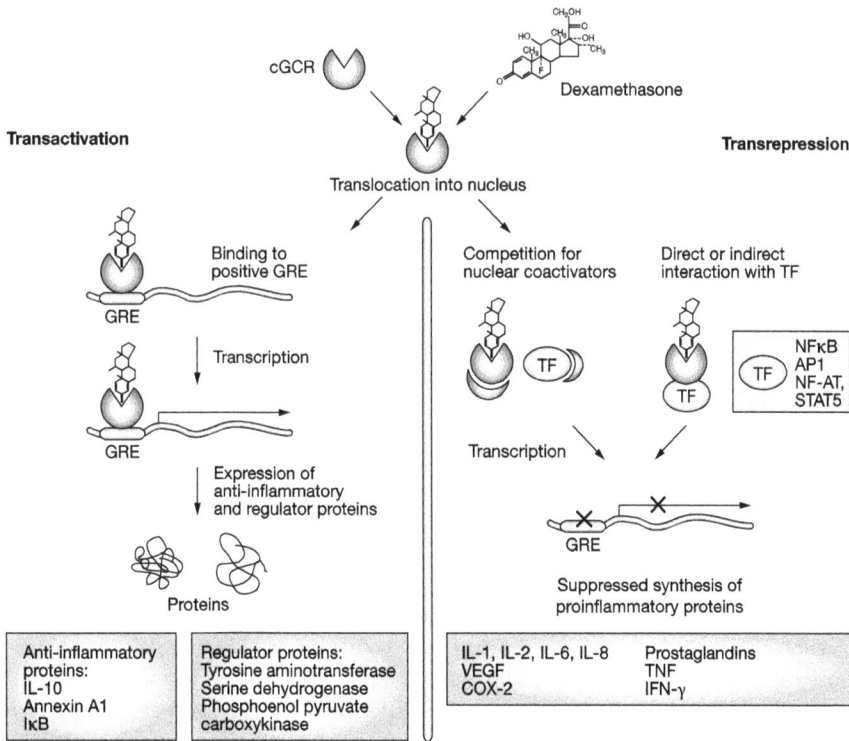

Figure 2. The genomic effect of glucocorticoids is in the form of transactivation or transrepression. In transactivation, the transcription of genes encoding certain anti-inflammatory or regulatory proteins is upregulated, while in transrepression the transcription of certain genes encoding proinflammatory proteins is up regulated. Abbreviations: AP1, activator protein 1; cGCR, cytosolic glucocorticoid receptor; COX-2, cyclooxygenase 2; GRE, glucocorticoid response element; IkB, inhibitor of NFkB; IFNγ interferon IL, interleukin; NF-AT, nuclear factor of activated T cells; NFkB, nuclear factor kB; STAT5, signal transducer and activator of transcription 5; TF, transcription factor; TNF, tumor necrosis factor; VEGF, vascular endothelial growth factor. Reprinted by permission from Macmillan Publishers Ltd: Nature Reviews Rheumatology. Cindy Stahn and Frank Buttgereit. Vol. 4(10):Page 529, copyright 2008.

Binding of glucocorticoid receptors to their GRE activates the transcription of certain genes encoding anti-inflammatory proteins, like IL-10 and IkB, and regulatory proteins. This process is called *transactivation* (figure 2). Some of the glucocorticoids adverse effects like glaucoma and hyperglycemia are mediated through this pathway (Schacke et al, 2002). On the other hand, binding of glucocorticoid receptors to pro-inflammatory transcription factors like nuclear factor kappa B (NFkB) or activator protein 1 (AP-1), or their competition for nuclear coactivators; down regulates the transcription of certain genes encoding pro-inflammatory proteins like IL-1, IL-2, IL-6, and TNF. This process is called *transrepression* (De Bosscher et al, 2003) (figure 2). Most of the desired genomic actions of glucocorticoids in asthma are mediated through this pathway.

4.2. Non-genomic action

Non-genomic action of glucocorticoids includes all actions that do not directly alter gene expression and are not blunted by inhibitors of gene transcription (Losel & Wehling, 2003). This mode of action is characterized by its rapid onset (seconds to minutes) and short duration (60-90 min). These actions are dose dependent (Wanner et al, 2004). There are four types of non-genomic action of glucocorticoids (Alangari, 2010). Firstly, acting through the inhibition of the extraneuronal monoamine transporter-mediated uptake of norepinephrine. Asthmatic patients have increased blood flow in their airways (Kumar et al, 1998). IGC were shown to decrease blood flow in the airways within few minutes. This effect will last for 90 minutes only and therefore, cannot be explained by the genomic action (Kumar et al, 2000; Mendes et al, 2003). The proposed mechanism is that IGCs by a topical effect can block the extraneuronal monoamine transporter on the membrane of vascular endothelial cells, preventing their uptake of norepinephrine and thus making it more available in the synaptic cleft (Horvath & Wanner, 2006). Secondly, in high doses, glucocorticoids can induce physiochemical changes in the cell membrane by directly incorporating into the membrane. This can result in immune cell suppression (Buttgereit & Scheffold, 2002). Thirdly, glucocorticoids may interact with membrane bound GRs on mononuclear cells. These receptors are variants of cytosolic GRs and can mediate inhibition of Lck/Fyn kinases down stream form the T-cell receptor leading to immune suppression (Lowenberg et al, 2005; Lowenberg et al, 2007). Lastly, few in vitro studies showed that some protein components associated with GRs complex, which are released upon GR ligation can inactivate cytosolic phospholipase 2 and therefore inhibit the production of arachidonic acid and downstream components like prostaglandins and leukotriens (Croxtall et al, 2000; Croxtall et al, 2002). However this action was not shown to be of clinical significance.

5. Future directions and recommendations

We have seen through this chapter that glucocorticoids play an extremely important role in the current prophylactic treatment of patients with persistent asthma, in the treatment of acute asthma exacerbations post discharge from the ER and possibly in the acute management in the ER. The introduction of IGC has revolutionized the way we manage asthma and it seems that those medications will stay with us for a long while. Further research is greatly needed to shed more light on the use of IGC in the ER in patients coming with acute asthma exacerbation and on the safety of dispensing oral glucocorticoids for home use in case of asthma exacerbation. Training physicians to follow asthma management guidelines as well as education of patients and their families cannot be over emphasized and will save a lot of money.

Our improved understanding of the tertiary structure of glucocorticoids and their receptors and their mechanisms of action has led to the discovery and development of selective glucocorticoid receptor modulators (SGRM). Those are new agents that have the transrepression but little or no transactivation properties of glucocorticoids, which means that those compounds could deliver the desired anti-inflammatory action of glucocorticoids while avoiding most of their adverse effects (De Bosscher et al, 2010). Still under investigation, those agents could hold a lot of promise in the future. Moreover, it was recently shown that simultaneous activation of GRα and peroxisome proliferator-activated receptor alpha (PPARα), which are cytosolic receptors with many immunomodulatory functions and multiple natural ligands, can block the GRE mediated transactivating effects of glucocorticoids while potentiating their anti-inflammatory effects in mice (Bougarne et al, 2009). If this holds true in humans, combination therapy of a glucocorticoid and a PPARα agonist could be very promising.

Author details

Abdullah A. Alangari
Department of Pediatrics, College of Medicine, King Saud University, Saudi Arabia

Acknowledgement

I am very grateful to Prof. Dale Umetsu for reviewing this manuscript. This work was supported by a grant form the Program of Strategic Technologies of the National Plan for Science and Technology and Innovation, Saudi Arabia. Grant number 08-MED520-02.

6. References

Adams JY, Sutter ME, Albertson TE (2011) The Patient with Asthma in the Emergency Department. *Clin Rev Allergy Immunol*

Agertoft L, Pedersen S (2000) Effect of long-term treatment with inhaled budesonide on adult height in children with asthma. *N Engl J Med* 343(15): 1064-1069

Alangari AA (2010) Genomic and non-genomic actions of glucocorticoids in asthma. *Ann Thorac Med* 5(3): 133-139

Altamimi S, Robertson G, Jastaniah W, Davey A, Dehghani N, Chen R, Leung K, Colbourne M (2006) Single-dose oral dexamethasone in the emergency management of children with exacerbations of mild to moderate asthma. *Pediatr Emerg Care* 22(12): 786-793

Becker JM, Arora A, Scarfone RJ, Spector ND, Fontana-Penn ME, Gracely E, Joffe MD, Goldsmith DP, Malatack JJ (1999) Oral versus intravenous corticosteroids in children hospitalized with asthma. *J Allergy Clin Immunol* 103(4): 586-590

Bergeron C, Al-Ramli W, Hamid Q (2009) Remodeling in asthma. *Proc Am Thorac Soc* 6(3): 301-305

Bougarne N, Paumelle R, Caron S, Hennuyer N, Mansouri R, Gervois P, Staels B, Haegeman G, De Bosscher K (2009) PPARalpha blocks glucocorticoid receptor alpha-mediated transactivation but cooperates with the activated glucocorticoid receptor alpha for transrepression on NF-kappaB. *Proc Natl Acad Sci U S A* 106(18): 7397-7402

Brenner BE, Chavda KK, Camargo CA, Jr. (2000) Randomized trial of inhaled flunisolide versus placebo among asthmatic patients discharged from the emergency department. *Ann Emerg Med* 36(5): 417-426

Buttgereit F, Scheffold A (2002) Rapid glucocorticoid effects on immune cells. *Steroids* 67(6): 529-534

Camargo CA, Jr., Gurner DM, Smithline HA, Chapela R, Fabbri LM, Green SA, Malice MP, Legrand C, Dass SB, Knorr BA, Reiss TF (2010) A randomized placebo-controlled study of intravenous montelukast for the treatment of acute asthma. *J Allergy Clin Immunol* 125(2): 374-380

Camargo CA, Jr., Spooner CH, Rowe BH (2003) Continuous versus intermittent beta-agonists in the treatment of acute asthma. *Cochrane Database Syst Rev*(4): CD001115

CAMP T (2000) Long-term effects of budesonide or nedocromil in children with asthma. The Childhood Asthma Management Program Research Group. *N Engl J Med* 343(15): 1054-1063

Cates CJ, Crilly JA, Rowe BH (2006) Holding chambers (spacers) versus nebulisers for beta-agonist treatment of acute asthma. *Cochrane Database Syst Rev*(2): CD000052

Clark TJ (1972) Effect of beclomethasone dipropionate delivered by aerosol in patients with asthma. *Lancet* 1(7765): 1361-1364

Covar RA, Leung DY, McCormick D, Steelman J, Zeitler P, Spahn JD (2000) Risk factors associated with glucocorticoid-induced adverse effects in children with severe asthma. *J Allergy Clin Immunol* 106(4): 651-659

Croxtall JD, Choudhury Q, Flower RJ (2000) Glucocorticoids act within minutes to inhibit recruitment of signalling factors to activated EGF receptors through a receptor-dependent, transcription-independent mechanism. *Br J Pharmacol* 130(2): 289-298

Croxtall JD, van Hal PT, Choudhury Q, Gilroy DW, Flower RJ (2002) Different glucocorticoids vary in their genomic and non-genomic mechanism of action in A549 cells. *Br J Pharmacol* 135(2): 511-519

Cumming RG, Mitchell P, Leeder SR (1997) Use of inhaled corticosteroids and the risk of cataracts. *N Engl J Med* 337(1): 8-14

De Bosscher K, Haegeman G, Elewaut D (2010) Targeting inflammation using selective glucocorticoid receptor modulators. *Curr Opin Pharmacol* 10(4): 497-504

De Bosscher K, Vanden Berghe W, Haegeman G (2003) The interplay between the glucocorticoid receptor and nuclear factor-kappaB or activator protein-1: molecular mechanisms for gene repression. *Endocr Rev* 24(4): 488-522

Devidayal, Singhi S, Kumar L, Jayshree M (1999) Efficacy of nebulized budesonide compared to oral prednisolone in acute bronchial asthma. *Acta Paediatr* 88(8): 835-840

Donahue JG, Weiss ST, Livingston JM, Goetsch MA, Greineder DK, Platt R (1997) Inhaled steroids and the risk of hospitalization for asthma. *JAMA* 277(11): 887-891

Ducharme FM, Chalut D, Plotnick L, Savdie C, Kudirka D, Zhang X, Meng L, McGillivray D (2008) The Pediatric Respiratory Assessment Measure: a valid clinical score for assessing acute asthma severity from toddlers to teenagers. *J Pediatr* 152(4): 476-480, 480.e471

Ducharme FM, Lemire C, Noya FJ, Davis GM, Alos N, Leblond H, Savdie C, Collet JP, Khomenko L, Rivard G, Platt RW (2009) Preemptive use of high-dose fluticasone for virus-induced wheezing in young children. *N Engl J Med* 360(4): 339-353

Edmonds ML, Camargo CA, Saunders LD, Brenner BE, Rowe BH (2000) Inhaled steroids in acute asthma following emergency department discharge. *Cochrane Database Syst Rev*(3): CD002316

EPR3 (2007) Expert Panel Report 3: Guidelines for the Diagnosis and Management of Asthma

Fanta CH (2009) Asthma. *N Engl J Med* 360(10): 1002-1014

Fanta CH, Rossing TH, McFadden ER, Jr. (1983) Glucocorticoids in acute asthma. A critical controlled trial. *Am J Med* 74(5): 845-851

Fuhlbrigge A, Peden D, Apter AJ, Boushey HA, Camargo CA, Jr., Gern J, Heymann PW, Martinez FD, Mauger D, Teague WG, Blaisdell C (2012) Asthma outcomes: exacerbations. *J Allergy Clin Immunol* 129: S34-48

Garbe E, LeLorier J, Boivin JF, Suissa S (1997) Inhaled and nasal glucocorticoids and the risks of ocular hypertension or open-angle glaucoma. *JAMA* 277(9): 722-727

Gern JE, Busse WW (2002) Relationship of viral infections to wheezing illnesses and asthma. *Nat Rev Immunol* 2(2): 132-138

GINA (2011) Global Initiative for Asthma (GINA): Global Strategy for Asthma Management and Prevention.

Gorelick MH, Stevens MW, Schultz TR, Scribano PV (2004) Performance of a novel clinical score, the Pediatric Asthma Severity Score (PASS), in the evaluation of acute asthma. *Academic emergency medicine* 11(1): 10-18

Green RM, Custovic A, Sanderson G, Hunter J, Johnston SL, Woodcock A (2002) Synergism between allergens and viruses and risk of hospital admission with asthma: case-control study. *BMJ* 324(7340): 763

Gulliver T, Eid N (2005) Effects of glucocorticoids on the hypothalamic-pituitary-adrenal axis in children and adults. *Immunol Allergy Clin North Am* 25(3): 541-555, vii

Guttman A, Afilalo M, Colacone A, Kreisman H, Dankoff J (1997) The effects of combined intravenous and inhaled steroids (beclomethasone dipropionate) for the emergency treatment of acute asthma. The Asthma ED Study Group. *Acad Emerg Med* 4(2): 100-106

Haahtela T, Jarvinen M, Kava T, Kiviranta K, Koskinen S, Lehtonen K, Nikander K, Persson T, Reinikainen K, Selroos O, et al. (1991) Comparison of a beta 2-agonist, terbutaline, with an inhaled corticosteroid, budesonide, in newly detected asthma. *N Engl J Med* 325(6): 388-392

Harrison BD, Stokes TC, Hart GJ, Vaughan DA, Ali NJ, Robinson AA (1986) Need for intravenous hydrocortisone in addition to oral prednisolone in patients admitted to hospital with severe asthma without ventilatory failure. *Lancet* 1(8474): 181-184

Hasegawa T, Ishihara K, Takakura S, Fujii H, Nishimura T, Okazaki M, Katakami N, Umeda B (2000) Duration of systemic corticosteroids in the treatment of asthma exacerbation; a randomized study. *Intern Med* 39(10): 794-797

Holgate ST (2008) Pathogenesis of asthma. *Clin Exp Allergy* 38(6): 872-897

Horvath G, Wanner A (2006) Inhaled corticosteroids: effects on the airway vasculature in bronchial asthma. *Eur Respir J* 27(1): 172-187

Ito K, Chung KF, Adcock IM (2006) Update on glucocorticoid action and resistance. *J Allergy Clin Immunol* 117(3): 522-543

Jackson DJ, Evans MD, Gangnon RE, Tisler CJ, Pappas TE, Lee WM, Gern JE, Lemanske RF, Jr. (2011a) Evidence for a Causal Relationship between Allergic Sensitization and Rhinovirus Wheezing in Early Life. *Am J Respir Crit Care Med* 185(3): 281-285

Jackson DJ, Sykes A, Mallia P, Johnston SL (2011b) Asthma exacerbations: origin, effect, and prevention. *J Allergy Clin Immunol* 128(6): 1165-1174

Jones AM, Munavvar M, Vail A, Aldridge RE, Hopkinson L, Rayner C, O'Driscoll BR (2002) Prospective, placebo-controlled trial of 5 vs 10 days of oral prednisolone in acute adult asthma. *Respir Med* 96(11): 950-954

Kelly HW (2007) Levalbuterol for asthma: a better treatment? *Curr Allergy Asthma Rep* 7(4): 310-314

Khetsuriani N, Kazerouni NN, Erdman DD, Lu X, Redd SC, Anderson LJ, Teague WG (2007) Prevalence of viral respiratory tract infections in children with asthma. *J Allergy Clin Immunol* 119(2): 314-321

Khoo SM, Lim TK (2009) Effects of inhaled versus systemic corticosteroids on exhaled nitric oxide in severe acute asthma. *Respir Med* 103(4): 614-620

Krishnan JA, Davis SQ, Naureckas ET, Gibson P, Rowe BH (2009) An umbrella review: corticosteroid therapy for adults with acute asthma. *Am J Med* 122(11): 977-991

Kumar SD, Brieva JL, Danta I, Wanner A (2000) Transient effect of inhaled fluticasone on airway mucosal blood flow in subjects with and without asthma. *Am J Respir Crit Care Med* 161(3 Pt 1): 918-921

Kumar SD, Emery MJ, Atkins ND, Danta I, Wanner A (1998) Airway mucosal blood flow in bronchial asthma. *Am J Respir Crit Care Med* 158(1): 153-156

Lee-Wong M, Dayrit FM, Kohli AR, Acquah S, Mayo PH (2002) Comparison of high-dose inhaled flunisolide to systemic corticosteroids in severe adult asthma. *Chest* 122(4): 1208-1213

Levy ML, Stevenson C, Maslen T (1996) Comparison of short courses of oral prednisolone and fluticasone propionate in the treatment of adults with acute exacerbations of asthma in primary care. *Thorax* 51(11): 1087-1092

Li JT, Ford LB, Chervinsky P, Weisberg SC, Kellerman DJ, Faulkner KG, Herje NE, Hamedani A, Harding SM, Shah T (1999) Fluticasone propionate powder and lack of clinically significant effects on hypothalamic-pituitary-adrenal axis and bone mineral density over 2 years in adults with mild asthma. *J Allergy Clin Immunol* 103(6): 1062-1068

Lima JJ, Blake KV, Tantisira KG, Weiss ST (2009) Pharmacogenetics of asthma. *Curr Opin Pulm Med* 15(1): 57-62

Lin RY, Pesola GR, Bakalchuk L, Heyl GT, Dow AM, Tenenbaum C, Curry A, Westfal RE (1999) Rapid improvement of peak flow in asthmatic patients treated with parenteral methylprednisolone in the emergency department: A randomized controlled study. *Ann Emerg Med* 33(5): 487-494

Littenberg B, Gluck EH (1986) A controlled trial of methylprednisolone in the emergency treatment of acute asthma. *N Engl J Med* 314(3): 150-152

Losel R, Wehling M (2003) Nongenomic actions of steroid hormones. *Nat Rev Mol Cell Biol* 4(1): 46-56

Lowenberg M, Stahn C, Hommes DW, Buttgereit F (2008) Novel insights into mechanisms of glucocorticoid action and the development of new glucocorticoid receptor ligands. *Steroids* 73(9-10): 1025-1029

Lowenberg M, Tuynman J, Bilderbeek J, Gaber T, Buttgereit F, van Deventer S, Peppelenbosch M, Hommes D (2005) Rapid immunosuppressive effects of glucocorticoids mediated through Lck and Fyn. *Blood* 106(5): 1703-1710

Lowenberg M, Verhaar AP, van den Brink GR, Hommes DW (2007) Glucocorticoid signaling: a nongenomic mechanism for T-cell immunosuppression. *Trends Mol Med* 13(4): 158-163

Manser R, Reid D, Abramson M (2001) Corticosteroids for acute severe asthma in hospitalised patients. *Cochrane Database Syst Rev*(1): CD001740

Marquette CH, Stach B, Cardot E, Bervar JF, Saulnier F, Lafitte JJ, Goldstein P, Wallaert B, Tonnel AB (1995) High-dose and low-dose systemic corticosteroids are equally efficient in acute severe asthma. *Eur Respir J* 8(1): 22-27

Mendes ES, Pereira A, Danta I, Duncan RC, Wanner A (2003) Comparative bronchial vasoconstrictive efficacy of inhaled glucocorticosteroids. *Eur Respir J* 21(6): 989-993

Moore WC, Bleecker ER, Curran-Everett D, Erzurum SC, Ameredes BT, Bacharier L, Calhoun WJ, Castro M, Chung KF, Clark MP, Dweik RA, Fitzpatrick AM, Gaston B, Hew M, Hussain I, Jarjour NN, Israel E, Levy BD, Murphy JR, Peters SP, Teague WG, Meyers DA, Busse WW, Wenzel SE (2007) Characterization of the severe asthma phenotype by the National Heart, Lung, and Blood Institute's Severe Asthma Research Program. *J Allergy Clin Immunol* 119(2): 405-413

Morris CR, Becker AB, Pinieiro A, Massaad R, Green SA, Smugar SS, Gurner DM (2010) A randomized, placebo-controlled study of intravenous montelukast in children with acute asthma. *Ann Allergy Asthma Immunol* 104(2): 161-171

Murray CS (2008) Can inhaled corticosteroids influence the natural history of asthma? *Curr Opin Allergy Clin Immunol* 8(1): 77-81

Nuhoglu Y, Atas E, Nuhoglu C, Iscan M, Ozcay S (2005) Acute effect of nebulized budesonide in asthmatic children. *J Investig Allergol Clin Immunol* 15(3): 197-200

Parameswaran K, Belda J, Rowe BH (2000) Addition of intravenous aminophylline to beta2-agonists in adults with acute asthma. *Cochrane Database Syst Rev*(4): CD002742

Pelkonen A, Kari O, Selroos O, Nikander K, Haahtela T, Turpeinen M (2008) Ophthalmologic findings in children with asthma receiving inhaled budesonide. *J Allergy Clin Immunol* 122(4): 832-834

Peters SP, Jones CA, Haselkorn T, Mink DR, Valacer DJ, Weiss ST (2007) Real-world Evaluation of Asthma Control and Treatment (REACT): findings from a national Web-based survey. *J Allergy Clin Immunol* 119(6): 1454-1461

Pollack CV, Jr., Pollack ES, Baren JM, Smith SR, Woodruff PG, Clark S, Camargo CA (2002) A prospective multicenter study of patient factors associated with hospital admission from the emergency department among children with acute asthma. *Archives of pediatrics & adolescent medicine* 156: 934-940

Qureshi F, Pestian J, Davis P, Zaritsky A (1998) Effect of nebulized ipratropium on the hospitalization rates of children with asthma. *N Engl J Med* 339(15): 1030-1035

Rabe KF, Vermeire PA, Soriano JB, Maier WC (2000) Clinical management of asthma in 1999: the Asthma Insights and Reality in Europe (AIRE) study. *Eur Respir J* 16(5): 802-807

Ratto D, Alfaro C, Sipsey J, Glovsky MM, Sharma OP (1988) Are intravenous corticosteroids required in status asthmaticus? *JAMA* 260(4): 527-529

Rodrigo C, Rodrigo G (1994) Early administration of hydrocortisone in the emergency room treatment of acute asthma: a controlled clinical trial. *Respir Med* 88(10): 755-761

Rodrigo G (2006) Rapid Effects of Inhaled Corticosteroids in Acute Asthma: An Evidence-Based Evaluation. *Chest* 130(5): 1301-1311

Rodrigo G, Rodrigo C (1999) Corticosteroids in the emergency department therapy of acute adult asthma: an evidence-based evaluation. *Chest* 116(2): 285-295

Rodrigo GJ (2005) Comparison of inhaled fluticasone with intravenous hydrocortisone in the treatment of adult acute asthma. *Am J Respir Crit Care Med* 171(11): 1231-1236

Rodrigo GJ, Castro-Rodriguez JA (2005) Anticholinergics in the treatment of children and adults with acute asthma: a systematic review with meta-analysis. *Thorax* 60(9): 740-746

Rodrigo GJ, Rodrigo C (2002) Continuous vs intermittent beta-agonists in the treatment of acute adult asthma: a systematic review with meta-analysis. *Chest* 122(1): 160-165

Rowe BH, Bota GW, Fabris L, Therrien SA, Milner RA, Jacono J (1999) Inhaled budesonide in addition to oral corticosteroids to prevent asthma relapse following discharge from the emergency department: a randomized controlled trial. *JAMA* 281(22): 2119-2126

Rowe BH, Edmonds ML, Spooner CH, Diner B, Camargo CA, Jr. (2004) Corticosteroid therapy for acute asthma. *Respir Med* 98(4): 275-284

Rowe BH, Spooner C, Ducharme FM, Bretzlaff JA, Bota GW (2001) Early emergency department treatment of acute asthma with systemic corticosteroids. *Cochrane Database Syst Rev*(1): CD002178

Scarfone RJ, Fuchs SM, Nager AL, Shane SA (1993) Controlled trial of oral prednisone in the emergency department treatment of children with acute asthma. *Pediatrics* 92(4): 513-518

Scarfone RJ, Loiselle JM, Wiley JF, 2nd, Decker JM, Henretig FM, Joffe MD (1995) Nebulized dexamethasone versus oral prednisone in the emergency treatment of asthmatic children. *Ann Emerg Med* 26(4): 480-486

Schacke H, Docke WD, Asadullah K (2002) Mechanisms involved in the side effects of glucocorticoids. *Pharmacol Ther* 96(1): 23-43

Schneider SM, Pipher A, Britton HL, Borok Z, Harcup CH (1988) High-dose methylprednisolone as initial therapy in patients with acute bronchospasm. *J Asthma* 25(4): 189-193

Schuh S, Dick PT, Stephens D, Hartley M, Khaikin S, Rodrigues L, Coates AL (2006) High-dose inhaled fluticasone does not replace oral prednisolone in children with mild to moderate acute asthma. *Pediatrics* 118(2): 644-650

Schuh S, Reisman J, Alshehri M, Dupuis A, Corey M, Arseneault R, Alothman G, Tennis O, Canny G (2000) A comparison of inhaled fluticasone and oral prednisone for children with severe acute asthma. *N Engl J Med* 343(10): 689-694

Schuh S, Willan AR, Stephens D, Dick PT, Coates A (2009) Can montelukast shorten prednisolone therapy in children with mild to moderate acute asthma? A randomized controlled trial. *J Pediatr* 155(6): 795-800

Sharek PJ, Bergman DA (2000) The effect of inhaled steroids on the linear growth of children with asthma: a meta-analysis. *Pediatrics* 106(1): E8

Stahn C, Buttgereit F (2008) Genomic and nongenomic effects of glucocorticoids. *Nat Clin Pract Rheumatol* 4(10): 525-533

Subbarao P, Mandhane PJ, Sears MR (2009) Asthma: epidemiology, etiology and risk factors. *CMAJ* 181(9): E181-190

Subcommittee on clinical trials in asthma MRC (1956) CONTROLLED trial of effects of cortisone acetate in status asthmaticus. *Lancet* 271(6947): 803-806

Suissa S, Ernst P, Benayoun S, Baltzan M, Cai B (2000) Low-dose inhaled corticosteroids and the prevention of death from asthma. *N Engl J Med* 343(5): 332-336

Sung L, Osmond MH, Klassen TP (1998) Randomized, controlled trial of inhaled budesonide as an adjunct to oral prednisone in acute asthma. *Acad Emerg Med* 5(3): 209-213

Szefler SJ, Phillips BR, Martinez FD, Chinchilli VM, Lemanske RF, Strunk RC, Zeiger RS, Larsen G, Spahn JD, Bacharier LB, Bloomberg GR, Guilbert TW, Heldt G, Morgan WJ, Moss MH, Sorkness CA, Taussig LM (2005) Characterization of within-subject responses to fluticasone and montelukast in childhood asthma. *J Allergy Clin Immunol* 115(2): 233-242

Todi VK, Lodha R, Kabra SK (2010) Effect of addition of single dose of oral montelukast to standard treatment in acute moderate to severe asthma in children between 5 and 15 years of age: a randomised, double-blind, placebo controlled trial. *Arch Dis Child* 95(7): 540-543

Travers AH, Rowe BH, Barker S, Jones A, Camargo CA, Jr. (2002) The effectiveness of IV beta-agonists in treating patients with acute asthma in the emergency department: a meta-analysis. *Chest* 122(4): 1200-1207

Upham BD, Mollen CJ, Scarfone RJ, Seiden J, Chew A, Zorc JJ (2011) Nebulized budesonide added to standard pediatric emergency department treatment of acute asthma: a randomized, double-blind trial. *Acad Emerg Med* 18(7): 665-673

Wanner A, Horvath G, Brieva JL, Kumar SD, Mendes ES (2004) Nongenomic actions of glucocorticosteroids on the airway vasculature in asthma. *Proceedings of the American Thoracic Society* 1(3): 235-238

Zorc JJ, Pusic MV, Ogborn CJ, Lebet R, Duggan AK (1999) Ipratropium bromide added to asthma treatment in the pediatric emergency department. *Pediatrics* 103(4 Pt 1): 748-752

Glucocorticoid Therapy in Systemic Lupus Erythematosus – Clinical Analysis of 1,125 Patients with SLE

Hiroshi Hashimoto

Additional information is available at the end of the chapter

1. Introduction

Systemic lupus erythematosus (SLE), which is an inflammatory disease of unknown cause, is a representative autoimmune disease. Although SLE has multisystem organ involvement with a predilection for females, the disease varies from mild to severe and/or from active to inactive. The severity and activity of the disease affect SLE prognosis [1]. Glucocorticosteroids (steroids) have anti-inflammatory and immunosuppressive effects, although the biological effects of steroids are multiple. The anti-inflammatory effect of steroids is powerful and acts rapidly, and the immunosuppressive effect after administration of large doses of steroids is also strong. Therefore, steroids play a major and essential role in the treatment and management of SLE patients, especially those having severe and active SLE. However, the effectiveness and usefulness of steroids are limited because of their severe side effects, unresponsiveness and resistance to steroids. In these situations, additional therapies such as immunosuppressive agents or plasmapheresis, etc. are usually used in conjunction with steroids.

This paper will present clinical data related to steroid therapy from 1,125 patients with SLE who were examined and treated in Juntendo University Hospital between 1955 and 2002. It will show the benefits and risks of treatment with steroids and/or combined therapy with steroids and immunosuppressants.

2. Clinical presentation of 1,125 patients with SLE

2.1. Clinical findings

One thousand one hundred and twenty-five SLE patients fulfilling four or more of the revised ACR (American College of Rheumatology) criteria [2] were examined and treated at the Department of Internal Medicine and Rheumatology in Juntendo University School of Medicine between 1955 and 2002. In all patients, the diagnosis and treatment procedures were conducted during a period when the use of steroids and immunosuppressive agents was common. Computerized analysis of clinical manifestations, laboratory and immunological findings, treatments, complications, causes of death and prognosis was conducted.

The distribution of age at diagnosis and the difference in gender, showing that mean age at diagnosis was 27.1 years old and the male to female ratio was 1:9. In children and adults over the age of 50, the incidence of SLE demonstrated only a slight female predominance, however, for those in their twenties, thirties and forties, close to 90% of patients were women. The frequencies of major clinical manifestations and laboratory findings from observations together with the data from other investigators [3-6] are shown in Table 1.

Manifestations	Harvey, et al. [4] 105 cases 1954	Dubois, et al. [5] 520 cases 1964	Pistiner, et al. [6] 464 cases 1991	Hashimoto, et al. 1125 cases 2002
I. Systemic				
fever	86	84	41	79
weight loss	71	51	-	-
adenopathy	34	59	10	28
II. Musculoskeletal				
arthritis/arthralgia	90	92	91	89
myalgias	-	48	79	31
aseptic bone necrosis	-	5	5	10
III. Cutaneous-vascular				
butterfly area lesions	39	57	34	70
alopecia	3	21	31	48
photosensitivity	11	33	37	40
discoid lesion	-	29	23	17
urticaria	7	7	4	25
oral/nasal ulcer	14	9	19	42
subcutaneous nodules	10	5	-	5
Raynaud's phenomenon	10	18	25	48
IV. Renal				
proteinuria/abnormal sediment	65	46	31	95
nephrotic syndrome	-	23	14	17
V. Cardiopulmonary				
cardiomagaly	15	16	-	-
pericarditis	45	31	2	7
myocarditis	40	8	12	2
heart murmur	44	20	12	14
Libman-Sacks valvlitis	32	-	1	(10/45) 22
hypertension	14	25	25	38
pleurisy	56	45	31	11
lupus pneumonitis	22	1	6	4
pulmonary hypertension	-	-	-	(11/487) 2
VI. Nervous system				
psychosis	19	12	5	21
seizures	17	14	6	8
peripheral neuritis	-	12	5	7
cytoid bodies	24	10	4	(8/63) 13

Manifestations	Harvey, et al. [4] 105 cases 1954	Dubois, et al. [5] 520 cases 1964	Pistiner, et al. [6] 464 cases 1991	Hashimoto, et al. 1125 cases 2002
VII. Gastrointestinal				
abdominal pain	10	19	1	5
ascites	-	11	-	2
peritonitis	-	-	-	1
hepatomegaly	-	-	-	11
splenomegaly	-	-	-	4
VIII. Laboratory findings				
anemia	78	57	30	63
hemolytic anemia	-	-	8	11
leukopenia	-	43	51	62
thrombocytopenia	26	7	16	34
elevated IgG	-	-	-	(634/1011) 63
elevated IgM	-	-	-	(438/1010) 43
elevated IgA	-	-	-	(154/1010) 15
low CH50	-	-	-	(660/1025) 64
low C3	-	-	39	(712/940) 76
low C4	-	-	-	(659/939) 70
false positive STS	15	11	-	(78/510) 15
anti-cardiolipin antibody	-	-	38	(177/349) 51
lupus anticoagulant	-	-	-	(151/349) 43
LE cell	82	82	42	(448/957) 47
antinuclear antibody	-	-	96	97
anti-DNA antibody	-	-	40	(645/935) 69
anti-U1RNP antibody	-	-	14	(314/876) 36
anti-Sm antibody	-	-	6	(645/935) 20
anti-SSA antibody	-	-	19	(371/814) 46
RAHA test	-	-	-	(308/739) 42
RAPA test	-	-	-	(195/557) 35
RA test	-	-	-	(352/908) 39

Table 1. Cumulative percentage incidence of clinical and laboratory manifestations in SLE

2.2. Treatment according to disease severity

Clinical subsets of SLE were divided into three groups according to disease severity that related to prognosis [7]. They were severe, moderate and mild diseases. Severe disease included organ-threatening conditions: lupus nephritis; rapidly progressive glomerulonephritis (RPGN), diffuse proliferative glomerulonephritis (DPGN), nephrotic syndrome, neuropsychiatric lupus (NPLE); acute confusional state or organ brain syndrome, while pulmonary manifestations included acute lupus pneumonitis, alveolar hemorrhage, etc. Moderate disease: lupus nephritis without renal failure, pleuritis, pericarditis, meningitis, hemolytic anemia, thrombocytopenic purpura, etc. Mild disease: arthralgia/arthritis, myopathy, skin rash, etc.

Nonsteroidal anti-inflammatory drugs	800/1125 (71%)
Steroids (initial dose of steroids) (n=1125)	
no	99 (9%)
PSL ≦ 39mg/day	769 (68%)
PSL 40-59mg/day	133 (12%)
PSL ≧ 60mg/day	124 (11%)
Pulse therapy	171 (15%)
Immunosuppressants	300/1125 (27%)
azathioprine	160 (53%)
6-mercaptoprine	26 (9%)
cyclophosphamide	70 (23%)
mizoribin	32 (11%)
others	12 (4%)
Plasmapheresis	105/953 (11%)
Hemodialysis	25/1125 (2%)

PSL:prednisolone

PSL ≦39mg/day was used for patients with mild or moderate diseases.
PSL 40-59mg/day was used for patients with moderate or severe diseases.
PSL ≧60mg/day was used for patients with severe diseases. Pulse therapy was used for patients with severe diseases followed by large doses of steroids.

Table 2. Treatments of 1125 SLE patients

Treatments including steroids and immunosuppressive agents are shown in Table 2. Steroids were a mainstay of treatment for SLE. Although there are several kinds of steroids, prednisolone (PSL) is commonly used to treat SLE. The initial dose of steroids was usually determined according to the severity and activity of the disease. The above severe diseases required large doses of steroids usually of 1 mg/kg/day of PSL or more. Sometimes steroid pulse therapy (methylprednisolone 0.5-1g/day, intravenously administration, for 3days) was used followed by large doses of steroids. The above moderate to mild diseases usually required 0.5-1mg/kg/day and less than 0.5mg/kg/day of PSL, respectively. When a satisfactory response was achieved, the daily dose was reduced by 5 to 10% over 2 or 3 weeks until reaching a maintenance dose of 0.2 to 0.3mg/kg/day.

Steroids have sometimes little or no effect because of impaired bioavailability due to reduced steroid absorption, increased steroid metabolism, induction of activating protein 1(AP-1) which is mutually antagonistic with steroid receptors for trans-activation effects [8], and insensitive steroid-mediated apoptosis of T cells [9], etc. Furthermore, steroids characteristically have a high risk of serious side effects such as infection, gastric ulcer, diabetes mellitus, osteoporosis, etc. Therefore, the effectiveness and usefulness of steroids were limited because of severe side effects, unresponsiveness and resistance to steroids. In these situations, immunosuppressive agents such as cyclophosphamide, azathioprine, mizoribine, tacrolimus and/or plasmapheresis or other innovative therapies were usually used in conjunction with steroids. Recently, belimumab (anti-BLyS antibody), the first targeted biological drug, was approved for treatment of SLE by the FDA [10]. Targeted biological and small-molecule therapies in SLE are going to begin to take the place of steroids that have been used as the major drug in SLE for more than 50 years.

2.3. Prognosis and causes of death

In this paper, the survival rate was 93% at 5years, 89% at 10years and 69% at 20years after diagnosis. One hundred and fifty-one out of 1,125 patients (13%) died. The causes of death were renal failure (30%), cerebrovascular diseases (23%), infection (19%), and others. Infections which led to causes of death included sepsis or bacteremia due to E. coli, methicillin resistant Staphylococcus aureus (MRSA), candidiasis, asprgilosis, Klebsiella, Pseudomonas, etc., and tuberculosis, pneumocyctis carini pneumonia, Cryptococcus meningitis, listeria meningitis, cytomegalovirus infection, etc. In the last 2 or 3 decades it has been noted that the prognosis of SLE has improved [11-13]. Changes in the mortality rate in accordance with the cause of death in SLE patients were also observed, showing a significant reduction in death due to renal failure.

3. Steroid therapy in principal organ involvement in SLE

3.1. Lupus nephritis (LN)

3.1.1. Clinical analysis of LN

LN is one of the diseases influencing the prognosis of SLE. The diseases of LN vary from mild to severe and from active to inactive. The clinical pictures of LN and the types of the World Health Organization (WHO) classification according to histopathological findings [14] in this study are shown in Table 3.

Persistent proteinuria of more than 0.2g/day and less than 3.5g/day was observed in approximately 37% of cases and profuse proteinuria of more than 3.5g per day was observed in approximately 17% of cases. Patients without proteinuria accounted for 16%. Abnormal urinary sediments including erythrocytes, leukocytes and casts were observed frequently. An increasing serum creatinine level was observed in 41% of cases. The WHO classification according to histopahological findings of LN by renal biopsy was used in this study, although the classification of LN by the International Nephrology/Renal Pathology Society (ISN/RPS) was proposed in 2003[15]. Diffuse proliferative glomerulonephritis (DPGN) of Type IV, which has a poor prognosis, could be seen in 55 of 216 cases (25%), which underwent renal biopsy. Membranous glomerulonephritis (MGN) of Type V characteristic of nephrotic syndrome, was observed in 18% of cases. Types I and II, which are thought to have better prognosis, were observed in 23% and 16% of cases, respectively. Advanced Type VI, which indicates end stage GN, could be seen in 12% of cases.

A. Urinalysis, Renal function	n=1125 (%)
No proteinuria	176 (16)
Proteinuria	949 (84)
Intermittent	431 (45)
Persistent	354 (37)
Profuse (>3.5g/day)	164 (17)
Microhematuria	1066 (95)
Urine casts	838 (74)
Elevated BUN	659/1063 (62)
Elevated S-creatinine	429/1047 (41)
B. Histopathological findings (WHO classification)	n=216 (%)
I. Minimal change (MC) or Normal	49 (23)
II. Mesagial alteration	34 (16)
III. Focal segmental glomerulonephritis (FGN)	35 (16)
IV. Diffuse proliferative glomerulonephritis (DPGN)	55 (25)
V. Membranous glomerulonephritis (MGN)	39 (18)
VI. Advanced	4 (12)

Table 3. Lupus nephritis in 1125 cases

3.1.2. Treatment of LN

The available therapeutic procedures include steroids, immunosuppressive agents, plasmapheresis, anticoagulants and hemodialysis, etc. Steroids were the first choice for treatment of LN. However, doses of steroids were determined according to urinary findings, renal function and renal histopathological findings evaluating the activity and severity of LN. The patients with active and /or severe LN, including persistent or profuse proteinuria, renal dysfunction, DPGN of type IV, rapidly progressive glomerulonephritis (RPGN) or MGN of Type V in conjunction with low serum complement levels and high titers of anti-dsDNA antibodies, were initially treated with large doses of steroids (PSL 1-1.5mg/kg/day) as induction therapy for remission. Steroid pulse therapy was often administered at first. It led to more rapid recovery which might be result of a rapid nongenomic physicochemical effect. The patients with intermittent proteinuria, abnormal urine sediments, and Type II or III, were initially treated with PSL less than 0.5-1mg/kg/day. After PSL administration for 3-6 weeks, the dosage of PSL was then reduced by nearly 10% every 2–3 weeks according to the improvement in proteinuria, urinary sediments, abnormal renal function, low serum complement levels and high titers of anti-dsDNA antibodies. If PSL had no or incomplete response, the dosage was increased by 20% or steroid pulse therapy was conducted again. In the patients with DPGN or RPGN, intravenous pulse therapy of cyclophosphamide (IVCY) (500-750mg, monthly for 3 to 6 months), as immunosuppressive agent, was used. Alternative induction therapies included combined therapies with steroids and immunosuppressive agents such as daily oral cyclophosphamide, azathioprine, tacrorimus, mizoribine, and cyclosporine, etc. If an incomplete response after 2 months treatment with

PSL alone was also observed, immunosuppressant agents were administered in addition to PSL. If the patients had high titers of anti-dsDNA antibodies and/or immune complexes, plasmapheresis was conducted in conjunction with the above steroid and immunosuppressant agent treatment. In patients who achieved remission showing less than 0.5g/day of proteinuria, inactive urine sediment, normal complement levels and /or quiescent extrarenal lupus activity, they continued maintenance treatment with a maintenance dosage of steroids of PSL 5–15mg/day. Thereafter, the PSL dosage was tapered to discontinuance in an extremely gradual manner.

3.1.3. Outcome and prognosis of LN

During the past half century, the prognosis of SLE has significantly improved. One of the major factors in this improvement is the significant reduction in renal death. This is assumed to be partially due to early diagnosis and early treatment with the development of diagnostic procedures, as well as the development of treatments including the implementation of hemodialysis [1,11-13]. However, the remission rate of lupus nephritis was not so high.

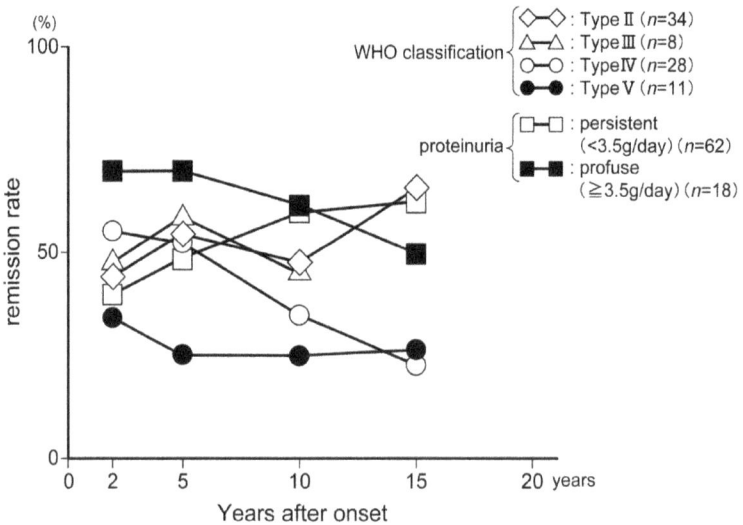

Figure 1. Remission rate of lupus nephritis according the WHO classification type and degree of proteinuria

Figure 1 shows the remission rate after onset according to the WHO classification type and degree of proteinuria. The remission rates of patients with Type IV (DPGN) and profuse peroteiniria or nephrotic syndrome tended to decrease during the course of the disease, while the remission rates of patients with Type II and persistent proteinuria tended to increase. Patients with Type V (MGN) had a low remission rate through out the course of the disease, but no decrease in the remission rate was observed until later on. Furthermore, in the outcome of 32 patients who were treated over the long-term for over 20 years, the complete remission rate was 27%, the incomplete remission rate was 37.8%, and the worsening rate was 21.6 %. As for the treatments used, those that contributed to remission could not be specified. This fact suggests that the underlying disease types had a greater influence on the remission rate than the treatment method.

3.2. Neuropsychiatric manifestations of SLE (NPLE)

3.2.1. Clinical analysis of NPLE

The frequencies of various neuropsychiatric manifestations of SLE (NPLE) have been reported to vary from 28 to 59%. In our study, NPLE could be observed in 47.6% of 1,125 cases as shown in Table 4.

Total SLE patients	1125
The number of patients with NPLE	535 (48%)
1. Neurological manifestations	
1) seizure, unconsciousness	146 (13%)
2) cerebrovascular disease	158 (14%)
3) neuropathy, cranial	45 (4%)
4) myelopathy	45 (4%)
5) aseptic meninngitis	45 (4%)
6) peripheral neuropathy	79 (7%)
7) headache	101 (9%)
2. Neuropsychological syndromes	236 (21%)

Table 4. Frequencies of neuropsychiatric manifestations (NPLE) in 1125 lupus patients

The American College of Rheumatology (ACR) proposed new criteria for the classification of neuropsychiatric syndrome of systemic lupus erythematosus (NPSLE) in 1999 [16]. NPLE is divided into psychiatric and neurological manifestations. The frequency of psychiatric manifestations was higher than that of neurological manifestations. The former included acute confusional state or organ brain syndrome, cognitive dysfunction, anxiety disorders and psychosis, etc., while the latter included seizure, cerebrovascular disease, myelopathy, aseptic meningitis, headache, and peripheral neuropathy, etc.

Although no single pathogenetic process could explain all these manifestations, it was assumed that other potential causes of these manifestations, such as side effects from treatment, complications including infections, etc., had been excluded except for causes due to lupus itself. Many NPLE cases were considered to be caused by lupus itself, excluding obvious causes such as antiphospholipid antibody syndrome (APS), necrotizing angiitis, and complications.

NPLE is one of the diseases that influence the prognosis of SLE as well as LN. Especially, patients with acute confusional state or organ brain syndrome (OBS), cognitive dysfunction, recurrent seizure, and cerebrovascular disease, etc., had poor prognosis. Acute OBS exhibits characteristic malfunctions such as consciousness disorders (i.e. delirium), disorientation, memory disorders, and cognitive dysfunction. Acute OBS showed an 85% correlation with SLE activity and exacerbation, which was greater than that of the psychiatric illness group (57%) and the psychosyndrome group (23%) [17].

Although acute OBS was correlated with active SLE lesions, correlations with high titers of anti-dsDNA antibodies and low complement levels, which were seen in active LN, were not necessarily observed. Serologically, acute OBS correlated with the serum anti-liposomal P antibody, interferon α and IL-6 in cerebrospinal fluid (CSF) [18-19].

On the other hand, acute neurologic syndrome has been reported to correlate with the anti-asialo GM1 antibody, anti-liposomal P antibody, anti-lymphocyte antibody, and anti-neurocyte antibody, as well as the anti-PCNA antibody and anti-Sm antibody [7,20].

Psychiatric symptoms often required differentiation from steroidal psychiatric symptoms. Differentiation from secondary psychiatric symptoms due to uremia and/or infection was also important. Although quite a number of cases were difficult to determine, the following information might have been helpful:

a.   The actual incidence of steroid-induced psychosis is small, probably about 5%, which is less than that of lupus-induced psychosis [21].
b.   The psychiatric side effects of steroids include, most commonly, mild to moderate mood changes such euphoria, sleeplessness, or depression rather than unconsciousness disorders, although there are also perceptual changes, hallucinations, anxiety, insomnia and confusion.
c.   Steroid-induced psychosis appears half a month to one month after administration of steroids. It has been reported that the incidence of steroid-induced psychosis increases when over 40mg/day of PSL is administered [22].
d.   Although lupus psychosis may not always be improved by increasing of the dosage of PSL, deterioration of lupus psychosis after increasing the dosage of PSL is rare.
e.   High levels of IgG index and IL-6 in CSF can be seen in lupus psychosis [23].

The evaluation of NPLE should always include an assessment of whether SLE is active or not. In addition, patients with both focal and diffuse syndromes should have various examinations including CSF, electroencephalogram (EEG), and an imaging studies (such as computed tomography (CT) and magnetic resonance imaging (MRI)), cerebral blood flow by angiography or single photon emission computerized tomography (SPECT), etc. The more serious the NPLE, the more aggressive immunosuppressive therapy, including steroids, is needed.

3.2.2. Treatment of NPLE

If NPLE was active and there was severe major organ involvement, steroid therapy was indicated. In particular, patients with an acute confusional state or organic brain syndrome, and recurrent convulsive seizures were treated with high steroid doses (PSL 1–2 mg/kg/day) in conjunction with steroid pulse therapy. However, when improvement could not be seen within 48 hours after treatment, 250 to 500mg of hydrocortone was administered every 12 hours. If improvement could not be seen after treatment of steroids alone, IVCP pulse therapy or oral administration of CP in conjunction with steroids and/or plasmapheresis was given.

When signs of clinical manifestations were stable for more than 6 weeks and acute phase reactants or tests of organ function were improved or stable for 6 weeks, the dose of PSL was reduced by approximately 10 to 20% every two weeks. When the dose of PSL reached about 15mg/day, it was slowly tapered and reduced by 1mg every week.

When the patients showed panic or marked agitation and their hallucinations and delusions were threatening, several antipsychotic drugs in conjunction with steroids were also used.

3.2.3. Outcome and prognosis of NPLE

Almost all patients with NPLE improved after immunosuppressive therapies including steroids, immunosuppressive drugs and /or plasmapheresis.

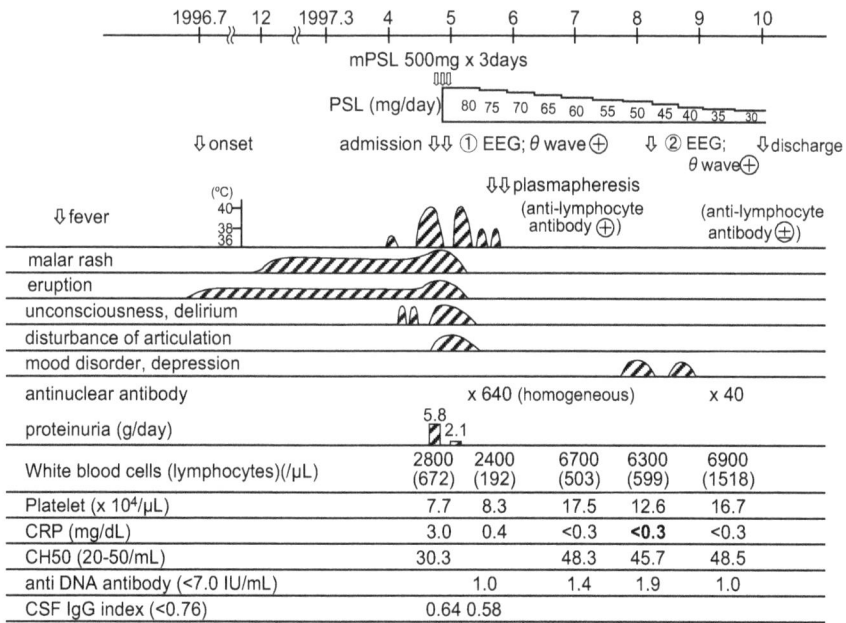

PSL: prednisolone, mPSL: methylprednisolone, EEG: electroencephalogram, CSF: cerebrospinal fluid.

Figure 2. The clinical course of SLE patient (46 years old, female) with organic brain syndrome (OBS)

Figure 2 shows the clinical course of an SLE patient with OBS who was a 46-year old female. She was diagnosed as SLE with malar rash, eruption, leucopenia, thrombocytopenia, proteinuria and positive anti-nuclear antibodies, etc. in March 1997. In April 1997, she had recurrent unconsciousness with delirium, disturbance of articulation with high fever and a worsening malar rash. Although anti-DNA antibodies and low complemetemia could not be seen, she was diagnosed as OBS or acute confusional state and treatment with steroid pulse therapy followed by a PSL dose of 80mg/day. Plasmapheresis was also conducted to remove anti-lymphocyte antibodies. Although mood disorder and depression were observed in August, 1997, her disease improved without increasing doses of steroids or additional treatment with immunosuppressive agents.

As for prognosis of lupus patients with NPLE according to the different treatment, patients treated with combined therapy of steroid pulse therapy and other therapies was significantly more favorable than those treated with steroids alone (PSL>40mg/day) and those treated with combined therapy of immunosuppressive agents and steroids.

3.3. Pulmonary manifestations

3.3.1. Pleuritis

Pleuritis is by far the most common pulmonary manifestation, occurring at some time in the course in 40 to 50% of lupus patients. However, the frequency of pleuritis in Japanese SLE patiens was lower than that in European countries and the United States. The frequency of pleuritis was 11% in this study. . Clinically, fever, chest pain, cough, dyspnea etc. could be seen in patients with pleuritis. On chest X-rays, slight to moderate pleural effusion caused by pleural inflammation could be observed bilaterally in approximately half of cases.

Pleuritis mostly improved after administration of PSL (20-40mg/day). However, in cases with a large amount of pleural effusion , thoracic drainage was needed.

3.3.2. Interstitial pneumonitis

Lupus pneumonitis is classified as acute lupus pneumonitis and chronic interstitial pneumonitis/pulmonary fibrosis. Acute lupus pneumonitis was relatively rare with an occurrence of 0.5–11.7% [24-25]. It was observed in 6 of 1,125 patients (0.5%) in this study. As clinical symptoms, fever, chest pain, dry cough, severe dyspnea, and occasional hemoptysis were noted. Bibasilar Velcro rales were noted in all instances. The majority of patients were hypoxic, requiring supplemental oxygen or intubation for assisted ventilation. Acute lupus pneumonitis was diagnosed by several examinations including X-ray, CT scan, KL-6 and/or SP-D as biomarkers, and various kinds of infectious examination to exclude infectious diseases.

All 6 patients with acute lupus pneumonitis were treated with steroid pulse therapy following 1-2mg/kg/day of PSL. Half of the patients drastically improved, but the remaining

3 patients died of pulmonary hemorrhage despite combined therapy with steroid and immunosuppressant agents and /or plasmapheresis.

Chronic interstitial pneumonitis in SLE is also rare, showing a low frequency of 3-5%. Six patients with chronic interstitial pneumonitis were observed in this study and they were treated with maintenance therapies including low doses of steroids and/or immunosuppressant agents. In one patient, chronic interstitial pneumonitis deteriorated to acute interstitial pneumonitis during the course of the disease and a large dose of steroids was needed

3.3.3. Alveolar hemorrhage

Alveolar hemorrhage in SLE is relatively rare, and it has been reported to occur in 1.4–1.7% of SLE patients in Europe and the United States [26].

It is a serious complication and results in poor prognosis. It was observed in 8 out of 1,125 patients (0.7%) in this study.

SLE patients with alveolar hemorrhage had hemoptysis and hypoxemia and rapid progression of anemia in conjunction with active LN and/or NSLE disease.

All patients with alveolar hemorrhage were treated with steroid pulse therapy following large doses of PSL, but it was also necessary to concomitantly use other immunosuppressive tharapies such as cyclophosphamide including IVCY, and plasmapheresis. Unfortunately, all of the patients with alveolar hemorrhage died, comfirming that the prognosis was very poor.

3.4. Cardiac manifestations

3.4.1. Pericarditis

The most common cardiac abnormality was pericarditis, which occured in 8-25% [27], but it was relatively rare in Japan, with a frequency of 7% (47 out of 1,125cases) in this study. Pericarditis is often one of the first manifestations. Most of the cases with pericarditis improved with administration of PSL 0.5–1 mg/day, but cases with cardiac tamponade, which was rare in this study, needed large doses of PSL over 1mg/day and/or steroid pulse therapy.

3.4.2. Myocarditis

Myocarditis was rarely observed in 2% in this study. In cases with myocarditis, positive CRP, elevated CK, IgG class anti-dsDNA antibodies, hematuria, etc., in conjunction with tachycardia, cardiac enlargement, congestive heart failure could often be observed. A myocardial biopsy was performed in order to confirm the diagnosis in one patient. The patients with myocarditis associated with congestive heart failure were treated with large-dose administration of steroids (PSL 1–1.5 mg/kg/day, divided into 3~4 dosages). All of the patients with myocarditis improved after steroid therapy.

3.4.3. Myocardial infarction and coronary artery disease

Coronary artery disease due to arteriosclerotic changes is more common in SLE patients. Death from myocardial infarction late in the course of the disease is one of the most frequent causes of death after 10 to 30 years of SLE [28]. Eleven lupus patients with myocardial infarction could be seen in this study. The average age at diagnosis of SLE was 37 years old (26–63 years old), and the average age at development of myocardial infarction was 51 years old (41–66 years old) in these patients. There were two death cases, including one case of death from cardiac rupture.

Several risk factors that cause myocardial infarction due to atherosclerosis in SLE are considered. They are renal involvement, hypertension, hyperlipidemia, long-term administration of steroids, diabetes mellitus, anti-phospholipid syndrome, smoking, etc. In this study, 4 patients had hypertension, hyperlipemia and diabetes mellitus as risk factors. Furthermore, positive antiphospholipid antibodies were observed in 5 cases. Death from myocardial infarction due to inflammation of the coronary arteries has been reported in SLE patients dying early in the course of their disease, but this is a rare event [28].

Regarding the treatment in this study, conservative medical management without large doses of steroids was used in most cases. PTCA and AC bypass procedures were also occasionally conducted.

3.5. Intestinal vasculitis

Acute abdomen caused by intestinal vasculitis is often observed. Occasionally, surgery is needed. According to a report by Zizic, et al. [29], acute abdomen was observed in 15 of 140 cases, and caused death in 53% of cases. Vasculitis was observed in 9 of 11 cases with abdominal surgery, and intestinal perforation was observed in 6 cases. In this study, 4 patients had intestinal vasculitis and 3 died of intestinal perforation. Intestinal bleeding and peritoneal bleeding due to vasculitis were often observed. In cases with mesenteric arteritis, acute abdomen with severe abdominal pain in conjunction with nausea/vomiting, diarrhea, ascites, gastrointestinal bleeding, and fever, etc., were observed. Those symptoms may be masked by steroids or immunosuppressive drugs used for treatment, thus resulting in a delayed diagnosis.

Patients with intestinal vasculitis and/or mesenteric arteritis were treated with large dose steroids including steroid pulse therapy.

When a rapid improvement was not obtained, intermittent IVCY therapy was simultaneously used. In cases associated with bowel infarction or perforation, treatment for infection was also needed.

3.6. Hematologic manifestations

Hematologic manifestations in SLE include normochromic-normocytic anemia caused by chronic inflammation, autoimmune hemolytic anemia (AIHA), iron-deficiency anemia, leukocytopenia, lymphocytopenia, thrombocytopenia, thrombocytopenic purpura (TP), thrombotic thrombocytopenic purpura (TTP), and antiphosphlipid syndrome (APS), etc. The diseases, which needed high doses of steroids were AIHA, TP, and TTP.

3.6.1. AIHA

AIHA was observed in 11% of patients in this study. AIHA is rare in Japanese SLE patients in comparison to those in Europe and the United States. Steroids were the mainstay of the treatment for AIHA and a response was achieved in about 75% of patients. PSL was given initially at a dose of 1.0 to1.5mg/kg and continued at that level for at least 4 to 6 weeks. Following a satisfactory response, the dose was reduced gradually by 10% every week. The reticlocyte count was a reliable indicator of both responsiveness to treatment and relapse. In cases of severe fulminant hemolysis, steroid pulse therapy was conducted. Patients with AIHA who failed to respond to steroids were treated with immunosuppressant agents and/or splenectomy. Plasmapheresis, high-dose intravenous gammagloburin therapy (IVIg), and danazole were also used for some refractory cases.

3.6.2. TP

Thrombocytopenia lower than 150,000 was observed in 34% of cases in this study. However, thrombocytopenia lower than 50,000 was relatively rare, and it occured in approximately 10% of cases. Thrombocytopenia in SLE is usually due to antiplatelet autoantibodies (platelet associate-IgG; PA-IgG, platelet binding-IgG; PB-IgG). In some cases, thrombocytopenia was associated with antiphospholipid antibodies. In rare case, so-called Evans syndrome, in which AIHA and TP coexist, was observed. Some cases did not tend to bleed until platelet counts were less than 20,000/ul. Patients with thrombocytopenia less than 20,000 were treated with large doses of steroids. The initial dose of PSL was usually 1-2mg /kg/day. After an increase in platelet count occurred in response to steroids, the dose was gradually reduced after 4 weeks. If thrombocytopenia did not respond to steroids with bleeding from the major organs such as gastrointestinal tract, kidney, bladder, other mucosal surface, steroid pulse therapy was used. IVIg was useful to achieve a temporary improvement in thrombocytopenia in surgical operations such as splenectomy, which was often conducted in steroid resistant cases. .In steroid resistant cases, immunosuppressive drugs such as azathioprine, cyclophosphamide, and cyclosporine, danazol, and vincristine, etc., were also used.

3.6.3. TTP

TTP usually consists of a pentad of TP, microangiopathic hemolytic anemia, fever, renal failure, and neurologic manifestations. TTP has been reported in association with various other diseases, including SLE, most of which are characterized by some degree of vasculitis of the small vessels and circulating immune complexes [30]. The main cause of acquired TTP including SLE is assumed to be an autoantibody that is an inhibitor (IgG inhibitor) of von Willebrand factor cleaving protease [31]. It has been clarified that congenital TTP is caused by a mutation in the *ADAMTS-13* gene of cleaving protease. TTP must be differentiated from DIC or catastrophic antiphospholipid syndrome, but coexistence of both are often observed.

Regarding treatment, plasmapheresis using fresh frozen plasma, and transfusion therapy of normal plasma are used. In addition, large-doses of steroids including steroid pulse therapy, immunosuppressive drugs, IVIg therapy, and anti-platelet drugs, etc. are simultaneously used.

3.7. Pregnancy and birth

When an SLE patient wished to conceive and give birth, a medical determination as to whether pregnancy would be possible was considered. Basically, there were presumed to be almost no problems in pregnancy when the patient was in remission with a maintenance dosage of steroids, and when serious organ failure was not observed. Moreover, even if the patient had active disease, pregnancy was allowed after the disease improved with treatment.

3.7.1. Treatment and management during pregnancy

It was important for the physician and the gynecologist to be in close communication for the treatment and management during pregnancy. Usually, it was unnecessary to change the maintenance dose of the steroid during pregnancy. When mild deterioration was observed in the early stage of pregnancy, an increased steroid dosage was attempted according to the clinical manifestations. If the clinical manifestations required administration of a large-dose of steroids, considering the risks to the mother and the effect of the steroids on the fetus, an artificial abortion was performed at an early stage. Although the level of serum cortisol in the fetus decreases during the steroid administration, cortisol secretion and response to ACTH are believed to remain normal [32]. If a mother is treated with prednisolone or hydrocortisone, these steroids are assumed to have a minimal effect on the fetus because they are inactivated by 11-β-dehydrogenase in the placenta. However, the use of dexamethasone and betamethasone is avoided because these steroids are difficult for the enzyme to inactivate and were assumed to have an adverse effect on the fetus.

3.7.2. Treatment and management during and after deliverly

3.7.2.1. Prevention of exacerbation

The mother was hospitalized prior to the expected delivery date for management of the mother and fetus. If pregnancy remained steady, and SLE activity was not observed, the dose of steroids was increased immediately after delivery to prevent any exacerbation of SLE. The dose of steroids was usually increased to two or three times the pre-delivery dose. The dose was reduced by 10% every 4 to 7 days while confirming no exacerbation, and continually observed until eventually reducing it to the dosage at the time of delivery. If an exacerbation of SLE such as active LN or serositis was observed in the late stage of pregnancy, the delivery of the fetus was attempted as early as possible in order to start treatment of the mother's clinical manifestations.

3.7.2.2. Breast-feeding

Because the amount of steroids was increased upon delivery, breast-feeding was prohibited until the dose was reduced to less than 20 mg of PSL, considering the rate of transfer of steroids (0.1–0.3%/day) to the mother's milk [33].

3.8. Adverse effects and complications due to steroid treatment

Side effects of prolonged treatment with oral steroids are well known. Changes in the physical appearance could usually be seen. They were acne, hirsutism, moon face, buffalo hump, obesity, and abdominal striae, etc. Although reversible with a discontinuation or reduction in dose, hypertension, peptic ulcer, diabetes mellitus, pancreatitis, osteoporosis, psychosis, etc. were also induced. Thinning of the skin, cataracts, glaucoma, osteoporosis, and osteonecrosis could be observed as irreversible side effects.

Infections were major complications in SLE and one of the major causes of death. Susceptibility to infection, particularly bacterial infection, was increased with steroid use. Staples et al. found that the infection rate in hospitalized patients increased from 0.43 to 1.63 per 100 hospital days with an increase in steroid dose from zero to more than 50mg/day [34]. Although infection rarely occurs with a small dose of PSL (2–10 mg/day), the SLE patients treated with PSL of more than 20mg/day have a higher risk of infection due to the higher dose of PSL, especially after 14 days of administration. PSL was also noted to be a major risk factor for the development of opportunistic infection, with the most common organisms including Salmonella, Candida, Strongyloides, and Aspergillus.sp according to a case controlled study of 797 SLE patients [35].

It has been noted that systemic administration of steroids could be linked to the higher occurrence of vascular diseases such as coronary artery disease, stroke, peripheral vascular disease than the expected occurrence in SLE. However, it is unclear whether this reflects pro-atherogenic effects of the underlying disease process or adverse metabolic effects associated with steroid use [36]. Recently, the number of patients with complications such as myocardial infarction/angina pectoris, cerebral infarction, diabetes mellitus, hypertension, and aseptic bone necrosis, has tended to increase over a long-term observation period due to a favorable SLE prognosis.

Table 5 shows the frequencies of these complications at the time of occurence in 97 SLE patients who had been observed for over 20 years. The number of patients with myocardial infarction/angina pectoris, diabetes, cerebral infarction increased from the ninth year of the observation period. Hypertension and aseptic osteonecrosis were seen from the onset of SLE. Most of the above complications were thought to be due to treatment including steroids, as well as aging. It was also noted that GC-associated damage accumulated over time to constitute most of the damage at 15 years, although disease –activity related damage occurred early [37].

Years after diagnosis (yrs)	1-2	3-4	5-8	9-12	13-16	17-20	>21
Myocardial infarction				1			3
Angina pectoris			1		1		2
Diabetes mellitus				3	1	3	5
Cerebral infarction				1	3	3	4
Hypertension	10	9	5	8	4	5	10
Aseptic osteonecrosis	1	3	5	1	4	3	3

yrs: years, number: cases

Table 5. Frequencies of complications related to vascular diseases according to the year (s) of the occurrence in 97 SLE patients who had been observed for over 20 years

Steroid use contributes significantly to risk of osteoporosis in women with SLE. Ramsey-Goldman et al. surveyed the frequency of fractures and associated risk factores in702 women with SLE who had been followed for 5951 person-years and found that fractures occurred in 12.3% of patients, an almost fivefold increase compared with a background population [38]. Older age at diagnosis and longer duration of steroid use were important valuables. Sinigaglia, et al. reported that osteoporosis in 22.6% of 84 premenopousal patients with SLE according to bone mineral density (BMD) was observed, and both disease duration and glucocorticoids were associated risks [39]. Steroid–induced osteoporosis leading to fracture, particularly vertebral collapse, was a major problem.

Aseptic osteonecrosis (AON) was observed in approximately 10% of SLE, with the femoral head being a common site. It also appeared in the femoral condyle, caput humeri, proximal end and distal end of the tibia, etc.. It has been suggested that increased doses of steroids (especially in the first year of treatment) and the duration of steroid therapy are correlated with a grater risk of AON in SLE patients [40]. In a prospective survey of SLE patients with administration of high-dose steroids (more than 30 mg/day of PSL for more than one month), AON occurred in 15% (9/62 patients) and the average period from the administration of a large dose of steroids to onset of AON was 640 days [41].

4. Conclusion

In this paper, steroid therapy for SLE based on the clinical analysis of 1,125 cases, especially for principal organ involvement that required large doses of steroids, was evaluated. Although there is no doubt that steroids contribute to a significant improvement in the prognosis in SLE, the effectiveness and usefulness of steroids are limited because of severe side effects, unresponsiveness and resistance to steroids.

Now, new biological agents that target B cells, T-B cell interaction, co-stimulatory pathways, intracellular molecules, etc. are being developed and are going to begin to revolutionize nonspecific therapy to a more specific pathophysiological tharapy in SLE.

Author details

Hiroshi Hashimoto
Professor Emeritus,
Aiwakai Medical Corporation, Bajikouen Clinic, Rheumatology, Tokyo, Japan

5. References

[1] Wallace DJ, Dubois EL (1987) Prognostic subsets, natural course, and causes of death in systemic lupus erythematosus, In: Wallace DJ, Dubois EL editors. Dubois' Lupus Erythematosus, 3rd ed. Lea & Febiger, Philadelphia, pp580

[2] Hochberg MC (1997) Updating the American College of Rheumatology revised criteria for the classification of systemic lupus erythematosus. Arthritis Rheum 40:1725 (letter)

[3] Wallace DJ (2007) The clinical presentation of systemic lupus erythematosus. In: Wallece DJ, Hahn BH editors. Dubois' Lupus Erythematosus. 7th ed. Lippincott Williams & Willkins, Philadelphia, pp638

[4] McGehee HA, Shulman LE, Tumulty AP, et al (1954) Systemic lupus erythematosus: review of the literature and clinical analysis of 138 cases. Medicine 33: 291-437

[5] Dubois EL, Tuffanelli DL (1964) Clinical manifestations of systemic lupus erythematosus. Computer analysis of 520 cases, JAMA 190: 104-111

[6] Pistiner M, Wallace DJ, Nessim S, et al (1991) Lupus erythematosus in the 1980s: a survey of 570 patients. Semin Arthritis Rheum 21: 55-64

[7] Hashimoto, H, Hirose S, Kano S, et al (1992) Studies on clinical subsets and severity of systemic lupus erythematosus based on a 1987 questionnaire conducted in Japan-Clinical analysis of the outcome and treatments in clinical subsets. Rhumachi 32: 27-38

[8] Wilder BL (1997) Glucocorticoids, In: Koopman WJ, editor. Arthritis and Allied Conditioins. 13th ed. Wiliams & Willkins, Baltimore, pp731

[9] Seki M, Ushiyama C, Seta N, et al (1998) Apoptosis of lymphocytes induced glucocorticoids and relationship to therapeutic efficacy in patients with systemic lupus erythematosus. Arthritis Rheum 41: 823-830

[10] Navarra SV, Guzman RM, Gallacher AE, et al (2011) Efficacy and safety of belimumab in patients with active systemic lupus eryhematosus: a randomized, placebo-controlled, phase 3 trial. Lancet 9767: 721-731

[11] Gladman DD, Urowitz MB (2007) Prognosis, mortality and morbidity in systemic lupus erythematosus. In: Wallace DJ, Hahn BH, editors. Dubois' Lupus Erythematosus, 7th ed. Lippincott Williams & Willkins, Philadelphia, pp1333

[12] Hashimoto H, Shiokawa Y (1978) Changing pattern of clinical features and prognosis in systemic lupus erythematosus. Scand J Rheumatol 7: 219-224

[13] Hashimoto H, Sugawara M, Tokano Y, et al. (1993) Follow up study on the changes in the clinical features and prognosis of Japanese patients with systemic lupus erythematosus during the past 3 to 4 decades. J Epidemiol 3:19-27

[14] D'Agati VD, Appel GB (2007) Lupus nephritis: pathology and pathogenesis. In: Wallace DJ, Hahn BH, editors, Dubois' Lupus Erythematosus, 7th ed.Lippincott Williams & Wilkins, Philadelphia, pp1094

[15] Weening JJ, D'Agati VD, Schwartz MM, et al (2004) The classification of glomerulonephritis in systemic lupus erythematosus revisited. Kidney Int 65: 521-530

[16] ACR Ad Hoc Committee on Neuropsychiatric Lupus Nomenclature (1999) The American College of Rheumatology nomenclature and case definitions for neuropsychiatric lupus syndromes. Arthritis Rheum 42: 599-608

[17] Akazawa S (1986) Psychiatric syndrome in systemic lupus erythematosus-study on 82 cases. Seishinigaku 28: 661-670(in Japanese)

[18] Schneebaum AB, Singleton JD,West SG, et al(1991)Association of psychiatric manifestations with antibodies to ribosomal-P proteins in systemic lupus erythematosus. Am J Med 90: 54-62

[19] Hirohata S, Iwamoto S, Sugiyama H, et al(1988) A patient with systemic lupus erythematosus presenting both central nervous system lupus and steroid induced psychosis. J Rheumatol 15: 706-710

[20] Bertsias G, Loannidis JPA, Bombardieri S, et al. (2008) EULAR recommendations for the management of systemic lupus erythematosus. Report of a task force of the EULAR standing committee for international clinical studies including therapeutics. Ann Rhum Dis 67:195-205

[21] Hall RCW, Popkin MK, Kirkpatrick B, et al (1978) Tricyclic exacerbation of steroid psychosis. J Nerv Ment Dis 166: 738-742

[22] Hall RCW, Popkin MK, Stickney SK, et al (1979) Presentation of steroid psychosis. J Nerv Ment Dis 167:229-236

[23] Hirohata S, Kanai Y, Mitsuo A, et al.(2009) Accuracy of cerebrospinal fluid IL-6 testing for diagnosis of lupus psychosis. A multienter retrospective study. Clin Rheumatol 28: 1319-1323

[24] D'Cruz D, Khamashta MA, Hughes G (2007) Pulmonary manifestations of systemic lupus erythematosus. In: Wallace DJ, Hahn BH, editors. Dubois' Lupus Erythematosus, 7th ed. Lippincott Williams & Wilkins, Philadelphia, pp678

[25] Matthay RA, Schwartz MI, Petty TL, et al (1975) Pulmonary manifestations of systemic lupus erythematosus: review of twelve cases of acute lupus pneumonitis. Medicine 54:397-409

[26] Baulware DW, hedgpeth MT (1989)Lupus pneumonitis and anti-SSA(Ro) antibodies . J Rheumatol 16: 479-481

[27] Bulkley BH, Roberts WC (1975) The heart in systemic lupus erythematosus and the changes induced in it by corticosteroid therapy. A study of 36 necropsy patients. Am J Med 58: 243-264

[28] Rothfield NF (1996) Cardiac aspects. In; Shur PH, ed. The Clinical Management of Systemic lupus Erythematosus, 2nd ed. Lippincott-Raven, Philadelphia, pp83

[29] Zizic TM, Classen JN, Stevens MB (1982) Acute abdominal complications of systemic lupus erythematosus and polyarteritis nodosa. Am J Med 73: 525-531

[30] Shoenfeld Y, Ehrenfelt M(1996) Hematological manifestations. In;Shur PH, ed.The Clinical Management of Systemic lupus Erythematosus, 2nd ed. Lippincott-Raven, Philadelphia, pp95

[31] Tsai HM, Lian ECY(1998) Antibodies to von Willebrand factor-cleaving protease in acute thrombotic thrombocytopenic purpura. N Eng J Med 339: 1585-1594

[32] Blanford AT, Murphy BE (1977) In vitro metabolism of prednisolone, dexamethasone, betamethasone, and cortisol by the human placenta. Am J Obstet Gynecolo 127: 264-267

[33] Katz FH, Duncan BR (1975)Letter: entry of prednisone into human milk. N Engl J Med 293:1154

[34] Staples PJ, Gerding DN, Decker JL, et al (1974) Incidence of infection in systemic lupus erythematosus. Arthritis Rheum 17: 110

[35] Ritchin C, Dobro J, Senie R, etl. (1989) Opportunistic infections in patients with systemic lupus erythematosus (abstract). Arthritis Rheum 32(Suppl):S115

[36] Wei L, MacDonald T, Walker B (2004) Taking glucocorticoids by prescription is associated with subsequent cardiovascular disease. Ann Intern Med 141:764-770,

[37] Gladman DD, Urowitz MB, Rahman P, et al. (2003) Accrual of organ damage over time in patients with systemic lupus erythematosus. J Rheumatol 30:1955-1959

[38] Ramsey-Goldman R, Dunn JE, Huang CF, et al (1999) Frequency of fractures in women with systemic lupus erythematosus: comparison with United States population data. Arthritis Rheum 42: 882-890

[39] Sinigaglia L, Varenna M, Binelli L, et al (1999) Determinations of bone mass in systemic lupus erythematosus: a cross sectional study on premenopausal women. J Rheumatol 26: 1280-1284

[40] Weiner ES, Abeles (1989) Aseptic necrosis and glucocorticosteroids in systemic lupus erythematosus: reevaluation. J Rheumatol 16: 604-608,

[41] Ono K, Tohjima T, Komazawa T(1992) Risk factors of avascular necrosis of the femoral head in patients with systemic lupus erythematosus under high-dose corticosteroid therapy. Clin Orthop 277: 89-97

Chapter 8

Glucocorticoid Resistance in the Upper Respiratory Airways

Fabiana C.P. Valera, Edwin Tamashiro and Wilma T. Anselmo-Lima

Additional information is available at the end of the chapter

1. Introduction

The nasal mucosa is known to be the first important barrier against inhalants of the respiratory tract. In contrast to initial opinion, this tissue actively interacts with external factors, producing a wide combination of mediators in response to aggressor agents [1]. In this respect, it is easy to understand why the nasal mucosa is predisposed to the development of several chronic inflammatory diseases, with rhinitis and rhinosinusitis being the most common disorders.

According to the ARIA guideline [2], the prevalence of allergic rhinitis has increased in the last years and has been found to be around 25% in Europe [3]. The prevalence of symptoms related to chronic rhinosinusitis is about 15% in the USA, being the second most prevalent chronic condition in the American population [4].

The most common and studied cause of chronic rhinitis is allergic rhinitis (AR) [2]. AR is a nasal inflammatory disease in which the allergen induces IgE-mediated inflammation. The mediators released by the nasal mucosa will finally lead to intense inflammatory cell recruitment (predominantly eosinophils) [5], epithelial metaplasia (more pronounced in perennial AR) [6], and noticeable stromal edema, especially due to the action of matrix metalloproteinases [7]. This response to allergens will finally induce the classical symptoms of AR, such as sneezing, itching, nasal discharge and nasal obstruction. These symptoms considerably impair the quality of life, affecting sleep quality, concentration during work/school, and other daily activities [2].

Chronic rhinosinusitis can be subdivided into two forms: chronic rhinosinusitis without nasal polyps (CRSsNP) and with nasal polyps (CRSwNP). These two entities are almost clinically identical, and it is very difficult to differentiate them based only on nasal symptoms [8]. Both forms present variable degrees of facial pain, decreased sense of smell, nasal discharge and nasal congestion. Clinically, the differentiation of these two entities is made by the detection of nasal polyps by nasal endoscopy. However, the major differences between CRSsNP and CRSwNP concern histology and molecular biomarkers [9]. CRSsNP is characterized by neutrophil recruitment, light edema, increased remodelling [9] and a Th1-subset profile. In contrast, CRSwNP is characterized by an eosinophil recruitment, intense oedema, loose connective tissue and a Th1/Th2 mixed –subset profile, but with remarkable Th2 polarization [8-10].

2. Cellular and molecular knowledge in nasal inflammatory diseases

2.1. Allergic Rhinitis

The development of signs and symptoms that characterize allergic rhinitis (AR) depends on three events: sensitization to an allergen, degranulation of inflammatory mediators after re-exposure to the allergen (early phase) and infiltration of inflammatory cells into the tissue (late phase).

The respiratory nasal mucosa is continuously exposed to several particles that are deposited on the mucous blanket that covers the respiratory epithelium. These antigens are processed by antigen-presenting cells (APCs) such as Langerhans cells, that are later presented to a naïve lymphocyte through a major histocompatibility complex (MHC) class II molecule [11]. For reasons not completely elucidated, naïve lymphocytes (Th0) differentiate into Th2 lymphocytes and produce and release a pool of cytokines characteristic of the Th2 response pattern (IL-3, IL-4, IL-5, IL-9, IL-10, IL-13, GM-CSF). Moreover, the differentiated Th2 lymphocytes stimulate the production of specific IgE by plasmocytes through IL-3 and IL-4, and inhibit the differentiation of Th0 lymphocytes into Th1, as well as its messenger molecules. This selective environment polarized to a Th2 response is typically seen in allergic mechanisms, such as AR, asthma and atopic dermatitis, and in helminthic infections. B cells that recognize the processed antigen and receive appropriate contact signals (CD40-CD40) and molecular stimuli (IL-4, IL-6, IL-10, IL-13) start to produce specific IgE. In the presence of continuous antigen stimulation, B-cells switch from the production of a low-affinity IgE molecule to the production of a high-affinity one [11].

Once high-affinity IgE circulates in the plasma and interstitial fluid, it binds to the Fc receptors. These receptors are present on the surface of mast cells and basophils, and are responsible for activating these cells when exposed to the binomial antibody-pathogen. After mast cells leave the post-capillary venules, they are able to reside in the stroma of the nasal submucosa and intraepithelially, probably by the production of several proteases. Resident mast cells are also able to produce some cytokines related to Th2 polarization (IL-4, IL-5), which in turn can cause an increased cell proliferation and survival time. In allergic mucosa, for instance, mast cells proliferate at a higher rate compared to a non-allergic environment, probably by the effect of Th2 cytokines [12, 13].

In a second phase, after sensitization and priming of resident mast cells with IgE, the respiratory mucosa becomes susceptible to a new exposure. When the specific inspired allergen binds to the complex IgE-mediator cell, massive degranulation of allergic molecules (either already existent and newly synthetized) are released in the extracellular compartment. Histamine is the main molecule released and involved in the early phase of symptoms of AR, but other mediators such as leukotriene, bradykinin, prostaglandins, platelet activating factor, and even some proteases (tryptase and chymase) and cytokines (TNF-α, IL-4, IL-5) also have a role in the development of allergic symptoms [14]. These mediators lead to the classical early symptoms of sneezing, itching, rhinorrhea, and nasal congestion that occur within a few minutes after allergen exposure (5-30 minutes). These symptoms are the consequence of direct actions of these mediators on different resident cells [15]. Glands are stimulated by leukotrienes and chymases to produce and release mucous secretions. Endothelial cells of post-capillary venules are affected by histamine, bradykinin, platelet activating factor and leukotrienes, inducing vasodilatation, increased vascular permeability and cell adhesion. Peripheral sensory endings are stimulated by histamine type 1 receptors on nociceptive type C fibers that generate an uncomfortable sensation of pain and pressure, sneezing and itching [16]. As the nasal mucosa is constantly assaulted by physical and chemical agents, the disruption of some areas facilitates the exposure of allergens to allergic mediator cells.

After the IgE-mediated inflammatory burst triggered by the allergen, some individuals present total clearance of mediators and have complete resolution of symptoms after some minutes. However, a significant percentage (60-70%) of the allergic population develops the late AR response due to the recruitment of inflammatory cells into the nasal mucosa. The increased vascular permeability added to the expression of adhesion molecules (ICAM-1) and production of chemokines, recruits a variety of inflammatory cells that include eosinophils and basophils and, to a lesser extent, neutrophils and other leukocytes.

The late phase typically occurs 4-6 hours after the allergen contact and is clinically represented by the nasal obstruction and congestion caused by mucosal edema. Toxic products of eosinophils, such as eosinophil cationic protein (ECP), major basic protein (MBP), eosinophil-derived neurotoxin and eosinophil peroxidase, are evident during the late phase and are proportional to the eosinophil recruitment. These highly charged proteins bind to proteoglycans and hyaluronic acid and cause cell damage and epithelial detachment. Other important inflammatory mediators involved in the late phase are leukotrienes, histamine, and cytokines of the Th2 response (IL-5, IL-6, GM-CSF) [17, 18]. Interestingly, the recruited eosinophils are able to promote an auto-positive feedback to prolong their survival and recruitment into the tissue, which ultimately leads to an independent eosinophilic inflammation (Figure 1). IL-3, IL-5, and GM-CSF are Th2 cytokines that reduce apoptosis and prolong eosinophil cell survival. Besides, IL-5, eotaxin and RANTES produced by eosinophils and other infiltrated cells recruit even more eosinophils to the inflammatory site, explaining the reason why a chronic allergic inflammation can be seen even when the allergen is not present [19].

Lymphocytes are another group of cells that may play an important role in the late phase of AR. Memory T cells, T-cytotoxic and B cells have been demonstrated to be increased in AR compared to other forms of non-allergic rhinitis and to controls [20].

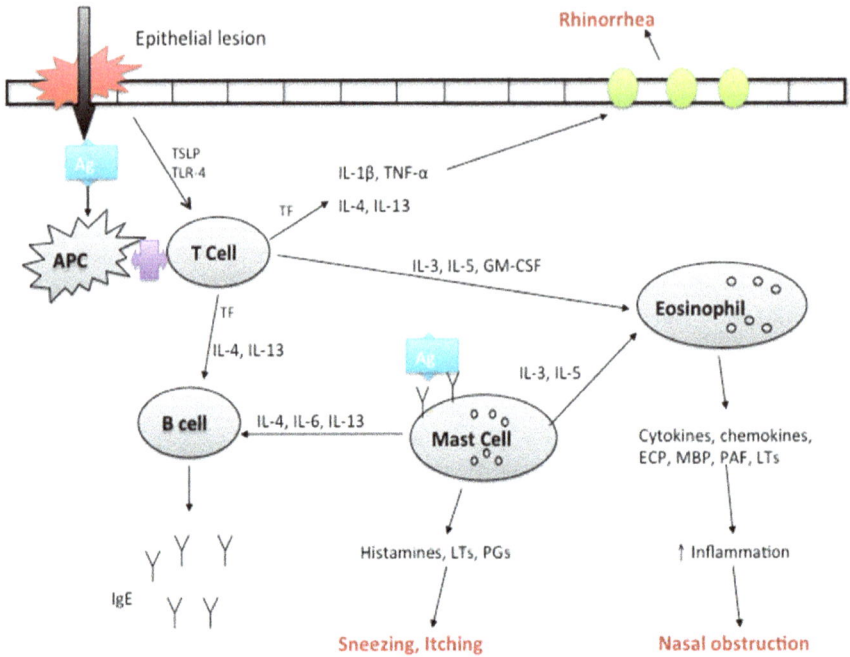

Figure legend: Ag: antigen; APC: antigen presenting cell; TSLP: thymic stromal lymphopoietin; TLR: toll-like receptor; IL: interleukin; TNF: tumor necrosis factor; TF: transcriptor factor; Ig: immunoglobulin; GM-CSF: granulocyte macrophage colony-stimulating factor; LT: leukotriene; PG: prostaglandin; ECP: eosinophil cationic protein; MBP: major basic protein; PAF: platelet activating factor

Figure 1. Cellular and molecular events involved in the early and late phase response of AR. Initially, the antigen invades the cell, and either binds to the APC (antigen presenting cell) or activates innate immune response through TSLP or TLR-4. These mechanisms together will activate adaptive immune response, and T cells are triggered to Th2 response, producing cytokines as IL-4, IL-5 and IL-13. These cytokines will induce epithelial cells to produce rhinorrhea and will recruit inflammatory cells (as eosinophils) to nasal mucosa. Eosinophils will produce several cytokines that will lead to nasal obstruction. B cells are activated and produce IgE, which, among the antigen itself, will induce the mast cell to secrete histamine, leukotrienes and prostaglandins, among others, finally leading to the symptoms of sneezing and itching.

Resident cells may also participate in the late phase and development of chronic allergic inflammation. Nasal epithelial cells express an increased number of pro-inflammatory cytokines such as IL-1α, IL-1β, IL-6, IL-8 and GM-CSF in allergic patients [21, 22]. Also, epithelial cells are the main source of thymic stromal lymphopoietin (TSLP) on the nasal mucosa, an important cytokine that drives T cells to produce Th2 cytokines [23] and is increased in AR patients compared to controls [24]. Submucosal glands located in the lamina propria are substantially increased in allergic patients (25%) compared to non-allergic individuals (15%), consistent with the chronic state of increased production of nasal secretions [25]

In summary, the cellular and molecular mechanisms of AR involve B cell production of IgE and mast cell/basophil priming, activation of resident cells, recruitment of inflammatory cells and, in some circumstances, induction of a persistent inflammatory reaction maintained by a positive feedback.

2.2. Chronic Rhinosinusitis (CRS)

Chronic Rhinosinusitis (CRS) is clinically defined as the persistence of signs and symptoms such as nasal obstruction, nasal congestion, rhinorrhea, facial pain, cough, and loss of smell for more than 12 weeks, confirmed by nasal endoscopy or computed tomography. It is related to an inflammatory process of the mucoperiosteal pavement of the sinonasal cavity, whose etiology can be clearly defined in a few subgroups of patients, involving mechanical obstruction, immunodeficiency, cystic fibrosis, and ciliary dyskinesia. However, in the majority of cases, the etiology of CRS cannot be determined. Some investigators have raised different hypotheses for the pathogenesis of CRS such as disruption of the epithelial barrier, allergy, exposure to pollutants, maintenance of mucosal inflammation due to underlying osteitis, persistence of bacterial biofilms, and overreaction to staphylococcal superantigens or fungus. It is interesting to note that individually these theories do not apply to all patients but may explain the pathogenicity in some cases. Despite the unrevealed etiopathogenesis, recent advances have been made in the elucidation of the cellular and molecular events involved in different situations of CRS. Based on molecular phenotyping studies, the classification of CRS into two different clinical subsets has been currently accepted: CRS without nasal polyps (CRS *sine* NP, CRSsNP) and CRS with nasal polyps (CRSwNP) [8, 26]. Clinically, the symptoms of both types are very similar to each other, with slight differences in the severity of nasal congestion, nasal obstruction, rhinorrhea, postnasal drip, change in the sense of smell, cough, and facial pain. In terms of physical examination, they differ by the presence or absence of nasal polyps extruding from the middle meatus of the nasal cavity. This simple difference noted by nasal endoscopy involves profound differences in cellular and molecular aspects that might be related to the prognosis and treatment of these two subsets of CRS.

Histologically, both forms of CRS are marked by niches of denuded respiratory epithelium with associated metaplasia, basal membrane thickening, and goblet cell hyperplasia. The histology of submucosal stroma demonstrates clear differences between CRSwNP and CRSsNP. In CRSwNP, the submucosal stroma usually is found with robust edema and low cellularity, in contrast to CRSsNP that characteristically involves more pronounced fibrosis and less edema [9].

In CRSwNP, eosinophilic infiltration is the hallmark of chronic inflammation. For reasons not fully elucidated, there is an increased expression of pro-inflammatory cytokines (IL-1β) mediated by transcription factors. These cytokines mediate the recruitment of inflammatory cells (eosinophils, lymphocytes, neutrophils, mast cells) through the up-regulation and expression of adhesion molecules (ICAM-1, VCAM-1) and chemokines (IL-8, eotaxin, and RANTES). In CRSwNP, the striking influx of inflammatory cells, especially eosinophils, into the stroma, leads to a positive feedback recruitment similar to allergic rhinitis [27]. In the

Caucasian CRS population, nasal polyps are remarkably characterized by a mixed expression of Th1 (INF-γ, IL-8) and Th2 cytokines, with an imbalance favoring the Th2 response. Th2 cytokines (IL-3, IL-5, GM-CSF) are produced by eosinophils and Th2 cells and increase eosinophil recruitment and survival, creating an autonomous inflammatory cycle even after the removal of the initial trigger. (Figure 2)

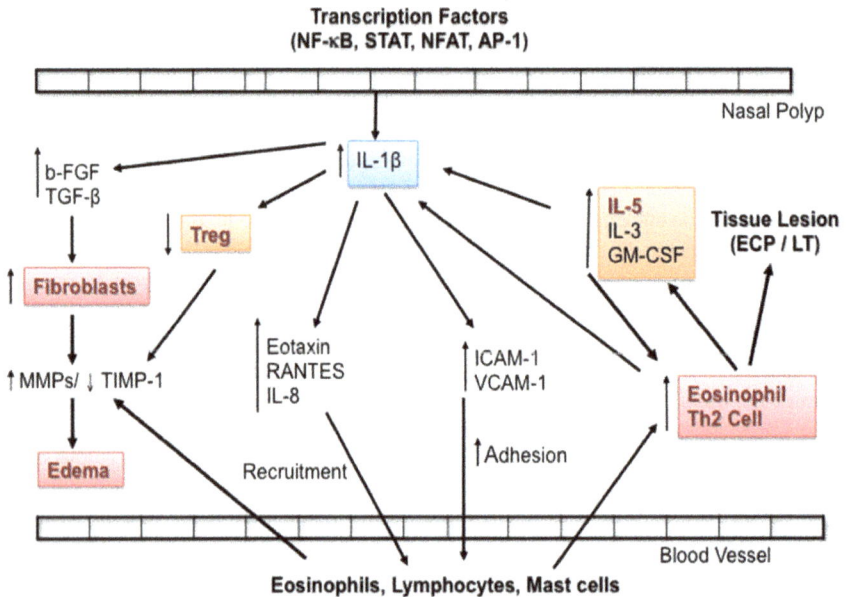

Figure legend: NF-κB: nuclear factor- κB; STAT: signal transducers and activators of transcription; NFAT: nuclear factor of activated T-cells; AP: activator protein; IL: interleukin; FGF: fibroblast growth factor; TGF: transforming growth factor; Treg: regulatory T cell; GM-CSF: granulocyte-macrophage colony-stimulating factor; ECP: eosinophil cationic protein; LT: leukotriene; MMP: matrix metalloproteinase; TIMP: tissue inhibitor of metalloproteinase; RANTES: regulated on activation, normal T cell expressed and secreted; ICAM: intercellular adhesion molecule; VCAM: vascular cell adhesion molecule; Th: T helper cell

Figure 2. Cellular and molecular events involved in the pathogenesis of CRSwNP.

Despite the similarities to allergic rhinitis and contrary to some speculations raised in the first studies, the eosinophilic infiltration and activation found in CRSwNP is not dependent on allergic mechanisms mediated by IgE [28, 29]. In the Chinese population, however, CRSwNP has been characterized by a different Th pattern of inflammation. A mixed Th1/Th17 has been found instead of the Th1/Th2 pattern, with a significantly lower GATA-3 (Th2 specific) expression and higher IL-17 levels in the polyp tissue. The Th17 response drives a more neutrophilic infiltration rather than an eosinophilic recruitment [30].

Another important feature of CRSwNP is the impaired regulatory modulation promoted by Treg cells, which balances the T helper cell response. Low levels of Treg cell biomarkers (transforming growth factor-β1 -TGF-β1- and forkhead box protein P3 -FOXP3) together with high expression of T-bet (Th1) and GATA-3 (Th2) demonstrate the deficiency of Treg control in CRSwNP patients [31].

In terms of molecular markers, among Caucasians, IL-5 is the most important cytokine found in CRSwNP. IL-5 is related to eosinophil infiltration and activation, and is significantly related to recurrence of nasal polyps after surgical removal [32]. Activated eosinophils also release several inflammatory mediators, such as leukotrienes, and other toxic products (Eosinophil Cationic Protein – ECP, Major Basic Protein – MBP, neurotoxin eosinophil protein). Besides the damage induced by infiltrated inflammatory cells, resident fibroblasts also play a role in the structural modification of the stroma. Stimulated by fibroblast growth factor (FGF) and TGF-β, fibroblasts are recruited, proliferate, and express matrix metalloproteinases (MMP), which degrade extracellular proteins (collagen, laminin, fibronectin, elastin) and favor tissue edema and albumin deposition. Other cells such as eosinophils and neutrophils are also able to produce MMP and may play a role in tissue remodeling [33]. Furthermore, fibroblasts suppress the expression of tissue inhibitors of metalloproteinases (TIMP) which increase the activity of MMP. Taken together, these features explain the main histopathological and molecular findings in CRSwNP, i.e., eosinophilic infiltration, tissue edema, and Th2 skewing polarization.

On the other hand, CRSsNP present some different features compared to CRSwNP. Although mixed inflammatory cells are found in CRSsNP, neutrophils are the predominant cells in this subset of CRS and, together with Th1 cells. seem to play the main cellular role in the pathogenesis of the disease. Neutrophil markers of activation such as myeloperoxidase and IL-8 are found in high levels in CRSsNP compared to controls and CRSwNP. Besides, the levels of Th1 cytokines (INF-γ, IL-8) found in CRSsNP are unbalanced with Th2 cytokines, revealing Th1 polarization. In contrast to CRSwNP, FOXP3 and TGF-β are not decreased in CRSsNP, demonstrating that Treg function is not altered in CRSsNP [31]. The up-regulated TGF- β signaling pathways are believed to be an important marker that reflects the fibrosis/albumin deposition remarkably seen in CRSsNP. (Figure 3)

In conclusion, in contrast to CRSwNP, the cellular and molecular findings in CRSsNP are characterized by neutrophilic infiltration, tissue fibrosis, and Th1 skewing polarization.

3. Glucocorticoid action on nasal mucosa

Glucocorticoid (GC) has a broad anti-inflammatory effect, regulating both innate and adaptive immune responses in a wide variety of cells, such as epithelial cells, fibroblasts, eosinophils and T cells [1, 12, 34]. This is the main reason why GC is considered to be the medication of choice to treat chronic rhinitis [2] and rhinosinusitis [8].

This wide anti-inflammatory effect of GC is explained by several events induced by it, from the signaling event to post-translational mechanisms. Basically, GC is a lipophilic compound which diffuses though the membrane and binds to its cytoplasmic receptor, called glucocorticoid receptor (GR) [35].

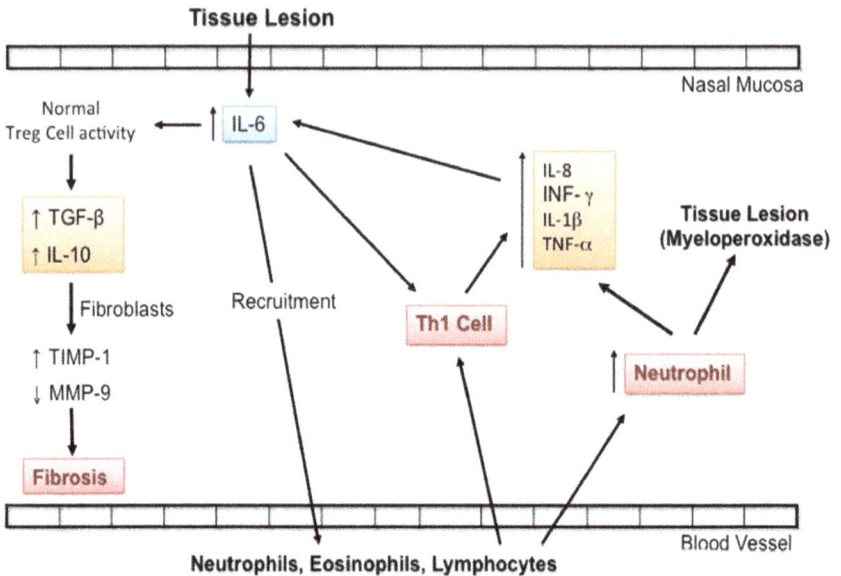

Figure legend: Treg: regulatory T cell; IL: interleukin; INF: interferon; TNF: tumor necrosis factor; Th: T helper cell; TGF: transforming growth factor; TIMP: tissue inhibitor of metalloproteinase; MMP: metalloproteinase

Figure 3. Cellular and molecular events involved in the pathogenesis of CRSsNP.

GR belongs to a large superfamily of steroid receptors. When inactivated, this receptor stays in the cytosol bound to heat shock proteins (hsp) [36]. When GC binds to GR, phosphorylation occurs to this receptor, which dissociates GR from hsp. The dimer GC-GR is able to translocate into the nucleus and then act as a transcription factor. In this respect, the GC-GR dimer can bind directly to a specific palindromic DNA consensus sequence, called glucocorticoid response elements (GREs), and consequently induces or inhibits (in case of nGREs) the transcription of several genes [35]. Nevertheless, it is recognized that the main anti-inflammatory action of GC at the transcriptional level is mediated by a direct interaction of GC-GR with other transcription factors (TF), inhibiting their action. This inhibition, called "DNA-independent transrepression" affects several pro-inflammatory TF, the most important ones being activator protein-1 (AP-1) and nuclear fator-κB (NF-κB) [1, 35-39] (Figure 4). This connection inhibits gene transcription by direct binding to DNA or by inducing histone deacetylation. Although the non-genomic effect of GC is widely known in the literature [2, 17], there is no report on its effect on chronic upper respiratory diseases, and only few studies have reported controversial results regarding asthma [40, 41].

The final effect of GC on nasal diseases is the inhibition of pro-inflammatory cytokines (IL-1β, TNF-α, GM-CSF, IL-3, IL-5, IL-6), chemokines (IL-8, RANTES, eotaxin) and adhesion molecules (VCAM-1, ICAM-1) [1, 13, 42]. Glucocorticoids also have a favorable effect on tissue remodeling (reducing MMP expression) [43, 44], reduce mucin production [45], increase cell apoptosis [46, 47], and decrease mast cell recruitment and activation [48].

Finally, glucocorticoids inhibit the expression of some cytokine receptors, among them IL-2 and IL-4 receptors.

Due to its holistic action, GC is considered to be the best medication for the treatment of chronic inflammatory diseases of the upper respiratory airways.

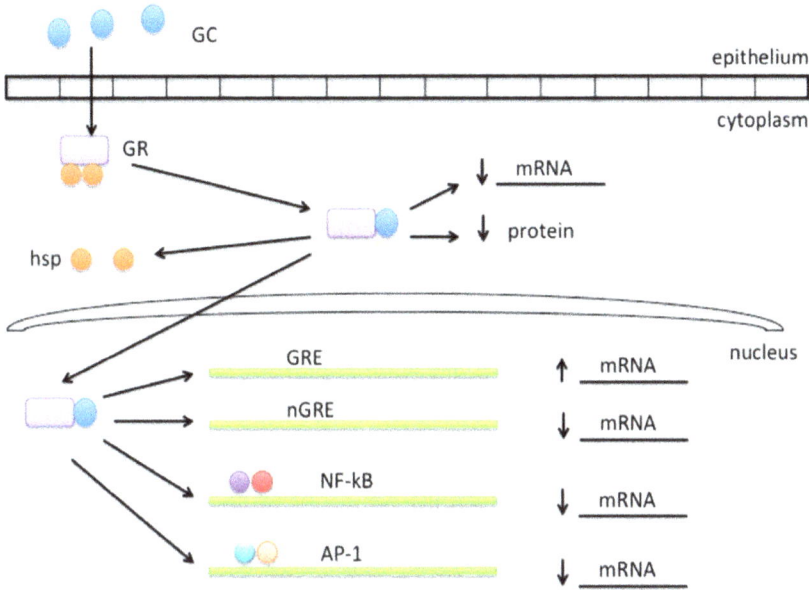

Figure 4. GC mode of action: binding to its cytoplasmic GR, and then translocating into the nucleus. GC: glucocorticoid; GR: glucocorticoid receptor; hsp: heat shock protein; GRE: glucocorticoid response element; NF-κB: nuclear factor κB; AP-1: activator protein-1

4. GR splicing

The GR gene is located in chromosome 5 and is composed of 9 exons. Alternative splicing in the ninth exon (hormone-binding domain) gives raise to several alternative GRs, GRα and GRβ being the most common [35-39].

GRα is the predominant GR isoform. It is transcriptionally active and, when ligated to GC, it can translocate into the nucleus, induce expression by binding to GRE, or repress expression by either binding to nGRE or by interacting with AP-1 and NF-κB [1, 35, 36].

For instance, GRβ is expressed at much lower rates than GRα. It cannot bind to GC, and although it can bind to GRE, nGRE, AP-1 and NF-κB, it does not activate their transcriptional action. Some authors have shown that, when overexpressed, GRβ inhibits the effect of GRα on both transactivation and on AP-1 and NF-κB repression [49-51]. GRβ is thus considered to be the dominant negative of GRα; instead, a recent study has shown that a glucocorticoid antagonist, named RU-486, has the ability to bind to GRβ, regulating gene expression even in the absence of GRα [52].

There is no previous study regarding the influence of GRγ on nasal mucosa.

5. Resistance to GC

Although GC is the medication of choice in chronic upper respiratory diseases in general, the rate of CG therapy failure in CRSwNP is reported to be between 60 and 80% [8]. Although there is no report on GC resistance in chronic rhinitis, resistance is believed to be identical to that occurring in CRSwNP. The main reasons for GC failure are: limited action of topical GC in extensive diseases [53], poor compliance with treatment [54] , and cellular/molecular resistance to GC [36, 55]. Among cellular and molecular mechanisms of GC resistance, the main lines investigated are GRα- GRβ interaction and TF influence.

One of the most studied mechanisms is the GRα-GRβ imbalance. Although GRβ is able to interact directly with GRα within the nucleus, it has a low capacity to bind to GC. This is why GRβ is considered to be an endogenous inhibitor of GRα [36, 56]. GRα-GRβ imbalance has been reported to increase cell resistance in chronic immune-mediated diseases, among those affecting the upper [37, 57] and lower airways [58, 59].

Increased expression of GRβ has been widely reported in the literature on inflammatory respiratory diseases such as CRSwNP and asthma, when compared to control mucosa [36, 55, 60, 61]. This has led to the hypothesis that increased GRβ expression could impair the action of GC. Decreased expression of GRα has also been recently reported in CRswNP with the use of a more reliable quantitative method of analysis [56, 62, 63]. More important than the expression of each individual isoform, GRα-GRβ imbalance might be the most relevant determinant of GC resistance. It is important to mention that some studies have demonstrated that CG therapy in CRSwNP does not change GR isoform expression or the GRα-GRβ relation [56, 63, 64].

Higher expression of TF could also lead to GC resistance, because TF (mainly AP-1 and NF-κB) repress the binding of the translocated GC-GR complex to GRE. This mechanism of GC resistance has been reported in several inflammatory diseases, such as inflammatory bowel diseases. Nevertheless, this mechanism has been poorly reported in respiratory diseases.

AP-1 is a dimer predominantly consisting of c-Fos/c-Jun heterodimers. As is the case for most TF, they are located in the cytoplasm and, when activated, translocate into the nucleus and induce the expression of several pro-inflammatory genes which regulate cell inflammation, proliferation, differentiation and apoptosis [65]. Conflicting results have been reported regarding the presence of AP-1 in CRSwNP. c-Fos expression has been studied in two reports because it is more important regarding the transcriptional action. One study [66] has reported an increased presence of c-Fos in patients with CRSwNP than in control mucosa using qualitative PCR, while the other [56] has observed a similar expression in the two groups using quantitative RT-PCR. The latter study also did not observe any influence of c-Fos expression on the outcome of GC treatment.

NF-κB is also a heterodimer, mainly consisting of p50 and p65 isoforms. When activated, NF-κB translocates into the nucleus, and p65 directly binds to DNA, inducing gene expression of pro-inflammatory and anti-apoptotic genes [37, 65]. NF-κB is considered pivotal to the regulation of immune and inflammatory genes, and its absence is incompatible with life. It is important to mention that the most important pro-inflammatory cytokines (IL-1β and TNF-α), whose expression is considerably influenced by NF-κB, also activate NF-κB translocation, inducing perpetuation of the inflammatory process.

Two studies have reported increased expression of both isoforms (p50 and p65) of NF-κB in patients with CRSwNP when compared to control nasal mucosa [56, 67]. Also, a high expression of p65 was related to a poor clinical outcome in response to medical treatment in CRSwNP patients [56]. This finding suggests that NF-κB may also have a pivotal effect on GC resistance.

6. Conclusions

Chronic inflammatory nasal diseases are highly prevalent in the population, and therefore nasal TGC has been widely prescribed by physicians. Considering that a high percentage of these patients only partially benefit from TGC, or do not respond to TCG treatment at all, the understanding of possible mechanisms of GC resistance is essential for future treatments.

Today, it has been accepted that cellular and molecular mechanisms of resistance do exist in nasal mucosa. Future investigations are still required to recognize affected individuals and how this would influence medical treatment. This will be essential to develop new drugs that would replace or act synergistically with CG, in order to improve the clinical outcome.

Author details

Fabiana C.P. Valera, Edwin Tamashiro and Wilma T. Anselmo-Lima
Division of Otorhinolaryngology, Departament of Ophthalmology, Otorhinolaryngology, and Head and Neck Surgery. Faculty of Medicine of Ribeirao Preto-University of São Paulo, Ribeirao Preto-SP, Brazil

7. References

[1] Stellato, C., Glucocorticoid actions on airway epithelial responses in immunity: Functional outcomes and molecular targets. J Allergy Clin Immunol 2007. 120(6): p. 1247-63.

[2] Bousquet J, K.N., Cruz AA, Denburg J, Fokkens WJ, Togias A, et al, Allergic Rhinitis and its impact on asthma (ARIA) 2008. Allergy 2008. 63: p. 8-160.

[3]   Bauchau V, D.S., Prevalence and rate of diagnosis of allergic rhinitis in Europe. Eur R
      Espir J, 2004. 24: p. 758-764.
[4]   Collins, J., Prevalence of selected chronic conditions: United States 1990-1992. Vital
      Health Stat, 1997. 194: p. 1-89.
[5]   Bentley AM, J.M., Cumberworth V, Barkans JR, Moqbel R, Schwartz LB, et al. ,
      Immunohistology of the nasal mucosa in seasonal allergic rhinitis: increases in
      activated eosinophils and epithelial mast cells. J Allergy Clin Immunol, 1992. 89: p.
      877– 883.
[6]   Laliberte F, L.M., Lecart S, Bousquet J, Klossec JM, Mounedji N, Clinical and pathologic
      methods to assess the long-term safety of nasal corticosteroids. French Triamcinolone
      Acetonide Study Group. . Allergy, 2000. 55(718-722).
[7]   Shaida A, K.G., Devalia J, Davies RJ, MacDonald TT, Pender SL, Matrix
      metalloproteinases and their inhibitors in the nasal mucosa of patients with perennial
      allergic rhinitis. J Allergy Clin Immunol 2001. 108(5): p. 791–796.
[8]   Fokkens WJ, L.V., Mullol J, Bachert C, Cohen N, Cobo R, et al. European Position Paper
      on Nasal Polyps 2007. Rhinology 2007, 20: 1-139., European Position Paper on Nasal
      Polyps 2007. Rhinology, 2007. 20: p. 1-139.
[9]   Huvenne W, v.B.N., Zhang N, van Zele T, Patou J, Gevaert P, et al, Chronic
      Rhinosinusitis With and Without Nasal Polyps: What Is the Difference? Curr Allergy
      Asthma Rep, 2009. 9: p. 213–220.
[10] Jankowski R, B.F., Coffinet L, Vignaud JM, Clinical factors influencing the eosinophil
      infiltration of nasal polyps. Rhinology, 2002. 40: p. 173-8.
[11] Pawankar R, M.S., Ozu C, Kimura S, Overview on the pathomechanisms of allergic
      rhinitis. Asia Pac Allergy, 2011. 1(3): p. 157-167.
[12] Bradding P, O.Y., Howarth PH, Church MK, Holgate ST, Heterogeneity of human mast
      cells based on cytokines content. J Immunol, 1995. 155: p. 297-307.
[13] Kawabori Y, K.N., Tosho T, Proliferative activity of mast cells in allergic nasal mucosa.
      Clin Exp Allergy 1995. 25: p. 173-8.
[14] Baraniuk, J., Pathogenesis of allergic rhinitis. J Allergy Clin Immunol 1997. 99: p. S763-
      S772.
[15] Eccles, R., Pathophysyology of Nasal Symptoms. Am J Rhinol 2000. 14(5): p. 335-338.
[16] McDonald, D., Neurogenic inflammation in the respiratory tract: actions of sensory
      nerve mediators on blood vessels and epithelium of the airway mucosa. Am Rev Respir
      Dis, 1987. 136(6 Pt 2): p. S65-S72.
[17] Gosset P, M.F., Delnest Y, et al., Interleukin 6 and interleukin-1α production is
      associated with antigen induced late nasal response. J. Allergy Clin. Immunol., 1993.
      94(11777-11783).
[18] Naclerio RM, B.F., Kagey-Sobotka A, Lichtenstein LM, Basophils and eosinophils in
      allergic rhinitis. J Allergy Clin Immunol, 1994. 94(6 Pt 2): p. 1303-1309.
[19] Moqbel R, L.-S.F., Kay AB, Cytokine generation by eosinophils. J Allergy Clin Immunol
      1994. 94(6 Pt 2): p. 1183-9.

[20] Pawankar RU, O.M., Okubo K, Ra C, Lymphocyte subsets in the nasal mucosa in perennial allergic rhinitis. Am J Respir Crit Care Med, 1995. 152(6 Pt 1): p. 2049-58.

[21] Nonaka M, N.R., Jordana M, Dolovich J, GM-CSF, IL-8, IL-1R, TNF-alpha R, and HLA-DR in nasal epithelial cells in allergic rhinitis. Am J Respir Crit Care Med, 1996. 153(5): p. 1675-81.

[22] Kenney JS, B.C., Welch MR, Altman LC, Synthesis of interleukin-1 alpha, interleukin-6, and interleukin-8 by cultured human nasal epithelial cells. J Allergy Clin Immunol, 1994. 93(6): p. 1060-7.

[23] Ziegler SF, A.D., Sensing the outside world: TSLP regutates barrier immunity. Nat Immunol, 2010. 11: p. 289-293.

[24] Miyata M, N.Y., Shimokawa N, Ohnuma Y, Katoh R, Matsuoka S, Okumura K, Ogawa H, Masuyama K, Nakao A, Thymic stromal lymphopoietin is a critical mediator of IL-13-driven allergic inflammation. Eur J Immunol, 2009. 39(11): p. 3078-83.

[25] Masuda, S., Quantitative histochemistry of mucus-secreting cells in human nasal mucosa. . Pract Otol (Kyoto), 1990. 83: p. 1855-63.

[26] Van Zele T, C.S., Gevaert P, Van Maele G, Holtappels G, VanCauwenberge P, Bachert C, Differentiation of chronic sinus diseases by measurement of inflammatory mediators. Allergy 2006. 61(11): p. 1280–1289.

[27] Bachert C, G.P., Holtappels G, Cuvelier C, van Cauwenberge P, Nasal polyposis: from cytokines to growth. Am J Rhinol, 2000. 14(279–290).

[28] Min YG, L.C., Rhee CS, Kim KH, Kim CS, Koh YY, Min KU, Anderson PL, Inflammatory cytokine expression on nasal polyps developed in allergic and infectious rhinitis. Acta Otolaryngol, 1997. 117(2): p. 302-6.

[29] Lee CH, R.C., Min YG, Cytokine gene expression in nasal polyps. Ann Otol Rhinol Laryngol 1998. 107(8): p. 665-70.

[30] Zhang N, H.G., Claeys C, Huang G, van Cauwenberge P, Bachert C, Pattern of inflammation and impact of Staphylococcus aureus enterotoxins in nasal polyps from southern China. Am J Rhinol, 2006. 20(4): p. 445–450.

[31] Van Bruaene N, P.-N.C., Basinski TM, Van Zele T, Holtappels G, De Ruyck N, Schmidt-Weber C, Akdis C, Van Cauwenberge P, Bachert C, et al, T-cell regulation in chronic paranasal sinus disease. J Allergy Clin Immunol, 2008. 121(6): p. 1435–1441, 1441. 1441.e1–e3.

[32] Bachert C, W.M., Hauser U, Rudack C, IL-5 synthesis is upregulated in human nasal polyp tissue. J Allergy Clin Immunol, 1997. 99: p. 837–842.

[33] Delclaux C, D.C., D'Ortho MP, Boyer V, Lafuma C, Harf A, Role of gelatinase B and elastase in human polymorphonuclear neutrophil migration across basement membrane. Am J Respir Cell Mol Biol, 1996. 14: p. 288-295.

[34] Holm AF, F.W., Godthelp T, Mulder PG, Vroom TM, Rjintejes E, Effect of 3 month's nasal steroid therapy on nasal T cells and Langerhans cells in patients suffering from allergic rhinitis. Allergy 1995. 50: p. 204-209.

[35] Liberman AC, D.J., Perone MJ, Arzt E, Glucocorticoids in the regulation of transcription factors that control cytokine synthesis. Cytokine Growth Factor Rev, 2007. 18(1-2): p. 45-56.

[36] Pujols L, M.J., Picado C, Alpha and beta glucocorticoid receptors: relevance in airway diseases. Curr Allergy Asthma Rep, 2007. 7(2): p. 93-99.

[37] Adcock IM, C.G., Cross-talk between pro-inflammatory transcription factors and glucocorticoids. Immunol Cell Biol, 2001. 79: p. 376-384.

[38] Li Q, V.I., NF-[kappa]B regulation in the immune system. Nat Rev Immunol, 2002. 2: p. 725-734.

[39] McKay LI, C.J., Molecular control of immune/inflammatory responses: interactions between nuclear factor-kappaB and steroid receptor-signaling pathways. Endocr Rev, 1999. 20(4): p. 435-459.

[40] Stellato, C., Post-transcriptional and nongenomic effects of glucocorticoids Proc Am Thorac Soc, 2004. 1(3): p. 255-263.

[41] Urbach V, V.V., Grumbach Y, Bousquet J, Harvey BJ, Rapid anti-secretory effects of glucocorticoids in human airway epithelium. Steroids, 2006. 71(4): p. 323-328.

[42] Valera FCP, B.M., Castro-Gamero AM, Cortez MA, Rosane GP Queiroz, Luiz G Tone, Anselmo-Lima, In vitro effect of glucocorticoids on nasal polyps. Braz J Otorhinolaryngol, 2011. 77(5): p. 605-610.

[43] Kyo Y, K.K., Asano K, Hisamitsu T, Suzaki H, Supressive effect of fluticasone propionate on MMP expression in the nasal mucosa of allergic rhinitis patients in vivo. . In Vivo 2006. 20: p. 439-444.

[44] Yigit O, A.E., Gelisgen R, Server EA, Azizli E, Uzun H, The effect of corticosteroid on metalloproteinase levels of nasal polyposis. Laryngoscope 2011. 121(3): p. 667-673.

[45] Bal CH, S.S., Kim YD, Effect of glucocorticoid on the MUC4 gene in nasal polyps. Laryngoscope 2007. 117: p. 2169-2173.

[46] Bobic S, v.D.C., Callebaut I, Hox V, Jorissen M, Fokkens WJ, et al, Dexamethasone-induced apoptosis of freshly isolated human nasal epithelial cells concomitant with abrogation of IL-8 production. Rhinology 2010. 48: p. 401-407.

[47] Hirano S, A.K., Namba M, Kanai K, Hisamitsu T, Suzaki H, Induction of apoptosis in nasal polyps fibroblasts by glucocorticoids in vitro. Acta Otolaryngol, 2003. 123(1075-1079).

[48] Juluisson S, A.F.E.L.P.c.o.m.c.o.n.m.e.o.n.a.a.o.l.c.t.A., 50:15-22, Protease content of mast cells of nasal mucosa: effects of natural allergen and of local corticosteroid treatment. . Allergy 1995. 50: p. 15-22.

[49] Lu NZ, C.J., Grissom SF, Cidlowski JA, Selective regulation of bone cell apoptosis by translational isoforms of the glucocorticoid receptor. Mol Cell Biol, 2007. 27(20): p. 7143–7160.

[50] Bamberger CM, B.A., de Castro M, Chrousos GP, Glucocorticoid receptor β, a potential endogenous inhibitor of glucocorticoid action in humans. J Clin Invest, 1995. 95: p. 2435–2441.

[51] Gougat C, J.D., Gagliardo R, Henriquet C, Bousquet J, Demoly P, Mathieu M, Over-expression of the human glucocorticoid receptor α and β isoforms inhibits AP-1 and NF-κ B activities hormone independently. J Mol Med, 2002. 80: p. 309–318.

[52] Lewis-Tuffin LJ, J.C., Bienstock RJ, Collins JB, Cidlowski JA Human glucocorticoid receptor beta binds RU-486 and is transcriptionally active. Mol Cell Biol, 2007. 27(2266-2282).

[53] Valera FCP, A.-L.W., Evaluation of efficacy of topical corticosteroid for the clinical treatment of nasal polyposis: searching for clinical events that may predict response to treatment. . Rhinology 2007. 45(1): p. 59-62.

[54] Badia L, L.V., Topical corticosteroids in nasal polyposis. Drugs 2001. 61: : p. 573-578.

[55] Hamilos DL, L.D., Muro S, Kahn AM, Hamilos SS, Thawley SE, et al., GRβ expression in nasal polyp inflammatory cells and its relationship to the anti-inflammatory effects of intranasal fluticasone. J Allergy Clin Immunol, 2001. 108: : p. 59-68.

[56] Valera FCP, Q.R., Scrideli C, Tone LG, Anselmo-Lima WT, NF-κB expression predicts clinical outcome for nasal polyposis. Rhinology 2010. 48(4): p. 408-414.

[57] Valera FCP, Q.R., Scrideli C, Tone LG, Anselmo-Lima WT, Evaluating budesonide efficacy in nasal polyposis and predicting the resistance to treatment. Clin Exper Allergy, 2009. 39(1): p. 81-88.

[58] Gagliardo R, C.P., Vignola AM, Bousquet J, Vachier I, Godard P, Bonsignore G, Demoly P, Mathieu M, Glucocorticoid Receptor α and β in glucocorticoid dependent asthma. Am J Respir Crit Care Med, 2000. 162: p. 7-13.

[59] Barnes, P., Corticosteroid resistance in airway disease. Proc Am Thorac Soc 2004(1): p. 264-268.

[60] Pujolsa L, M.J., Picado C, Glucocorticoid Receptor in Human Respiratory Epithelial Cells. Neuroimmunomodul, 2009. 16(5): p. 290–299.

[61] Sousa AR, L.S., Cidlowski JA, Staynov DZ, Lee TH, Glucocorticoid resistance in asthma is associated with elevated in vivo expression of the glucocorticoid receptor β-isoform. J Allergy Clin Immunol, 2000. 105(5): p. 943-950.

[62] Li P, L.Y., Zhang X, Zhang G, Ye J, Sun Y, et al., Detection of glucocorticoid receptor-alpha mRNA expression using FQ-RT-PCR in nasal polyp. Lin Chuang Er Bi Yan Hou Ke Za Zhi, 2005. 19(769-771).

[63] Pujols L, A.I., Benítez P, Martínez-Antón A, Roca-Ferrer J, Fokkens WJ, Mullol J, Picado C, Regulation of glucocorticoid receptor in nasal polyps by systemic and intranasal glucocorticoids. Allergy 2008. 63(10): p. 1377-1386.

[64] Choi BR, K.J., Gong SJ, Kwon MS, Cho JH, Kim JH, et al, Expression of glucocorticoid receptor mRNAs in glucocorticoid-resistant nasal polyps. Exp. Mol. Med, 2006. 38: p. 466-473.

[65] Necela BM, C.J., Mechanisms of glucocorticoid receptor action in noninflammatory and inflammatory cells. Proc Am Thorac Soc, 2004. 1(3): p. 239-246.

[66] Baraniuk JN, W.G., Ali M, Sabol M, Troost T, Glucocorticoids decrease c-fos expression in human nasal polyps in vivo. Thorax 1998. 53: p. 577- 582.

[67] Takeno S, H.K., Ueda T, et al, Nuclear factor-kappa B activation in the nasal polyp epithelium: relationship to local cytokine gene expression. Laryngoscope 2002. 112(1): p. 53-58

Chapter 9

Assessment of Glucocorticoids – Induced Preclinical Atherosclerosis

Amr Amin and Zeinab Nawito

Additional information is available at the end of the chapter

1. Introduction

In 1948, the US rheumatologist Philip Hench and his associates at the Mayo Clinic first administered hydrocortisone to a patient with rheumatoid arthritis and discovered its clinical benefits [1]. Two years later, Hench, together with biochemists Edward Kendall and Tadeus Reichstein, shared the Nobel Prize in Medicine. Today, glucocorticoids are among the most frequently prescribed class of anti-inflammatory medications [2]. They are part of the standard treatment for a wide range of disorders which feature inflammation and/or immune activation, such as asthma, chronic obstructive pulmonary disease, hypersensitivity reactions, autoimmune diseases, and in organ transplantation. However, even early on, the euphoria generated by the discovery of corticosteroids was rapidly tempered by the realization that clinicians were, in a sense, engaging in a Faustian pact between its impressive anti-inflammatory benefits and its potentially devastating Cushingoid side effects [3, 4].

From a cardiovascular standpoint, the propensity of glucocorticoids to produce hyperglycemia, hypertension, dyslipidemia, and central obesity has long produced concern regarding possible adverse cardiovascular events [5]. Glucocorticoids administration increases blood pressure in a dose dependent fashion. The mechanisms of glucocorticoids-mediated hypertension are incompletely understood but appear to be principally related to increased peripheral vascular resistance rather than to mineralocorticoid receptor mediated effects of increased sodium retention and plasma volume expansion [6]. Dyslipidemia in the context of long term glucocorticoids use is characterized by increased total cholesterol, low density lipoprotein cholesterol, and triglycerides. Corticosteroid treatment increases the risk of glucose intolerance in patients without known diabetes and is associated with deterioration of glycaemic control in diabetic patients [7]. Glucocorticoids treatment therefore contributes to the exacerbation of a cluster of cardiovascular risk factors that are central to the metabolic syndrome. However, as inflammation plays a central role in the pathogenesis of atherosclerosis [8], it is also possible that glucocorticoids may exert some anti-atherosclerotic effects.

There was a significant association between ever use of oral glucocorticoids and any cardiovascular or cerebrovascular outcome. The association was stronger for current use of oral glucocorticoids than for recent or past use. Among current users, the highest odds ratios were observed in the group with the highest average daily dose, although the dose–response relation was not continuous. Current use was associated with an increased risk of heart failure, which was consistent between patients with rheumatoid arthritis, patients with chronic obstructive pulmonary disease, and patients without either of the two conditions. Also, current use was associated with a smaller increased risk of ischaemic heart disease [9].

RA population has an increased cardio-vascular mortality and premature death rate, but why does these patients have a higher incidence of atherosclerosis? There are several factors which are known risks in the development of atherosclerosis. Steroids may play a role in the increased mortality from vascular disease. Some reports have suggested that prolonged treatment with steroids accelerates the development of atherosclerosis. Steroids have atherogenic properties that are known to enhance the development of atherosclerosis and they induce vascular injury. In addition, they produce a state of hypercoagulability. In Moreland and O'Dell study, they found an increased atherosclerotic burden in the patients who were on long-term steroids. This suggests that steroid treatment may be a contributor to the higher rate of atherosclerosis seen in them [10]. Del Rincón et al. studied the carotid and lower-limb arteries in a sample of RA patients, and found that the extent of cumulative glucocorticoids dose was significantly associated with arterial incompressibility. This association displayed a gradient in which the proportion of incompressible arteries increased with higher glucocorticoids exposure. This pattern was independent of age at RA onset, sex, disease duration, CV risk factors, and manifestations of RA [11].

2. Historical background

Calcification of the arterial atheroma occurs in the coronary tree as it does in the remainder of the arterial tree. Such calcified coronary arteries are occasionally noted on routine chest radiographs but are difficult to distinguish from normal mediastinal structures and are confused with calcification in the chest wall, lungs, or other intracardiac structures [12]. Calcification of the coronary arteries is a common autopsy finding and is generally present in 80 to 90% of post-mortem studies. Despite this common pathologic finding, description of coronary calcification was rare until the work of Lenk [13] in 1927, who noted calcification of the left coronary artery on a posteroanterior chest radiograph in a 61-year-old male with left ventricular aneurysm. In 1964 Beadenkopf et al. [14] reported their findings in 904 consecutive autopsies; their results indicated that as the number of coronary arteries with calcification increased, coronary artery wall thickness increased. Tampas and Soule [15] in 1965 using radiographs in 1097 patients over the age of 40 found an incidence of 15% coronary calcification with a male to female ratio of 3 to 2 that was associated with increasing age. They suggested that coronary calcification might be an alarm signal of potential ischemic heart disease. Currently, it is generally recognized that the incidence of Coronary artery disease (CAD) was greater in patients with coronary calcification and atherosclerosis than in those without calcification [16].

3. Value of assessment of preclinical atherosclerosis

The presence of preclinical atherosclerosis increases global cardiovascular risk; therefore, it can be considered an emerging determinant in assessing such a risk. Single or multiple risk factors increase cardiovascular risk in an exponential manner, meanwhile the presence of one or more risk factors for atherosclerosis is associated with the development of cardiovascular disease. *A specific issue is defined as risk factor when it is possible, on the basis of a strong statistical association, to relate it to the incidence of new cases of disease and if it is clinically demonstrated that new disease cases can be reduced by correcting the same risk factor.*

Atherosclerosis is defined as a progressive structural remodeling of a vessel wall towards definitive plaque formation and possible related complications. According to new data, the disease begins as an endothelium functional disorder [dysfunction] inducing loss of vascular homeostasis and related functional reserve that initially can become clinically evident only in conditions in which there is a need to increase tissue metabolic requirements (as for instance effort Angina, transient Ischemic Attack, intermittent Claudication) while, after more time, they can become symptomatic at rest because even basal perfusion [blood flow] is impaired (acute coronary syndrome, stroke, critical leg ischemia, and even cardiovascular death) [12].

Coronary atherosclerosis is the leading cause of death in industrialized western countries. In up to 50% of its victims the first manifestation of CAD is sudden death or acute myocardial infarction. The cost of lost human value and approximate dollars spent ($90 billion annually) due to coronary artery disease in the western society is of great concern and is the reason for increased efforts for its prevention and its consequences as well. The detection of CAD in its asymptomatic stage is highly desirable because it is an increasingly treatable disease, but till now it has been hindered by the lack of sensitive and specific tests [13].

4. Methodology of assessment

4.1. Clinical background and limitations

In evaluating atherosclerosis the following demographic and clinical data are needed; sex, age, cigarette smoking, alcohol consumption, physical activity and life style, socioeconomic status, previous diseases, family history, BMI, WHR [waist to hip ratio] and blood pressure assessments in the standard way.

Chronic subclinical inflammation is thought to be part of the metabolic syndrome [MetSyn]. The latter is characterized by a clustering of atherosclerotic CVD risk factors. The WHO definition of MetSyn [14] requires the presence of insulin resistance plus 2 other of central obesity, hypertension, or dyslipidemia. Insulin resistance is thought to be the most prominent pathophysiological process underlying MetSyn. Recent studies of coronary artery calcification (CAC) in asymptomatic samples have shown an association of MetSyn and insulin resistance with the burden of coronary atherosclerosis [13]. Lakka et al. [15] found a 2- to 4-fold increased risk of cardiovascular death with MetSyn in a sample of 1209 Finnish men free from diabetes and CVD at baseline. MetSyn predicted atherosclerosis progression and CVD events in 888 subjects in the Bruneck study, whereas most individual components of the syndrome were not significantly associated with CVD out-comes [16] supporting the concept that MetSyn provides information that is "more than the sum of its parts."[17].

4.2. Laboratory methods

In more than 15 large prospective studies, C-reactive protein (CRP) has emerged as an independent predictor of an incident cardiovascular event in initially healthy subjects and outcome after acute coronary syndrome [18]. More importantly, its high levels have been demonstrated to be an even stronger predictor of cardiovascular events than LDL cholesterol levels. CRP represents only one of several new inflammatory biomarkers to be associated, independent of lipid profile, with future cardiovascular events. Among these, serum amyloid A (SAA), soluble vascular cell adhesion molecule-1 (VCAM-1), soluble intercellular adhesion molecule 1 (ICAM-1), lipoprotein associated phospholipase A2 (Lp-PLA2), homocysteine and monocyte chemoattractant protein-1 (MCP-1) are the best characterized. Interestingly, from the most recent epidemiological trials, evidence has consistently emerged that these biomarkers are independent from cholesterol levels, but also unrelated to each other. For instance, in healthy middle-aged men, CRP levels were found to correlate only marginally to Lp-PLA2 and MCP-1. The direct evidence that inflammatory biomarkers contribute to atherogenesis would be validated from the utilization of novel specific inhibitors for each of the soluble molecules which should prevent atherogenesis and coronary artery disease [18].

4.3. Sonographic modalities

Atherosclerosis is a chronic inflammatory disorder that often progresses silently for decades before becoming clinically evident. In this section we will preview sonographic noninvasive imaging of the vascular changes that occur in the atherosclerosis disease process including assessment of its inflammatory component. Because inflammation participates in plaque initiation and progression, a method capable of imaging the extent of vascular inflammation could potentially provide powerful predictive information on both early disease presence and future risk for disease progression.

4.3.1. Intima-Media Thickness (IMT) or Asymptomatic Carotid Plaque (ACP)

Echocolordoppler scanning evaluation of the carotid wall is a non invasive, low cost, and highly reproducible procedure even if, like most parts of the echographic analysis, it is strongly operator dependent. The Doppler mode permits the visualization of vessels and an evaluation of flow disturbance that helps to quantify stenosis severity. It measures the IMT and size and number of atheromatous plaques. According to the European Society of Cardiology; 2007-Guidelines on the Management of arterial Hypertension, normal IMT is the distance between the media-adventitia and the intima-media interfaces and is interpreted as follows:

- under 0,9 mm of the entire vascular wall; normal
- between 0.9 and 1.5 mm is an increased IMT,
- While all conditions in which it is greater than 1.5 mm can be considered an ACP.

Increased IMT (or ACP) is related to the presence, number, intensity and duration of atherosclerosis risk factors as well as endothelial dysfunction [24, 25]. Also, IMT is a potent and independent predictor of future cerebro- and cardiovascular events, as proven by several studies (Finnish, American Rotterdam groups) [17].

4.3.2. Ankle Brachial Pressure Index (ABI)

Normally, ankle systolic arterial pressure (posterior or anterior tibial artery) is just a little higher than brachial pressure measurements so that their ratio always is always > 1.0. This parameter is called the Ankle-Brachial pressure Index (ABI) and can reflect altered pressure values. It is reduced < 0.90 if atherosclerosis induced arterial system impairment is present; hence the patient is considered to have an asymptomatic peripheral artery disease. It is a simple, non-expensive procedure and can also be practiced by general practitioners [17]. Several population trials evidenced an important correlation between decreased ABI, carotid or coronary atherosclerosis and future cardiac or cerebrovascular events (27).

4.3.3. Endothelial function evaluation

A new, non-invasive technique was introduced to evaluate brachial artery flow-mediated dilatation (FMD). The evaluation through a sonographic assessment of brachial artery in basal condition and after 5 minutes of occlusion using pneumonic cuff (250 mm Hg) determined a reactive hyperemia and therefore, FMD. A low FMD is a marker of multifocal atherosclerosis and severity of the disease where the progressive reduction of FMD is associated with more extensive coronary tree involvement and future cardiovascular events [28, 29].

4.3.4. Targeted Ultrasound Detection of Vascular Cell Adhesion Molecule-1 (VCAM-1)

VCAM-1 is expressed by activated endothelial cells and participates in leukocyte rolling and adhesion primarily by interacting with its counterligand VLA-4 (α4 β1) on monocytes and lymphocytes. VCAM-1 expression on the vessel endothelial surface or the underlying vasa vasorum plays an important role in atherosclerotic plaque development by monocyte and T-lymphocyte recruitment. It is an ideal target for molecular imaging because there is little constitutive expression and its upregulation occurs at the earliest stages of atherogenesis. It was hypothesized that molecular imaging with *targeted contrast enhanced ultrasound* **[CEU]** could be used to evaluate the degree of vascular inflammation in atherosclerosis. CEU have multiple practical considerations; low cost, short duration [10 Minutes], good sensitivity and balance between spatial resolution and sensitivity for targeted contrast agent detection. It can potentially be useful in the early diagnosis of atherosclerosis and in monitoring the efficacy of therapeutic interventions.

4.4. Radiological modalities

4.4.1. Fluoroscopy

The detection of coronary calcification on chest films is not easy and the accuracy is only 42% compared with fluoroscopy, which itself is not sensitive. Fluoroscopy has frequently been used to detect calcification in the coronary arteries [31]. Data from the Duke registry of 800 patients by Margolis et al. [32] showed that patients with fluoroscopic evidence of calcium in the coronary arterial tree had a remarkably high prevalence of significant disease (94%). Only 6% of patients with coronary calcification had normal coronary angiograms. Among those without demonstrable calcification, 87% survived for more than 5 years compared to 58% with coronary calcification. Hence the latter implies a greater risk of future cardiac events. Fluoroscopy is widely available but it has several disadvantages [18]:

1. Although it can detect moderate to large calcifications; its ability to identify small calcifications is low.
2. Fluoroscopic detection of calcification is dependent on the skill and experience of the operator as well as the number of views studied.
3. Other important factors include variability of the equipment, patient's body habitus, and calcifications in other structures such as valves and vertebrae and overlying anatomic structures.
4. Finally with fluoroscopy, quantification of calcium is not possible and film documentation is not commonly obtained.

4.4.2. Computed tomography (CT)

Conventional CT is extremely sensitive in detecting vascular calcification. CT showed 50% more calcified vessels than did fluoroscopy. Its limitations are slow scan times resulting in motion artifacts, breathing misregistration, and inability to quantify amount of plaque. *Helical CT* has considerably faster scan times than conventional CT and overlapping sections improves calcium detection. *Double-helix CT scanners* appear to be more sensitive and now termed *electron beam (EBCT)* to distinguish them from conventional CT scanners.

Only *EBCT* can quantitate the amount or volume of calcium. The absence of calcific deposits on an EBCT scan implies the absence of significant angiographic coronary narrowing; however, it does not imply the absence of atherosclerosis, including unstable plaque. One of the most appealing features of EBCT is the potential to detect progression or regression of coronary atherosclerotic disease non-invasively and quantification with the use of calcium-volume score. Although the ACC/AHA [American College of Cardiology (ACC) and the American Heart Association (AHA)] guidelines affirm the strong negative predictive value of a normal EBCT they are not supportive for its widespread use in asymptomatic patients [18].

4.4.3. Magnetic Resonance Imaging [MRI]

Imaging techniques are needed that allow earlier and more refined diagnosis, guide targeted treatment in individual patients and monitor response to that treatment. MRI is well-suited to these tasks as it can provide anatomical, structural, and functional data of the arterial wall. Its capabilities are further enhanced by the use of a range of increasingly sophisticated contrast agents that target specific molecules, cells, and biological processes. Currently, it is considered to identify biologically relevant targets involved in the pathogenesis of atherosclerosis along its different stages [33].

For assessment of lesions that encroach on the vessel lumen inducing ischemia as in angina; angiography provides excellent resolution for the affected vascular territory with possible therapeutic intervention. However, atherosclerosis commonly develops within the walls of arteries without impinging on the vessel lumen; even established disease can be concealed from lumenographic methods. Unfortunately, even these non-stenotic lesions can rupture or erode precipitating intra-arterial thrombosis and acute ischemic events.

Distinct from alternative imaging modalities, MRI can provide data on a large range of vascular parameters that includes measures of vascular physiology (compliance, pulse wave velocity, and flow-mediated vasodilatation), cellular imaging, molecular imaging [adhesion molecule expression (VCAM-1), fibrin and platelets targeting] and functional anatomical data such as wall sheer stresses and density of neovascularization [33].

4.5. Radionuclide evaluation

4.5.1. Tc-99m sestamibi lower extremity muscle scan

Amin et al. [34] stated that Tc-99m sestamibi lower extremity muscle scan is a technique that can be effectively used to diagnose preclinical atherosclerosis in rheumatoid arthritis disease by measuring the so called perfusion reserve [PR]. They reported that it has a place as a screening tool considering the fact; whenever the diagnosis, the better it is the result, however, it could be used for detecting preclinical atherosclerosis even in apparently healthy subjects.

4.5.2. Technique

Prior to the administration of Tc-99m sestamibi for measurement of PR in lower limbs, each subject moved her right foot to produce maximal dorsal and plantar flexion 30–40 times in the sitting position (exercising side). 185 mBq of Tc-99m sestamibi was injected through intravenous line at least 10 sec before exercise termination. Posterior images of each calf were obtained 10 min post-injection. The processing phase was carried out by drawing symmetrical and equal regions of interest (ROI) over both exercising and resting calves. The total counts (Cts) in each (ROI) were obtained through a closed program inherent to the computer system [figure 1]. The percentage of increase of Cts in the exercising right calf was calculated, and the percentile increase obtained was considered as the perfusion reserve using the following formula [normal PR is approx. 50%]:

Perfusion reserve (%) =

[Cts in the exercising calf - Cts in the resting calf/ Cts in resting calf] x 100

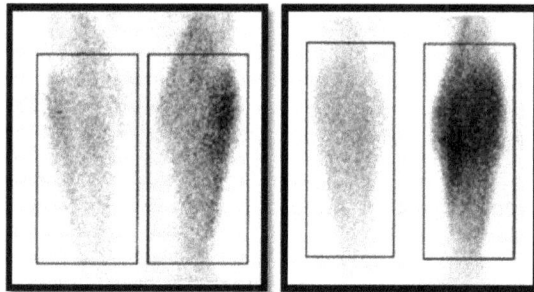

Figure 1. Tc-99m sestamibi muscle scans of an RA patient (PR 29.4%) [Left panel] and a control subject (PR 85%) [Right panel]

4.5.3. Myocardial sestaMIBI Gated-SPECT

Also, in our center a study was designed to evaluate usefulness of Dipyridamole pharmacological stress test in conjunction with Tc-99m sestamibi Gated-SPECT to screen the prevalence of subclinical coronary vascular dysfunction [SCED] in asymptomatic Egyptian Behçet's disease patients and to identify those at higher risk for the presence of such abnormalities as a predictor for preclinical atherosclerosis [*data are not published yet*]. Dipyridamole is an indirect coronary vasodilator that works by increasing intravascular adenosine through inhibition of phosphodiesterase that prohibits reuptake of endogenously produced adenosine into endothelial and red blood cells leading to arteriolar vasodilatation. This increases coronary arterial flow to approximately three times resting values in healthy endothelial state, however it is attenuated in diseased coronary arteries that cannot further dilate in response to adenosine. So, Dipyridamole infusion produces relative flow heterogeneity throughout coronary arteries, resulting in relatively more coronary blood flow in healthy arteries compared with the diseased-arteries inducing ischemia via a *"coronary steal phenomenon"* with subsequent perfusion defects ± abnormal left ventricular wall motion during radionuclide imaging. Hence, we used Dipyridamole stress in conjunction with Tc-99m sestamibi Gated-SPECT as a screening tool for SCED [Figure 2 and 3].

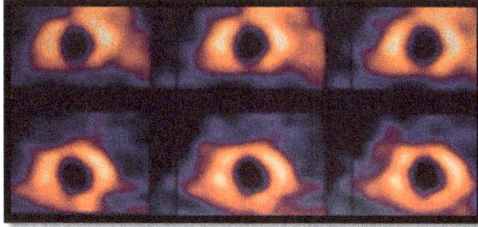

Figure 2. A 35-year-old male with stress induced reduced flow in LAD [anterior wall] and RCA vascular territories [inferior wall] with Complete recovery in the rest phase Coronary angiography was normal; [Stress; Upper row and Rest; Lower row- Short axis slices]

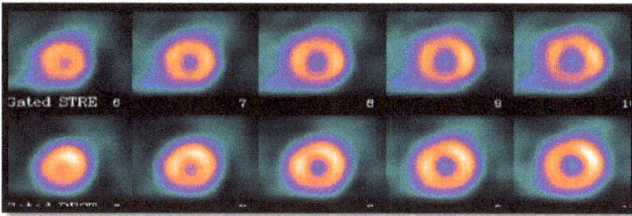

Figure 3. A 33-year-old negative Case for SCED [Stress; Upper row and Rest; Lower row-Short axis slices]

5. Special consideration

5.1. Premature lower limb atherosclerosis

Symptomatic lower extremity arterial occlusive disease in young adults is presumably rare provided that atherosclerosis is a natural consequence of ageing process. Several factors contribute to the "neglect" of premature lower extremity atherosclerosis (*PLEA*) among young population in clinical practice; including low public health awareness of this pathology, absence of large-scale epidemiologic studies, and overall low index of suspicion for vascular etiology of effort-induced lower extremity symptoms. A number of small clinical studies published in the last decade have strongly suggested that PLEA is the major cause for peripheral arterial disease (PAD) in young patients [35].

Levy report in 2002 identified 3 major clinical presentations of PLEA; the majority of patients had typical symptoms of effort-induced claudication, frequently misdiagnosed and attributed to arthritides, muscle spasms, and trauma. Approximately 20-25% present with "blue toe syndrome" caused by atheromatous embolization, most frequently originating from a segmental aortoiliac atherosclerotic lesion. The rest of patients presents with rapidly progressive symptoms of limb-threatening ischemia secondary to atherothrombosis. Also, they observed that many younger patients with isolated aortoiliac atherosclerotic disease had prolonged lower back pain on ambulation involving the spinal muscles who have been treated for several years for chronic low back pain by orthopedic surgeons, or neurosurgeons and some of them even had "unsuccessful" laminectomies before the diagnosis of PAD. In PLEA patients, clinical atherosclerotic disease was present in more than one anatomic location in approximately 60% including the coronary tree. Noninvasive studies are a mainstay of the PLEA diagnosis including ABI measurement and standardized lower extremity treadmill testing that has been developed to assess hyperemic blood flow response to exercise with repeat ABIs compared to the resting ABI with pulse-wave recordings. Also, Tc-99m sestamibi lower extremity muscle scan is suggested as a diagnostic test in PLEA patients [35].

6. Summary and conclusions

In summary, improved understanding of atherogenesis allowed the identification of a large number of molecules and processes. This will provide functional insights to aid diagnosis and to guide treatment with the introduction of new molecular imaging approaches that hold much promise for translation to the clinical practice. In fact, inflammatory biomarkers and imaging will combine structural and functional information to provide a comprehensive evaluation of vascular status at an early stage; hoping to be reversible.

Author details

Amr Amin
Nuclear Medicine, Cairo University, Egypt

Zeinab Nawito
Rheumatology & Rehabilitation, Cairo University, Egypt

Acknowledgement

To our parents and families for their patience, time and support they give all through our life time.

7. References

[1] Hench PS, Kendall EC, Slocumb CH, et al. The effect of a hormone of the adrenal cortex (17-hydroxy-11-dehydrocorticosterone, compound 8E) and of pituitary adrenocorticotrophic hormone on rheumatoid arthritis. Proc Staff Meet Mayo Clin 1949;24:181–97.

[2] Schacke H, Docke WD, Asadullah K. Mechanisms involved in the side effects of glucocorticoids. Pharmacol Ther 2002;96:23–43.

[3] Plotz CM, Knowlton AI, Ragan C. The natural history of Cushing's syndrome. Am J Med 1952;13:597–614.

[4] Plotz CM, Knowlton AI, Ragan C. Natural course of Cushing's syndrome as compared with the course of rheumatoid arthritis treated by hormones. Ann Rheum Dis 1952;11:308–9.

[5] Sholter DE, Armstrong PW. Adverse effects of corticosteroids on the cardiovascular system. Can J Cardiol 2000; 16:505–11.

[6] Kelly JJ, Mangos G,Williamson PM, et al. Cortisol and hypertension. Clin Exp Pharmacol Physiol Suppl 1998; 25:S51–6.

[7] Andrews RC, Walker BR. Glucocorticoids and insulin resistance: old hormones, new targets. Clin Sci (Lond) 1999;96:513–23.

[8] Libby P. Inflammation in atherosclerosis. Nature 2002; 420:868–74.

[9] Rheumatoid arthritis and macrovascular diseasJ. K. Alkaabi, M. Ho1 ,R.Levison,T.Pullar andJ.J.F.Belch Rheumatology 2003;42:292–297.

[10] Moreland LW, O'Dell JR. Glucocorticoids and Rheumatoid Arthritis Back to the Future? Arthritis Rheum. 2002; 46: 2553–63

[11] Del Rincón I, O'Leary DH, Haas RW, Escalante A. Effect of glucocorticoids on the arteries in rheumatoid arthritis. Arthritis Rheum. 2004; 50:3813-22.

[12] McCarthy JH, Palmer FJ: Incidence and significance of coronary artery calcification. Br Heart J 1974, 36:499–506.

[13] Lenk R: Rontgendiagnose der Koronarsklerose in vivo. Fortschr ad Geb D Rontgenstrahlen 1927, 35:1265–1268.

[14] Beadenkopf WG, Daoud AS, Love BM: Calcification in coronary arteries and its relationship to arteriosclerosis and myocardial infraction. Am J Roentgenol 1964, 92:865–871.

[15] Tampas JP, Soule AB: Coronary arterial calcification: its incidence and significance in patients over forty years of age. Am J Roentgenol 1966, 97:369–376.

[16] Fuseini M, Goodwin WJ, Ferris EJ, Mehta JL. Does electron beam computer tomography provide added value in the diagnosis of coronary artery disease? Curr Opin Cardiol. 2003; 18:385-93.

[17] Novo S, Amoroso G, Novo G. Cardiovascular Disease Prevention - Risk Assessment and Management. European society of cardiology 2007: Vol 6, No 10.

[18] Fuseini M, Goodwin WJ, Ferris EJ, Mehta JL. Does electron beam computer tomography provide added value in the diagnosis of coronary artery disease? Curr Opin Cardiol. 2003; 18:385-93.

[19] Alberti KG, Zimmet PZ. Definition, diagnosis and classification of diabetes mellitus and its complications, II: diagnosis and classification of diabetes mellitus provisional report of a WHO consultation. Diabet Med.1998;15:539–553.

[20] Lakka HM, Laaksonen DE, Lakka TA, Niskanen LK, Kumpusalo E, Tuomilehto J, et al. The metabolic syndrome and total and cardiovascular disease mortality in middle-aged men. JAMA. 2002;288:2709–2716.

[21] Bonora E, Kiechl S, Willeit J, Oberhollenzer F, Egger G, Bonadonna RC, et al. Carotid atherosclerosis and coronary heart disease in the metabolic syndrome: prospective data from the Bruneck study. Diabetes Care. 2003;26:1251–1257.

[22] Reilly MP, Rader DJ. The metabolic syndrome: more than the sum of its parts? Circulation. 2003; 108:1546–1551.

[23] Ferri N, Paoletti R, Corsini A. Biomarkers for atherosclerosis: pathophysiological role and pharmacological modulation. Curr Opin Lipidol. 2006; 17:495-501.

[24] Novo S, Pernice C, Barbagallo C M, Tantillo R, Caruso R, Longo B. Influence of risk factors and aging on asymptomatic carotid lesions. In: Advances in Vascular Pathology 1997, A. N. Nicolaides and S. Novo (Eds.), Elsevier Science, Excerpta Medica, Amsterdam, 1997, pp. 33-44.

[25] Corrado E, Bonura F., Tantillo R, Muratori I, Rizzo M, Vitale G, Mansueto S, Novo S. Markers of infection and inflammation influence the outcome of patients with baseline asymptomatic carotid lesions in a 5 years follow-up. Stroke 2006; 37: 482-6.

[26] Corrado E, Muratori I, Tantillo R, Contorno F, Coppola G, Strano A, Novo S. Relationship between endothelial dysfunction, intima media thickness and cardiovascular risk factors in asymptomatic subjects. Int Angiol. 2005; 24:52-8.

[27] Diehm C, Lange S, Darius H, Pittrow D, von Stritzky B, Tepohl G, Haberl RL, Allenberg JR, Dasch B, Trampisch HJ. Association of low ankle brachial index with high mortality in primary care. Eur Heart J. 2006; 27: 1743-9.

[28] Corrado E, Rizzo M, Coppola G, Muratori I, Carella M, Novo S. Endothelial dysfunction and carotid lesions are strong predictors of clinical events in patients with early stages of atherosclerosis: a 24-month follow-up study. Coron Artery Dis. 2008; 19(3):139-44.

[29] Landmesser U, Hornig B, Drexler H Endothelium Function: A Critical Determinant in Atherosclerosis. Circulation. 2004; 109 (suppl. II): II-27-II-33.

[30] Kaufmann BA, Sanders JM, Davis C, Xie A, Aldred P, Sarembock IJ, Lindner JR. Molecular imaging of inflammation in atherosclerosis with targeted ultrasound detection of vascular cell adhesion molecule-1. Circulation. 2007; 116:276-84.

[31] Souza AS, Bream PR, Elliot LP: Chest film detection of coronary artery calcification: the value of the CAC triangle. Radiology 1978, 129:7–10.

[32] Margolis JR, Chen JTT, Kong Y, et al.: The diagnostic and prognostic significance of coronary artery calcification. Radiology 137:609–616.

[33] Choudhury RP. Atherosclerosis and thrombosis: identification of targets for magnetic resonance imaging. Top Magn Reson Imaging. 2007 Oct;18(5):319-27.

[34] Amin AM, Nawito ZO, Atfy RA, El-Hadidi KT. Tc-99m sestamibi lower extremity muscle scan, is it a useful screening tool for assessment of preclinical atherosclerosis in rheumatoid arthritis patients? Rheumatol Int. 2012 Jul;32(7):2075-81.

[35] Levy PJ. . Premature lower extremity atherosclerosis: clinical aspects. Am J Med Sci. 2002; 323:11-6.

Chapter 10

The Role of Corticosteroids in Today's Oral and Maxillofacial Surgery

Mohammad Zandi

Additional information is available at the end of the chapter

1. Introduction

Corticosteroids are group of hormones with similar chemical formulas which are secreted by adrenal cortex. The very slight differences in molecular structure of various corticosteroids give them very different functions. The hormonal steroids are classified according to their biologic effects as glucocorticoids, which mainly affect intermediary metabolism and the immune system, and mineralocorticoids , which have principally a salt-retaining activity. Of large number of steroids released into the circulation by adrenal cortex, two are of greater importance – aldosterone, which is a mineralocorticoid, and cortisol, which is a glucocorticoid.

Mineralocorticoids promote sodium and water retention, and potassium loss by kidney, but have no anti-inflammatory or anti-allergic effect.

Cortisol, also known as hydrocortisone, is the major glucocorticoid in humans. It is synthesized by the cells of the zona fasciculata and zona reticularis of adrenal cortex; its secretion is regulated by the adrenocorticotropic hormone (ACTH) from anterior pituitary gland. Cortisol has a wide range of physiologic actions such as influencing carbohydrate, protein, and fat metabolism; regulation of blood pressure and cardiovascular function; and affecting immune system.

Corticosteroid drugs are the synthetic analogs of cortisol hormone. They bind to specific intracellular receptors upon entering target tissues, and mimic the effects of the naturally occurring hormones; the main differences are the relative glucocorticoid versus mineralocorticoid potency and the long half-life that the synthetic analogs have. The relative potencies and duration of action of representative corticosteroids are presented in Table 1.

Compound	Glucocorticoid potency	Mineralocorticoid potency	Duration of action
Cortisol	1	1	short
Cortisone	0.8	0.8	short
Fludrocortisone	10	125	Intermediate
Prednisone	4	0.8	Intermediate
Prednisolone	4	0.8	Intermediate
Methylprednisolone	5	0.5	Intermediate
Triamcinolone	5	0	Intermediate
Betamethasone	25	0	Long
Dexamethasone	25	0	Long

Short: 8-12 hours biologic half-life; Intermediate: 12-36 hours biologic half-life; Long: 36-72 hours biologic half-life. Adapted and modified from [1]

Table 1. Relative potencies and equivalent doses of representative corticosteroids

Glucocorticoids are used, either singly or in combination with other drugs, in the treatment of a wide variety of medical disorders. Some therapeutic indications for these drugs are as follows:

• Musculoskeletal and connective tissue diseases (rheumatoid arthritis, polymyositis, systemic lupus erythematosus, and vasculitis)
• Respiratory diseases (sarcoidosis and chronic bronchitis)
• Gastrointestinal diseases (ulcerative colitis and crohn's disease)
• Allergic disorders (asthma, hay fever, and allergic rhinitis)
• Skin conditions (pemphigus, eczema, and dermatitis)
• Eye diseases (conjunctivitis, uveitis, and optic neuritis)
• Oral and maxillofacial diseases (lichen planus, keloid formation, and Bell's palsy)

Although corticosteroids are widely used for treatment of diseases and conditions affecting oral and maxillofacial region, the scientific literature on this topic is limited and scattered throughout numerous journals and books. By gathering this scattered information, this chapter presents a concise review of various uses of corticosteroid drugs in the treatment of diseases affecting oral and maxillofacial region, and the role they have in reducing post-operative morbidities such as pain, edema and trismus after various maxillofacial surgical procedures. The relation between maternal corticosteroid use and congenital maxillofacial deformities are explained. Also discussed is the perioperative management of patients receiving long-term therapeutic doses of corticosteroids.

2. Uses of corticosteroids in the treatment of oral and maxillofacial diseases

Corticosteroids are widely used in the treatment of diseases, disorders and conditions affecting the oral and maxillofacial area and the adjacent and associated structures. The diseases of the oral and maxillofacial region may be either local or the manifestation of a systemic problem. Corticosteroids have their widest application in the management of acute and chronic conditions which have an allergic, immunologic, or inflammatory basis. Therefore, a group of corticosteroids which have predominantly a glucocorticoid activity and little or no mineralocorticoid action such as betamethasone, dexamethasone, triamcinolone, and prednisolone are used.

The following are the main therapeutic indications for glucocorticoids in oral and maxillofacial diseases.

2.1. Temporomandibular disorders (TMDs)

TMDs are clinical problems involving the temporomandibular joints (TMJs), the masticatory muscles, or both. TMDs affect a significant number of individuals, and are the most common musculoskeletal disorders that cause orofacial pain. [2] Trauma to the joint structures, especially microtrauma, accounts for the majority of patients who develop TMJ problems. However, a small number of joint diseases are caused by nontraumatic etiologic factors including benign and malignant neoplasms (osteoma, chondroma, and synovial sarcoma), congenital or developmental anomalies (condylar agenesis and heperplasia), arthritides (rheumatoid arthritis), and systemic diseases. The most common signs and symptoms of TMDs are pain, altered mandibular movements, and the elicitation of joint noise.

Treatment of TMDs varies according to their etiologic basis. Conservative managements (splint therapy, thermal application, pharmacotherapy, and physiotherapy), surgical treatments, or a combination of them may be required. A variety of medications have been used to relieve pain, inflammation, muscle spasm and other signs and symptoms associated with TMDs. They include nonsteroidal anti-inflammatory drugs (NSAIDs), corticosteroids, analgesics, and muscle relaxants.

Various glucocorticoids are used in the treatment of TMDs (Table 2). These drugs have dramatic effects on pain, hypomobility, and inflammation associated with acute TMJ problems. Oral corticosteroids are used mainly for treatment of acute TMJ discomforts or for diagnostic purposes. They should be used in a short term basis (tapering dose lasting 5 to 7 days), and repeated as infrequently as possible. Long term use of corticosteroids for the treatment of TMDs is contraindicated; it can result in a cushing's- like disease process, acute adrenal crisis, hypertension, electrolyte abnormalities, diabetes, and formation of osteoporosis including the TMJ. [2]

Drug	Alternative name	Usual dose
Hydrocortisone	Hydrocortone	20-240 mg/day
Prednisone	Deltasone, Orasone	5-60 mg/day
Prednisolone	Delta-Cortef	5-60 mg/day
Dexamethasone	Decadron	0.75-9.0 mg/day
Betamethasone	Celestone	0.6-7.2 mg/day

Adapted and modified from [2]

Table 2. Oral corticosteroids used in TMDs

Intracapsular injection of glucocortcoids has been reported to decrease pain in patients with both pain and limited mouth opening secondary to inflammatory disorders of the joint, such as arthritis and capsulitis. [3-5]

A number of mechanisms have been described for the anti-inflammatory actions of glucocorticoids. These drugs inhibit inflammatory mediator release from many cell types involved in inflammation such as macrophages, T-lymphocytes, mast cells, dendritic cells, and neutrophilic leukocytes. Glucocorticoids also reduce prostaglandin production by blocking the phospholipase A_2 enzyme.

The most striking effect of glucocorticoids is to inhibit the expression of multiple inflammatory genes encoding cytokines, chemokines, inflammatory enzymes, receptors and adhesion molecules. [6] Changes in gene transcription are regulated by proinflammatory transcription factors, such as nuclear factor-κB (NF-κB) and activator protein-1 (AP-1). These proinflammatory transcription factors switch on inflammatory genes via a process involving recruitment of transcriptional coactivator proteins and changes in chromatin modifications such as histone acetylation. Glucocorticoids exert their anti-inflammatory effect on responsive cells by binding and activating a cytoplasmic glucocorticoid receptor. The interaction between the activated glucocorticoid receptor and proinflammatory transcription factors may result in deacetylation of histones and repression of inflammatory genes. [7]

In chronic inflammatory disorders of TMJ, macrophages, T-lymphocytes, and other cell types involved in inflammation release many cytokines and chemokines which will induce expression of adhesion molecules, release of variable enzymes from fibroblasts and osteoclasts and result in bone erosion. IL-8, which is a chemokine, is known to cause the infiltration of neutrophils into synovial fluid and promote joint inflammation. It was detected in 80% of the synovial tissue specimens taken from the TMJs with internal derangement. Similarly, IL-11 has been involved in the pathogenesis of osteoarthritis and rheumatoid arthritis. It has been found in synovial fluids of diseased temporomandibular joint and other joints. [8]

Cytokines participate in various inflammatory processes and induce protease synthesis; their effects can be either synergic or inhibitory. In synovial joints, IL-1 α, IL-1 β and TNF-α induce synovitis and promote the production of proteinases resulting in degradation of cartilage, while IL-1ra works to block IL-1α and IL-1 β from binding to other cell receptors and has many beneficial effects on inflammatory diseases. [9] In a study by Nordahl et al. it was found that the local production of tumor necrosis factor-*alpha* (TNF-α) occured in the TMJ synovium of patients with chronic inflammatory connective tissue disease, and the severity of pain and tenderness of the TMJ was related to the level of TNF-α. [10] In a study by Frediksson et al., it was shown that the presence of TNF-α in the synovial fluid of TMJ predicted a positive treatment response to intra-articular glucocorticoid injection in patients with chronic TMJ inflammatory disorders. [11]

Long-term complications associated with intra-articular glucocorticoid injection cannot be determined from the limited investigations done to date and thus remained unclear. Wenneberg et al. in a study evaluating the long-term prognosis of intra-articular glucocorticoid injections for TMJ arthritis observed that this treatment modality was helpful, and there were no radiographically demonstrable side effects of the treatment. [12] In contrast, Haddad IK showed that intra-articular injections of corticosteroids (triamcinolone acetonide) cause damage to fibrous layer, cartilage, and bone of TMJ. [13]

Juvenile idiopathic arthritis (JIA) is a chronic rheumatologic disease of children which may involve TMJ region, and cause significant craniofacial growth disturbances. The treatment of TMJ arthritis is controversial. It has been shown that glucocorticoid injection of the TMJ reduces pain and inflammation, and improves the function of TMJ in children with JIA. [14] Other studies also confirmed that corticosteroid injection of the TMJ can be safely performed in children with JIA, and is effective. [15-18] Few studies have evaluated TMJ corticosteroid injection in JIA. In these studies the volume of corticosteroid injected was chosen empirically. Treatment protocols such as injection of 1 cc (40 mg) of triamcinolone acetonide, 1 cc (20 mg) of triamcinolone hexacetonidein, and 0.5 to 1 cc of the diluted (with 1% lidocaine HCL) triamcinolone hexacetonidein into each of the involved TMJs, all have been used in previous studies. [14-16] The peak effect occurs after approximately 6 weeks of treatment, and the expected duration is 6-17 months. The children may receive a second injection approximately 6 months after the first. [16]

Side effects of intra-articular steroid injection in children include immediate reactions, such as pain and headache, or delayed side effects, such as joint infection and loss of subcutaneous fat. [16] Because the mandibular endochondral growth zone is located at the head of condyle (at the site of corticosteroid injection), the concern is whether intra-articular corticosteroid injection per se may cause growth retardation. Stoustrup et al., in an animal study demonstrated that intra-articular glucocorticoid injection may result in even more pronounced mandibular growth reduction than that caused by the arthritis alone. [19] Schindler et al. reported a case of severe temporomandibular dysfunction and joint destruction after intra-articular injection of triamcinolone, and El-Hakim et al. showed TMJ resorption with active osteoclastic activity after intra-articular injection of a single dose of dexamethasone in rats. [20,21]

intra-articular corticosteroid injection has been used to improve mouth opening in patients with anterior disk displacement without reduction (ADDWOR), i.e., closed lock. [22]

2.2. Oral ulcerative and vesiculobullous lesions

Corticosteroids are successfully used for the treatment of several ulcerative and vesiculobullous lesions involving the oral cavity and perioral areas including recurrent aphthous stomatitis (RAS), Behcet's syndrome, pemphigus vulgaris, bullous pemphigoid, mucous membrane pemphigoid, erythema multiforme and Stevens-Johnson syndrome (Tables 3-5). [23]

Recurrent aphthous stomatitis: These superficial painful ulcers occur commonly in the oral cavity. Minor form of the disease has 1 to 5 ulcers at one episode. The ulcers which are under 1 cm in diameter persist 8 to 14 days, and heal spontaneously without sequelae. The major aphthous ulcers are larger than 1 cm, and persist for weeks to months. Corticosteroids either alone or in combination with other drugs have been used for treatment of these lesions. [24-28] Topical steroids, such as triamcinolone acetonide and prednisolone (2 times/day), are formulated as oral pastes. Therapeutic benefit can be derived from a mouthwash containing betamethasone. It should be noted that the long-term use of topical steroids may predispose patient to developing oral candidiasis. [28]

Topical and injectable (intralesional) corticosteroids are useful for large and painful lesions. Systemic administration of corticosteroids is reserved for severe cases to prevent lesion formation or to reduce the number of lesions. Systemic corticosteroids should be prescribed in short courses, and only for severe outbreaks or cases that don't respond to topical or injectable corticosteroids. [23]

Behcet's syndrome: The treatment of oral lesions of Behcet's syndrome is similar to the treatment of severe or major RAS. [23]

Pemphigus vulgaris: Pemphigus vulgaris is a severe, potentially life-threatening vesiculobullous disease that may affect skin and mucous membranes. Oral cavity is involved in nearly 80% of patients. In the past, corticosteroid therapy was the treatment of choice but later, combination therapy involving the use of systemic corticosteroids with immunosuppressive agents was introduced, in an attempt to achieve disease control with lower doses of steroids. [29-31]

The principal treatment of pemphigus vulgaris is systemic administration of corticosteroids at doses of 1 to 2 mg/kg/day. Maintenance of remission may be achieved with topical corticosteroids, allowing reduction of systemic drugs. Isolated lesions can be treated with injectable corticosteroids. [23]

Bullous and mucous membrane pemphigoid: The choice of drugs used for the treatment of pemphigoid is based upon the sites of involvement, clinical severity, and disease progression. For more severe disease, or with rapid progression, systemic corticosteroids are the agents of choice for initial treatment, combined with steroid-sparing agents for long-term maintenance. [32] Topical and injectable corticosteroids are useful for treatment of mild or localized oral lesions. [23]

Erythema multiforme (EM) and *Stevens-Johnson syndrome (SJS):* It has been shown that corticosteroids have a favorable influence on the outcome of EM and SJS, if administered in high doses, over a short period of time, early in the course of the disease, and with proper tapering of medication. [33-37] However, the dosing and route of administration that provides the most benefit for EMM and SJS patients is in question. Treatment protocols such as early therapy with systemic prednisone (0.5 to 1.0mg/kg/day) or pulse methylprednisolone (1mg/kg/day for 3 days), intravenous pulsed dose methylprednisolone (3 consecutive daily infusions of 20–30mg/kg to a maximum of 500mg given over 2 to 3 hours), and dexamethasone pulse therapy (1.5mg/kg IV over 30 to 60 minutes on 3 consecutive days), all have been shown to be effective. [33-35,37-39]

Drug	Triamcinolone (10 mg/ml) Dexamethasone (4 mg/ml)
Indications	Severe recurrent aphthous stomatitis, major aphthous stomatitis, erosive lichen planus
Usual dosage	Inject 0.1 cc/cm lesion
Contraindications	Hypersensitivity to corticosteroids, systemic fungal infection, live vaccines, active tuberculosis
Common side effects	Candidiasis, hyperglycemia
Unusual side effects	Peptic ulceration with perforation, osteoporosis, impaired wound healing, mucosal atrophy

Adapted and modified from [23].

Table 3. Injectable (intralesional) corticosteroids used for treatment of oral lesions

Drug	Beclomethasone	Betamethasone	Clobetasol	Halobetasol	Fluocinonide
Indications	Severe recurrent aphthous stomatitis, Behcet's syndrome, pemphigus vulgaris, pemphigoid				
Administration	Inhaler spray topically to mucosal lesions	Topical intraoral cream or gel, soluble tablets as mouth wash	Topical intraoral cream or gel	Topical intraoral cream or ointment	Topical intraoral cream
Usual dosage	50-100 µg sprayed onto oral lesion	0.1% cream or 0.05% gel applied thinly bid; 0.5 mg 2-4 times daily as mouth wash	0.05% cream or gel applied thinly bid	0.05% cream or ointment applied thinly bid	0.05% cream applied thinly bid
Contraindications	Untreated infections				
Common side effects	Oral candidiasis				
Unusual side effects	Adrenal suppression if doses exceeded				

Adapted and modified from [23].

Table 4. Topical corticosteroids used for treatment of oral lesions

Drug	Prednisone (tablets)
Indications	Severe recurrent aphthous stomatitis, Behcet's syndrome, pemphigus vulgaris, pemphigoid, erythema multiforme
Usual dosage	1. 30-40 mg daily after breakfast for 4-5 days 2. 1-2 mg/kg/day after breakfast until disease controlled 3. 1-2 mg/kg/day, then maintenance of 2.5-15 mg daily 4. 20-40 mg daily for 7-10 days at onset of lesions or until lesions resolve 5. 60 mg daily for 2 days, 50 mg daily for 2 days, 40 mg daily for 2 days, 30 mg daily for 2 days, 20 mg daily for 2 days, 10 mg daily for 2 days
Contraindications	Hypersensitivity to corticosteroids, systemic infection (unless specific antimicrobial therapy given), peptic disease (unless proton pump inhibitor given), live vaccines
Common side effects	Dyspepsia, candidiasis, myopathy, osteoporosis, adrenal suppression, Cushing's syndrome, euphoria, depression
Unusual side effects	Peptic ulceration with perforation, Cushingoid side effects increasingly likely with doses above 7.5 mg daily

Adapted and modified from [23].

Table 5. Systemic corticosteroids used for treatment of oral lesions

2.3. Keloid and hypertrophic scars

Keloid and hypertrophic scar (HS) represent pathologic overhealing conditions which are caused by excessive production of fibrous tissue following healing of skin injuries. Keloid produces significantly more collagen than HS. Their exact cause is unknown but inflammation, tension, and genetic background are mentioned as contributing factors. Keloid and HS have different clinical features. Keloids extend beyond the confines of the original wound, develop months after injury, and rarely regress. HS is a raised scar that remains confined to the area of the injury, usually form within weeks, and may regress without intervention.

Various treatment modalities have been used for prevention and treatment of keloid and HSs such as pressure therapy, silicone gel sheeting, topical flavonoids, corticosteroid therapy, radiotherapy, and surgery.

Topical and intralesional glucocorticoids are frequently used to treat existing keloid and HS or, prophylactically, to prevent their formation or recurrence after surgical removal. Topical administration of steroids doesn't appear to be as efficacious as intralesional injection of the drug. Intralesional steroid injection, either on its own or in combination with other treatment modalities is the most common treatment used for keloid and HSs. Glucocorticoids have a multiplicity of effects on scars including suppressive effects on the inflammatory process in the wound, diminishing collagen and glycosaminoglycan synthesis, inhibition of fibroblast growth, and enhancing collagen and fibroblast degeneration. [40,41] Triamcinolone acetonide is the most commonly used steroid for the treatment of HS and keloid. It is used in a concentration of 10-20 mg/ml, though it can be given at a dose of 40 mg/ml for a tough bulky lesion; the concentration depends upon the size and site of the lesion and age of the individual. [42] Side effects of steroid injection include hypopigmentation, dermal atrophy, telangiectasia, and cushingoid effects from systemic absorption. [41] Cushing's syndrome secondary to injection of triamcinolone acetonide for the treatment of keloids have been reported by several investigators. [43,44]

2.4. Central giant cell granuloma

Central giant cell granuloma of the jaws is a benign tumor which occurs most often in children and young adults. This tumor is made up of loose fibrous connective tissue stroma with many interspersed proliferating fibroblasts, aggregations of multinucleated giant cells, and foci of hemorrhage.

Various surgical and nonsurgical treatments have been advocated for this lesion. One of the nonsurgical treatments proposed is intralesional corticosteroid injections. Intralesional injection of triamcinolone acetonide has been shown to induce partial and in some cases complete resolution of central giant cell granuloma. However, there is no reasonably strong consensus in the literature regarding optimal dosage and duration of treatment that provides the most benefit. The mechanism of action of corticosteroids in the treatment of central giant cell granuloma is unknown. A rationale for its use has been the histologic resemblance of central giant cell granuloma to sarcoid. Because corticosteroids have been effective in the treatment of sarcoid, it was thought that they may have a similar therapeutic effect on central giant cell granuloma. In addition, corticosteroids may act by suppressing any angiogenic component of the lesion. [45]

2.5. Bell's palsy

Bell's palsy is an idiopathic inflammation of the facial nerve (the seventh of twelve paired cranial nerves) which occurs almost always on one side only. It is characterized by facial muscle weakness, hyperacusis, decreased tearing, and loss of taste on the anterior two thirds of the tongue. Because Bell's palsy results from inflammation and edema of the facial nerve, corticosteroids constitute the standard medicine in the treatment of this condition. [46-48] For adults, prednisolone at doses of 1 mg/kg/day for 7 to 10 days, taken in divided doses in the morning and evening, is suggested.

2.6. Management of post-operative morbidities associated with maxillofacial surgeries

Facial pain, edema, ecchymosis and limitation of mouth opening are the expected sequelae of oral and maxillofacial surgeries. These post-operative complications affect the ability of patient to interrelate and to return to the daily life and activities, and deteriorate the quality of life of patient. [49,50]

Many modalities are used to abate sequelae in the oral and maxillofacial surgery including use of ice pack, pressure dressing, surgical drain, and drugs.

Corticosteroids are commonly used to control post-operative morbidities and to provide comfort for patients. However, there are no definite protocols relative to molecules, doses, schedules, and routes of administration. [51] The most commonly administered types of corticosteroids are betamethasone, dexamethasone, and methylprednisolone, administered intravenously, orally or by injection into the masseter muscle. The morbidity-management protocol also varies depending upon the type of surgery being performed.

To decrease post-rhinoplasty edema, the administration of corticosteroids has been advocated for many years. In a study by Gurlek et al., it was shown that high dose methylprednisolone was effective in preventing and reducing both the periorbital ecchymosis and edema in open rhinoplasty. [52] In the same line, Kargi et al., and Kara and Gokalan showed that the perioperative use of corticosteroids reduced edema and ecchymosis associated with rhinoplasty surgery. [53,54] In contrast, Hoffmann et al. did not observe any increase either in the edema or the ecchymosis after rhinoplasty surgery. [55]

Regarding orthognathic surgery, several investigations demonstrated that perioperative corticosteroid administration significantly reduced post-operative inflammation and edema. [56-59] In contrast, Munro et al. did not observe any significant decrease in postoperative edema even with the highest doses and the longest durations of corticosteroid treatment. [56]

The effects of corticosteroids on post-operative edema after oral surgery have been widely investigated in the literature. Many prior studies demonstrated a significant decrease in post-operative edema after administration of corticosteroids. [60-63] In a study by Zandi, it was shown that steroids not only reduced the facial swelling, but also the severity of pain after surgery. [60] Similarly, several studies reported that corticosteroids significantly decreased post-operative edema and pain, indicating a strong correlation between edema and pain decreases. [62-64]

Even though the effects of corticosteroids on post-operative morbidities after various oral and maxillofacial surgeries have been widely investigated in the literature, methodological differences, variation in agents, doses, and routes of administration of the drugs have compromised the scientific conclusions.

2.7. Other uses of corticosteroids in oral and maxillofacial surgery

In addition to the aforementioned indications, corticosteroids are successfully used in the management of acute trigeminal nerve injuries, traumatic facial nerve paralysis, chronic facial pain, and allergic diseases involving maxillofacial area.

3. Corticosteroids contraindications

In prescribing corticosteroids, physicians must be aware that some patients are poor candidates for systemic, locally injected, or topical corticosteroid therapy.

Systemic corticosteroids must be used with the greatest of caution in patients with uncontrolled hypertension, diabetes, active peptic ulcer, heart diseases, infections, psychiatric disorders, osteoporosis, cataract, glaucoma, tuberculosis, mycobacterial diseases, herpes simplex infection, pregnancy, varicella zoster infection, immune deficiency, underactive thyroid, and mental disorders.

Injectable corticosteroid use is contraindicated in patients with hypersensitivity to corticosteroids, infections, and active tuberculosis.

Use of topical corticosteroids is absolutely contraindicated in the treatment of primary bacterial infections such as impetigo, furuncles, carbuncles, erysipelas, cellulitis, lymphangitis, and erythrasma. Topical corticosteroids are also contraindicated in patients with a history of hypersensitivity to any of the components of the preparation. Currently, little is known about the safety of topical corticosteroids in pregnancy. Although it has been reported that there is an association between very potent topical corticosteroids and congenital abnormalities including low birth weight and orofacial clefts, use of these drugs in pregnancy is not recommended unless the potential benefit justifies the potential risks to fetus. [65]

Ophthalmic use of topical corticosteroids is contraindicated in most viral, bacterial, and fungal diseases of ocular structures.

4. Corticosteroids side effects

Although corticosteroids have great potential in the treatment of various diseases and conditions affecting oral and maxillofacial region, they also carry the risk of many side effects. Therefore, benefits from corticosteroids should always be weighed against their potential risks. Side effects of corticosteroids vary depending on the type and dose of the medication, rout of administration, and length of treatment. Significant adverse effects are most likely to occur in patients using oral corticosteroids for a long period of time. These may include weight gain, impaired growth, adrenal insufficiency, electrolyte abnormalities, increased susceptibility to infection, myopathy, osteoporosis, osteonecrosis, cataract, glaucoma, psychological problems, fractures, hypertension, insomnia, moon face, diabetes, and peptic ulcer. [1,66]

Topical glucocorticoids may cause adverse effects such as skin atrophy, hypopigmentation, subcutaneous fat wasting, telangectasia, contact dermatitis, oral thrush, and cushingoid effects from systemic absorption. [28,41] Application of topical corticosteroids on eyelids has been reported to cause glaucoma. Adrenal suppression, growth retardation in children, and cushing's syndrome are rare adverse effects of long term topical corticosteroid use.

Intralesional glucocorticoids may cause sterile abscess, skin atrophy, hypopigmentation, panniculitis, and skin necrosis.

Although the frequency of side effects of inhaled corticosteroids is lower than systemic corticosteroids, high doses of inhaled corticosteroids have the potential to produce various local and systemic side effects. Systemic side effects associated with inhaled corticosteroids

include osteoporosis, retarded growth in children, cataracts, glaucoma, and skin thinning. Inhaled corticosteroids may cause local side effects including oropharyngeal candidiasis, dysphonia, reflex cough, bronchospasm, and pharyngitis. [67]

5. Perioperative management of patients with adrenal insufficiency

Insufficient adrenocortical function is a rare disorder resulting from endogenous deficiency (primary) or from the administration of exogenous corticosteroids (secondary). Adrenal suppression should be suspected in those patients receiving the equivalent of 20 mg of prednisone daily for one week or the equivalent of 7.5 mg of prednisone daily for one month within the past year. [2] In adrenal suppression the body is not able to appropriately manage the challenge of stresses such as medical illness, surgery, and trauma. This may precipitate an adrenal crisis, signaled by the onset of fever, restlessness, flank and abdominal pain, vomiting, lethargy, hypotension, or coma.

Any patient suspected of having adrenal insufficiency should be evaluated with an ACTH (cortrosyn) stimulation test or be given supplemental corticosteroids empirically perioperatively. Cortrosyn stimulation test measures how well the adrenal glands respond to a synthetic ACTH administered to the patient.

The currently recommended corticosteroid coverage for various surgical procedures is based on the magnitude of stress and the known glucocorticoid production rate associated with it, and includes the following: [2,68]

- Minor surgical stress such as tooth extraction, biopsy, periodontal surgery, genioplasty, etc: 25 mg of hydrocortisone equivalent, the day of surgery
- Moderate surgical stress such as panfacial fractures, two jaw surgery, etc: 50-75 mg of hydrocortisone equivalent for 1 to 2 days.
- Major surgical stress such as extensive head and neck resection and reconstruction, etc: 100-150 mg of hydrocortisone equivalent for 2 to 3 days.

In the case of postoperative complications such as fever and pain, it is recommended that the corticosteroid administration be continued consistent with the post-operative stress response. [68]

6. Maternal corticosteroid use and the risk of orofacial clefts in infants

Orofacial clefts are the most common congenital deformity affecting maxillofacial area. The etiology of facial clefting is complex and has been extensively investigated. There are both major and minor genetic influences involved, with variable interactions from environmental factors. [69] Several environmental factors such as maternal drug intake, trauma, smoking, and exposure to x-rays during the pregnancy period have been suggested to increase the chance of cleft development in infants. [70]

Pregnant women often use topical, inhaled, or systemic corticosteroid drugs for a variety of inflammatory and allergic conditions. Several investigations have reported that the use of corticosteroids during early pregnancy is associated with a 3- to 6-fold increased risk of orofacial clefts. [71-75] Although systemic corticosteroids are associated with a higher risk of orofacial clefts than topical corticosteroids, the latter is not without risk. It has been shown that application of hydrocortisone cream on eczematous skin is associated with significant increase in the level of plasma cortisol. [76] In a study by Edwards et al., a significant association between topical corticosteroids and orofacial cleft was observed. [77] Epidemiologic data have shown that low-to-moderate doses of inhaled corticosteroids taken during the first trimester of pregnancy are safe but raise concerns about high doses. [78]

The mechanism of cleft palate production by corticosteroids is uncertain; it is a complicated interference in a complex developmental program involving many genetic and biochemical processes. Glucocorticoids may cause cleft palate deformity by delaying palatal shelf elevation. [79] Corticosteroids can reduce the collagen content of connective tissue by inhibiting collagen synthesis, which could disrupt cell-cell interaction and tissue-tissue interactions. [71]

7. Conclusion

Glucocorticoids are used, either singly or in combination with other drugs, for the treatment of various diseases affecting oral and maxillofacial area. They are also frequently used to minimize expected post-operative morbidities such as pain and edema after oral and maxillofacial surgeries. Because of anti-inflammatory and anti-allergic actions of glucocorticoids, they have their widest application in the management of acute and chronic conditions which have allergic, immunologic, or inflammatory basis. However, corticosteroids carry the risk of potential side effects which are sometimes severe and life threatening. Therefore, benefits from corticosteroids should always be weighed against their potential risks in each patient.

Prescribing the minimal dose and the least potent type of corticosteroids necessary to produce a given therapeutic effect, simultaneous use of non-steroidal agents to reduce the dose of corticosteroids, and prescribing corticosteroids for a short period of time or sporadically are some strategies to minimize corticosteroids adverse effects.

Author details

Mohammad Zandi
Department of Oral and Maxillofacial Surgery,
Hamedan University of Medical Sciences, Hamedan, Iran
Researcher, Dental Research Center,
Hamedan University of medical sciences, Hamedan, Iran

Acknowledgement

The author wishes to express his deep appreciation to Dr. Mojgan Ahmadian for her extensive assistance in the preparation of this chapter.

8. References

[1] Brunton LL, Lazo JS, Parker KL (2005) Goodman & Gilman's The pharmacological basis of therapeutics. Eleventh edition. New York: McGraw-Hill.

[2] Fonseca RJ, Marciani RD, Turvey TA (2009) Oral and maxillofacial surgery. Second edition. Saunders.

[3] Kopp S, Akerman S, Nilner M (1991) Short-term effects of intra-articular sodium hyaluronate, glucocorticoid, and saline injections on rheumatoid arthritis of the temporomandibular joint. J Craniomandib Disord. 5: 231-238.

[4] Alstergren P, Appelgren A, Appelgren B, Kopp S, Lundeberg T, Theodorsson E (1996) The effect on joint fluid concentration of neuropeptide Y by intra-articular injection of glucocorticoid in temporomandibular joint arthritis. Acta Odontol Scand. 54: 1-7.

[5] Fredriksson L, Alstergren P, Kopp S (2005) Serotonergic mechanisms influence the response to glucocorticoid treatment in TMJ arthritis. Mediators Inflamm. 2005:194–201.

[6] Barnes PJ (1998) Anti-inflammatory actions of glucocorticoids: molecular mechanisms. Clin Sci. 94: 557–572.

[7] Adcock IM, Ito K, Barnes PJ (2004) Glucocorticoids: effects on gene transcription. Proc Am Thorac Soc. 1: 247-254.

[8] Gulen H, Ataoglu H, Haliloglu S, Isik K (2009) Proinflammatory cytokines in temporomandibular joint synovial fluid before and after arthrocentesis. Oral Surg Oral Med Oral Pathol Oral Radiol Endod. 107: e1-4.

[9] Kardel R, Ulfgren AK, Reinhold FP, and Holmlund A (2003) Inflammatory cell and cytokine patterns in patients with painful clicking and osteoarthritis in the temporomandibular joint. Int J Oral Maxillofac Surg. 32: 390-396.

[10] Nordahl S, Alstergren P, Kopp S (2000) Tumor necrosis factor-alpha in synovial fluid and plasma from patients with chronic connective tissue disease and its relation to temporomandibular joint pain. J Oral Maxillofac Surg. 58: 525–530.

[11] Fredriksson L, Alstergren P, Kopp S (2006) Tumor necrosis factor- alpha in temporomandibular joint synovial fluid predicts treatment effects on pain by intra-articular glucocorticoid treatment. Mediators Inflamm. 2006: 59425.

[12] Wenneberg B, Kopp S, Gröndahl HG (1991) Long-term effect of intra-articular injections of a glucocorticosteroid into the TMJ: a clinical and radiographic 8-year follow-up. J Craniomandib Disord 5: 11-18.

[13] Haddad IK (2000) Temporomandibular joint osteoarthrosis. Histopathological study of the effects of intra-articular injection of triamcinolone acetonide. Saudi Med J. 21: 675-679.

[14] Arabshahi B, Dewitt EM, Cahill AM, Kaye RD, Baskin KM, Towbin RB, Cron RQ (2005) Utility of corticosteroid injection for temporomandibular arthritis in children with juvenile idiopathic arthritis. Arthritis Rheum. 52: 3563-3569.

[15] Stoll ML, Good J, Sharpe T, Beukelman T, Young D, Waite PD, Cron RQ (2012) Intra-articular corticosteroid injections to the temporomandibular joints are safe and appear to be effective therapy in children with juvenile idiopathic arthritis. J Oral Maxillofac Surg. (Article in press).

[16] Cahill AM, Baskin KM, Kaye RD, Arabshahi B, Cron RQ, Dewitt EM, Bilaniuk L, Towbin RB (2007) CT-guided percutaneous steroid injection for management of inflammatory arthropathy of the temporomandibular joint in children. AJR Am J Roentgenol. 188: 182-186.

[17] Ringold S, Torgerson TR, Egbert MA, Wallace CA (2008) Intraarticular corticosteroid injections of the temporomandibular joint in juvenile idiopathic arthritis. J Rheumatol. 35: 1157-1164.

[18] Parra DA, Chan M, Krishnamurthy G, Spiegel L, Amaral JG, Temple MJ, John PR, Connolly BL (2010) Use and accuracy of US guidance for image-guided injections of the temporomandibular joints in children with arthritis. Pediatr Radiol. 40: 1498- 1504.

[19] Stoustrup P, Kristensen KD, Küseler A, Gelineck J, Cattaneo PM, Pedersen TK, Herlin T (2008) Reduced mandibular growth in experimental arthritis in the temporomandibular joint treated with intra-articular corticosteroid. Eur J Orthod. 30: 111-119.

[20] Schindler C, Paessler L, Eckelt U, Kirch W (2005) Severe temporomandibular dysfunction and joint destruction after intra-articular injection of triamcinolone. J Oral Pathol Med. 34: 184-186.

[21] El-Hakim IE, Abdel-Hamid IS, Bader A (2005) Temporomandibular joint (TMJ) response to intra-articular dexamethasone injection following mechanical arthropathy: a histological study in rats. Int J Oral Maxillofac Surg 34: 305-310.
[22] Samiee A, Sabzerou D, Edalatpajouh F, Clark GT, Ram S (2011) Temporomandibular joint injection with corticosteroid and local anesthetic for limited mouth opening. J Oral Sci. 53: 321-325.
[23] Greenberg MS, Glick M, Ship JA (2008) Burket's oral medicine. Eleventh edition. Hamilton: BC Decker Inc.
[24] Rodriguez M, Rubio JA, Sanchez R (2007) Effectiveness of two oral pastes for treatment of recurrent aphthous stomatitis. Oral Diseases. 13: 490-494.
[25] Holbrook WP, Kristmundsdottir T, Loftsson T (1998) Aqueous hydrocortisone mouthwash solution: clinical evaluation. Acta Odontol Scand. 56: 157-160.
[26] Lo Muzio L, Della Valle A, Mignogna MD, Pannone G, Bucci P, Bucci E, Sciubba J (2001) The treatment of oral aphthous ulceration or erosive lichen planus with topical clobetasol propionate in three preparations: a clinical and pilot study on 54 patients. J Oral Pathol Med. 30: 611-617.
[27] Gonzalez-Moles MA, Morales P, Rodriguez-Archilla A, Isabel IR. Gonzalez-Moles S (2002) Treatment of severe chronic oral erosive lesions with clobetasol propionate in aqueous solution. Oral Surg Oral Med Oral Pathol Oral Radiol Endod. 93: 264-270.
[28] Altenburg A, Zouboulis CC (2008) Current concepts in the treatment of recurrent aphthous stomatitis. Skin Therapy Lett. 13: 1-4.
[29] Chams-Davatchi C, Esmaili N, Daneshpazhooh M, Valikhani M, Balighi K, Hallaji Z, Barzegari M, Akhyani M, Ghodsi SZ, Seirafi H, Nazemi MJ, Mortazavi H, Mirshams-Shahshahani M (2007) Randomized controlled open-label trial of four treatment regimens for pemphigus vulgaris. J Am Acad Dermatol. 57: 622-628.
[30] Ionnides D, Chrysomallis F, Bystryn JC (2000) Ineffectiveness of cyclosporine as an adjuvant to corticosteroids in the treatment of pemphigus. Arch Dermatol 136: 868- 872.
[31] Beissert S, Werfel T, Frieling U, Böhm M, Sticherling M, Stadler R, Zillikens D, Rzany B, Hunzelmann N, Meurer M, Gollnick H, Ruzicka T, Pillekamp H, Junghans V, Luger TA (2006) A comparison of oral methylprednisolone plus azathioprine or mycophenolate mofetil for the treatment of pemphigus. Arch Dermatol 142: 1447- 1454.
[32] Neff AG, Turner M, Mutasim DF (2008) Treatment strategies in mucous membrane pemphigoid. Ther Clin Risk Manag. 4: 617-626.
[33] Michaels B (2009) The role of systemic corticosteroid therapy in erythema multiforme major and stevens-johnson syndrome: a review of past and current opinions. J Clin Aesthet Dermatol. 2: 51-55.
[34] Kardaun SH, Jonkman MF (2007) Dexamethasone pulse therapy for Stevens-Johnson syndrome/toxic epidermal necrolysis. Acta Derm Venereol. 87: 144–148.
[35] Patterson R, Dykewicz MS, Gonzalzles A, Grammer LC, Green D, Greenberger PA, McGrath KG, Walker CL (1990) Erythema multiforme and Stevens-Johnson syndrome. Descriptive and therapeutic controversy. Chest. 98: 331–336.

[36] Kakourou T, Klontza D, Soteropoulou F, Kattamis C (1997) Corticosteroid treatment of erythema multiforme major (Stevens-Johnson syndrome) in children. Eur J Pediatr. 156: 90–93.

[37] Martinez AE, Atherton DJ (2000) High-dose systemic corticosteroids can arrest recurrences of severe mucocutaneous erythema multiforme. Pediatr Dermatol. 17: 87–90.

[38] Scully C, Bagan J (2008) Oral mucosal diseases: erythema multiforme. Br J Oral Maxillofac Surg. 46: 90–95.

[39] Schneck J, Fagot JP, Sekula P, Sassolas B, Roujeau JC, Mockenhaupt M (2008) Effects of treatments on the mortality of Stevens-Johnson syndrome and toxic epidermal necrolysis: a retrospective study on patients included in the prospective EuroSCAR Study. J Am Acad Dermatol. 58: 33–40.

[40] Gauglitz GG, Korting HC, Pavicic T, Ruzicka T, Jeschke MG (2011) Hypertrophic scarring and keloids: pathomechanisms and current and emerging treatment strategies. Mol Med. 17: 113-25.

[41] Donkor P (2007) Head and neck keloid: treatment by core excision and delayed intralesional injection of steroid. J Oral Maxillofac Surg. 65: 1292-1296.

[42] Gupta S, Sharma VK (2011) Standard guidelines of care: Keloids and hypertrophic scars. Indian J Dermatol Venereol Leprol. 77: 94-100.

[43] Langston JR, Kolodny SC (1976) Cushing's syndrome associated with the intradermal injection of triamcinolone diacetate. J Oral Surg 34: 846–9.

[44] Ritota PC, Lo AK (1996) Cushing's syndrome in postburn children following intralesional triamcinolone injection. Ann Plast Surg 36: 508–511.

[45] Ferretti C, Muthray E (2011) Management of central giant cell granuloma of mandible using intralesional corticosteroids: case report and review of literature. J Oral Maxillofac Surg. 69: 2824-2829.

[46] Sheikh SB, Jacobus C (2012) Are steroids effective for treating Bell's palsy? Ann Emerg Med. 59: 33-34.

[47] Sherbino J (2010) Evidence-based emergency medicine: clinical synopsis. Do antiviral medications improve recovery in patients with Bell's palsy? Ann Emerg Med. 55: 475-476.

[48] Gilden D (2009) Treatment of Bell's palsy--the pendulum has swung back to steroids alone. Lancet Neurol, 7: 976-977.

[49] McGrath C, Comfort MB, Lo EC, Luo Y (2003) Changes in life quality following third molar surgery--the immediate postoperative period. Br Dent J. 194: 265-8.

[50] Colorado-Bonnin M, Valmaseda-Castellón E, Berini-Aytés L, Gay-Escoda C (2006) Quality of life following lower third molar removal. Int J Oral Maxillofac Surg. 35: 343-347.

[51] Sortino F, Cicciù M (2011) Strategies used to inhibit postoperative swelling following removal of impacted lower third molar. Dent Res J (Isfahan). 8: 162-171.

[52] Gürlek A, Fariz A, Aydoğan H, Ersöz-Oztürk A, Evans GR (2009) Effects of high dose corticosteroids in open rhinoplasty. J Plast Reconstr Aesthet Surg. 62: 650-655.

[53] Kargı E, Hosnuter M, Babuccu O, Altunkaya H, Altinyazar C (2003) Effect of steroids on edema, ecchymosis, and intraoperative bleeding in rhinoplasty. Ann Plast Surg. 51: 570-574.

[54] Kara CO, Gokalan I (1999) Effects of single-dose steroid usage on edema, ecchymosis, and intraoperative bleeding in rhinoplasty. Plast Reconstr Surg 104: 2213-2218.

[55] Hoffmann DF, Cook TA, Quatela VC, Wang TD, Brownrigg PJ, Brummett RE (1991) Steroids and rhinoplasty. A double-blind study. Arch Otolaryngol Head Neck Surg. 117: 990-993.

[56] Weber CR, Griffin JM (1994) Evaluation of dexamethasone for reducing postoperative edema and inflammatory response after orthognathic surgery. J Oral Maxillofac Surg. 52: 35-9.

[57] Peillon D, Bubost J, Roche C, Bienvenu J, Breton P, Carry PY, Freidel M, Banssillon V (1996) Do corticotherapy and hemodilution decrease postoperative inflammation after maxillofacial surgery?]. Ann Fr Anesth Reanim. 15: 157-61.

[58] Schaberg SJ, Stuller CB, Edwards SM (1984) Effect of methylprednisolone on swelling after orthognathic surgery. J Oral Maxillofac Surg 42: 356-361.

[59] Munro IR, Boyd JB, Wainwright DJ (1986) Effect of steroids in maxillofacial surgery. Ann Plast Surg 17: 440-444.

[60] Zandi M (2008) Comparison of corticosteroids and rubber drain for reduction of sequelae after third molar surgery. Oral Maxillofac Surg. 12: 29-33.

[61] Buyukkurt MC, Gungormus M, Kaya O (2006) The effect of a single dose prednisolone with and without diclofenac on pain, trismus and swelling after removal of mandibular third molars. J Oral Maxillofac Surg. 64: 1761-1766.

[62] Graziani F, D'Aiuto F, Arduino PG, Tonelli M, Gabriele M (2006) Perioperative dexamethasone reduces post-surgical sequelae of wisdom tooth removal. A split-randomized double-masked clinical trial. J Oral Maxillofac Surg. 35: 241-246.

[63] Esen E, Tasar F, Akhan O (1999) Determination of the antiinflammatory effects of methylprednisolone on the sequelae of third molar surgery. J Oral Maxillofac Surg. 57: 1201–1206.

[64] Dan AE, Thygesen TH, Pinholt EM (2010) Corticosteroid administration in oral and orthognathic surgery: a systematic review of the literature and meta-analysis. J Oral Maxillofac Surg. 68: 2207-2220.

[65] Chi CC, Wang SH, Kirtschig G, Wojnarowska F (2010) Systematic review of the safety of topical corticosteroids in pregnancy. J Am Acad Dermatol. 62: 694-705.

[66] Manson SC, Brown RE, Cerulli A, Vidaurre CF (2009) The cumulative burden of oral corticosteroid side effects and the economic implications of steroid use. Respir Med. 103: 975-994.

[67] Dahl R (2006) Systemic side effects of inhaled corticosteroids in patients with asthma. Respir Med. 100: 1307-1317.

[68] Salem M, Tainsh RE Jr, Bromberg J, Loriaux DL, Chernow B (1994) Perioperative glucocorticoid coverage. A reassessment 42 years after emergence of a problem. Ann Surg. 219: 416-25.

[69] Zandi M, Miresmaeili A (2007) Study of the cephalometric features of parents of children with cleft lip and/or palate anomaly. Int J Oral Maxillofac Surg. 36: 200-206.

[70] Zandi M, Heidari A (2011) An epidemiologic study of orofacial clefts in hamedan city, iran: a 15-year study. Cleft Palate Craniofac J. 48: 483-489.

[71] Carmichael SL, Shaw GM, Ma C, Werler MM, Rasmussen SA, Lammer EJ; National Birth Defects Prevention Study (2007) Maternal corticosteroid use and orofacial clefts. Am J Obstet Gynecol. 197: 585.e1-7.

[72] Pradat P, Robert-Gnansia E, Di Tanna GL, Rosano A, Lisi A, Mastroiacovo P (2003) First trimester exposure to corticosteroids and oral clefts. Birth Defects Res Clin Mol Teratol. 67: 968-970.

[73] Kallen B (2003) Maternal drug use and infant cleft lip/palate with special reference to corticoids. Cleft Palate Craniofac J. 40: 624-628.

[74] Park-Wyllie L, Mazzotta P, Pastuszak A, Moretti ME, Beique L, Hunnisett L, Friesen MH, Jacobson S, Kasapinovic S, Chang D, Diav-Citrin O, Chitayat D, Nulman I, Einarson TR, Koren G (2000) Birth defects after maternal exposure to corticosteroids: prospective cohort study and meta-analysis of epidemiological studies. Teratology. 62: 385-392.

[75] Edwards MJ, Agho K, Attia J, Diaz P, Hayes T, Illingworth A, Roddick LG (2003) Case-control study of cleft lip or palate after maternal use of topical corticosteroids during pregnancy. Am J Med Genet. 120: 459-463.

[76] Turpeinen M (1991) Absorption of hydrocortisone from the skin reservoir in atopic dermatitis. Br J Dermatol. 124: 358-360.

[77] Edwards MJ, Agho K, Attia J, Diaz P, Hayes T, Illingworth A, Roddick LG (2003) Case-control study of cleft lip or palate after maternal use of topical corticosteroids during pregnancy. Am J Med Genet A. 120: 459-463.

[78] Blais L, Beauchesne MF, Lemière C, Elftouh N (2009) High doses of inhaled corticosteroids during the first trimester of pregnancy and congenital malformations. J Allergy Clin Immunol. 124: 1229-1234.

[79] Goldman AS (1984) Biochemical mechanism of glucocorticoid-and phenytoin-induced cleft palate. Curr Top Dev Biol. 19: 217-239.

Chapter 11

Steroids in Asthma: Friend or Foe

Mahboub Bassam and Vats Mayank

Additional information is available at the end of the chapter

1. Introduction

Asthma is a common chronic inflammatory disease of the respiratory tract characterized by episodic exacerbations with a heterogeneous population distribution. The prevalence of asthma has increased substantially over the past 5 decades throughout the globe, yet the reasons for this increase remain unknown. The disease represents a substantial burden, not only in terms of morbidity, mortality and reduced quality of life of patients, but also imposing a huge cost on the healthcare facilities in all countries.

2. Burden of asthma

Approximately 300 million people worldwide currently have asthma, and its prevalence increases by 50% every decade, seeing a rise to 400 million by year 2025 (Braman, 2006; Masoli et al., 2004) The increasing number of hospital admissions for asthma, which are most pronounced in young children, reflect an increase in severe asthma, poor disease management, and poverty. Worldwide, approximately 180,000 deaths annually are attributable to asthma. Most asthma deaths occur in those >45 years old and are largely preventable, frequently being related to inadequate long-term medical care or delays in obtaining medical help during the attack.

The financial burden on patients with asthma in different western countries ranges from $300 to $1,300 per patient per year, disproportionately affecting those with the most severe disease. It is the most common chronic disorder in children and adolescents, with more than 3 million asthma attacks occurring in more than 5% of all children each year.

Asthma is a cause of concern due to under diagnosis, under investigated, under control and non-adherence to treatment (Barreto, 2006, National Institutes of Health, Bethesda, 2006, Woolcock, 1989, Bassam, 2012). A recent report from WHO suggests that 50% of patients from developed world with chronic diseases do not take their medications as recommended. In developing countries, the situation may be even worse when considering together all the issues related with poor access to health care, lack of appropriate diagnosis, and limited access to medicines. Poor adherence seriously threatens any effort to tackle such chronic illness (WHO, 2003, Horne, 2003).

Steroids V/S No Steroids in asthma: If ever there was a magic potion that should resolve the symptoms of an affliction, it is the use of glucocorticoids in asthma. Since their first clinical application, there has been uniform agreement that the anti-inflammatory activities of the corticosteroids make them ideal agents to stabilize asthma during all stages of asthma symptomatology ranging from chronic persistent phase to acute severe life threatening exacerbations.

Pathophysiology of asthma: Asthmatic inflammatory process results from inappropriate immune responses to common environmental antigens in a genetically susceptible individual (Wills-Karp 1999). These inappropriate immune responses are orchestrated by a subset of CD4+ T helper cells termed T helper 2 (Th2) cells.

Cytokines play a pivotal role in the development of asthma by regulating the expansion of Th2 cells and by mediating many of the Th2 effector functions that underlie the pathogenic events of an asthmatic response. Much effort has recently been placed in elucidating the pathways used by cytokines to mediate their actions. These studies have revealed that cytokine-mediated signals are primarily transduced by the Janus Kinase- Signal Transducer and Activator of Transcription (JAK-STAT) signaling cascade (Darnell, 1997). Recent advances have shown the important roles of JAK-STAT signaling pathway in the pathogenesis of asthma.

3. JAK-STAT signaling in Th1 and Th2 differentiation:

The two major subsets of CD4+ T helper cells, Th1 and Th2, secrete mutually distinct profiles of cytokines and thereby coordinate different classes of immune response. The cytokines IL-12 and IL-4 direct the differentiation of Th1 and Th2 cells, respectively, from naive T helper cells. Th1 cells secrete IL-2, IFN-γ, and TNF-β, whereas Th2 cells produce IL-4, IL-5, IL-6, IL-10, and IL-13.

Th1 cells are critically involved in the generation of delayed-type hypersensitivity responses, whereas Th2 cells can direct B cells to mount strong humoral responses. Polarization of immune response toward a Th2 phenotype and when directed against an otherwise innocuous environmental antigen result in the pathogenesis of allergic diseases like asthma.

The Th2 cytokines (IL-4, IL-5, and IL-13) control all the major components that characterize an inflammatory asthmatic response, including IgE isotype switching, mucus production, and the recruitment and activation of eosinophils and have been corroborated by studies in humans. The population of Th2 cells is notably expanded in the airways of asthmatic subjects, and presence of these cells correlates with airway hyper responsiveness (AHR) and airway eosinophilia (Rengarajan et al., 2000, Murphy et al., 2000).

IL-4 and IL-12 activate the Jak-Stat signaling cascade discussed elsewhere in this Perspective series. In this signaling pathway, binding of a cytokine to its receptor leads to the activation of members of the JAK family of receptor associated kinases. These kinases subsequently activate, via tyrosine phosphorylation, preexistent cytoplasmic factors termed Stats (signal transducer and activator of transcription). Tyrosine phosphorylation allows the Stat proteins to dimerize and translocate to the nucleus, where they mediate changes in gene expression by binding specific DNA elements. Although both IL-4 and IL-12 follow this basic signaling framework, the two cytokines differ in the specific Jak and Stat components that they activate (Wurster, A.L. et al 2000). IL-4 stimulates Jak1 and Jak3 to activate Stat6. In contrast, interaction of IL-12 with its receptor leads to the activation of Jak2 and Tyk2 and the subsequent phosphorylation of Stat4. Activation of Stat6 and Stat4 are thus critical events in the signaling cascades of IL-4 and IL-12, respectively.

Mechanism of Action of steroids: Glucocorticoids (GC's) are potent anti-inflammatory agents and are useful in the treatment of both allergic and idiosyncratic asthma. Although the mechanisms of corticosteroid action in asthma are poorly understood, several possible sites of action have been proposed which help reverse the pathologic process of bronchial asthma.

Glucocorticoid receptors (GRs) are specific cytoplasmic transcription factors that mediate the biological actions of corticosteroids (Beato M et al 1995). On ligand binding, GR translocates into the nucleus and binds to DNA at glucocorticoid response elements (GREs) in the promoter region of corticosteroid-responsive genes that induce transcription (Barnes PJ & Adcock IM 1998). GR activation may also influence antiinflammatory events by nongenomic pathways, forming inhibitory interactions within the nucleus with proinflammatory DNA-binding transcription factors, such as activator protein (AP)-1 or nuclear factor (NF)–_B, or by recruitment of co-repressors, and thereby repressing the actions of these important inflammatory proteins (Karin M. 1998, Ito K et al. 2000). GR nuclear translocation is, therefore, essential and necessary for corticosteroid action.

It has been well investigated that the novel mechanism of GC action is by blocking cytokine signaling via the JAK-STAT signaling pathway. Dexamethasone inhibited IL-2-induced DNA binding, tyrosine phosphorylation, and nuclear translocation of Stat5 in primary T cells. Inhibition of Stat5 correlated with inhibition of expression of IL-2-inducible genes and T cell proliferation. The mechanism of inhibition involved suppression of IL-2 receptor and Jak3 expression. Signaling by IL-4, IL-7, and IL-15, which use IL-2 receptor components, also was inhibited, indicating a block in T cell responses similar to that seen in immunodeficient patients lacking the IL-2 receptor gamma chain or Jak3.

IL-2 signaling also was blocked in patients after treatment with GC's, suggesting that inhibition of cytokine signaling contributes to the clinical efficacy of GC's. Hence inhibition of both cytokine production and Jak- stat signaling contribute to their therapeutic potency (Bianchi, 2000).

Corticosteroids enhance the beta-adrenergic response to relieve the muscle spasm. They also act by reversing the mucosal edema, decreasing vascular permeability by vasoconstriction, and inhibiting the release of Leukotrienes (LT) LT-C4 and LT-D4. Corticosteroids reduce the mucus secretion by inhibiting the release of secretagogue from macrophages. Corticosteroids inhibit the late phase reaction by inhibiting the inflammatory response and interfering with chemotaxis due to the inhibition of LT-B4 release. The eosinopenic effect of corticosteroids may help to prevent the cytotoxic effect of the major basic protein and other inflammatory mediators released from eosinophils. Corticosteroids have no effect on the immediate hypersensitivity reaction and have no direct role in bronchial reactivity. By blocking the late reaction, they prevent the increased airway reactivity observed with late bronchial reactions, all of which aid in the resolution of bronchospasm in asthmatic patients (**Figure 1**)

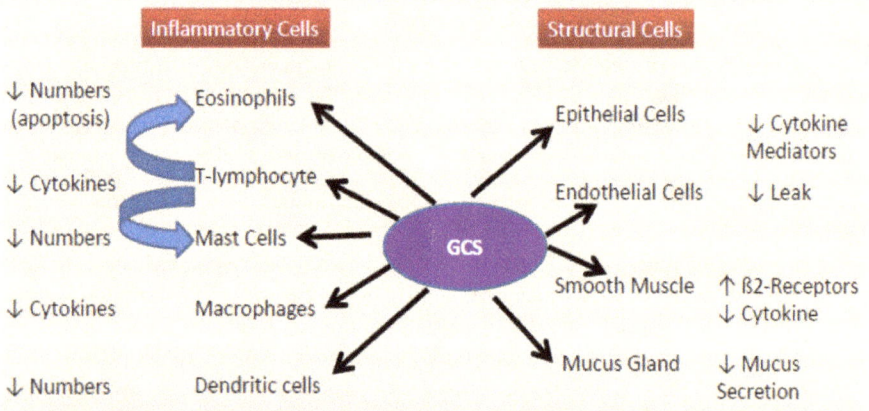

Figure 1. Mechanism of Action of Corticosteroids in asthma

Mode of Delivery: All levels of persistent asthma require daily anti-inflammatory treatment (with additional doses of oral or intravenous steroid based on the severity of symptoms). Inhaled corticosteroids (ICS's) are the safest and most effective anti-inflammatory treatment for patients with persistent asthma of all severity having a significant positive impact on outcomes. Although steroids may be given orally or systemically, and numerous non-steroidal medications are available for treating persistent asthma, ICS's are the treatment of choice considering their risk-benefit and cost-effectiveness ratio. Even when ICS's are given daily over prolong period of time, they have less toxicity than oral or systemic steroids administered only occasionally. A wide range of ICS's are available & the choice depends upon the availability, cost, physician and patient's preference, however it is important to use the equipotent doses of various ICS's while switching over the ICS's for control of asthma (**Table-1**)

In cases of acute severe asthma or patients requiring maintenance therapy with steroids for chronic persistent asthma intravenous or oral routes are to be preferred, it's important to know the equipotent doses of various type of steroid while starting or switching from one form to another or from one steroids to another in order to get the equivalent response and to avoid worsening of symptoms (if underdosing done) or side effects (if overdosing done). **Table 2** summarizes the equivalent doses of various types of intravenous or oral steroids. (http://www.globalrph.com/corticocalc.htm)

Drug	Low Daily dose (μgm)	Medicum Daily dose (μgm)	High Daily dose (μgm)
Beclomethasone Dipropionate	200-500	500-1000	1000-2000
Budesonide	200-400	400-800	800-1600
Ciclesonide	80-160	10-320	320-1280
Flunisolide	500-1000	1000-2000	>2000
Fluticasone Propionate	100-250	250-500	500-1000
Mometasone Furoate	200	400	800
Triamcinolone acetonide	400-1000	1000-2000	>2000

Table 1. Estimated Equipotent daily doses of all formulations of ICS in adults

Glucocorticoid	Approximate Equivalent dose (mg)	Half-life(Biologic) hours
Short-Acting		
Cortisone	25	8-12
Hydrocortisone	20	8-12
Intermediate-Acting		
Methylprednisolone	4	18-36
Prednisolone/ Prednisone	5	18-36
Triamcinolone	4	18-36
Long-Acting		
Betamethasone	0.6 - 0.75	36-54
Dexamethasone	0.75	36-54

Table 2. Estimated Equipotent daily doses of all formulations of glucocorticoids in adults

Steroids in Children: ICS are the first-line therapy for persistent asthma in children. Major safety concerns of long-term ICS therapy in children include suppression of adrenal function and impaired growth and bone development. Dosage, type of inhaler device used, patient technique, and characteristics of the individual drug influence systemic effects of ICS's. Systemic side effects can occur when continuous high-dose treatment is required for severe asthma or when prescribed dosage is excessive and compliance is unusually good.

It is very important to know that uncontrolled or severe asthma adversely affects growth and final adult height in children & no long-term controlled studies have reported any statistically or clinically significant adverse effects on growth of 100-200 μg/ day of ICS's however it may be seen with all ICS's when a high dose is administered for prolonged periods (dose dependent effect). Different age groups seem to differ in their susceptibility to the growth-retarding effects of ICS's, children aged 4 to 10 are more susceptible than adolescents, however Children with asthma treated with ICS's attain normal adult height (predicted from family members) but at a later age(Pedersen, 2001, Agertoft & Pedersen, 2000,. Sharek, & Bergman 2000). No studies have reported any statistically significant increase in risk of fracture in children taking ICS's.

Oral or systemic steroids increases the risk of fracture in children with a 32 % increase in 4 courses ever, however ICS's are safe in this regard. Controlled longitudinal studies of 2-5 yrs duration and several cross sectional studies found no adverse effect of ICS on bone mineral density (Agertoft & Pedersen , 1998, Hopp et al., 1995).

Suppression of Hypothalamic-pituitary-adrenal (HPA) axis: Though differences exist between the various ICS's and inhaler devices, treatment with ICS's doses of less than 200 μg budesonide or equivalent daily is normally not associated with any significant suppression of the HPA axis in children. At higher doses, small changes in HPA axis function can be detected with sensitive methods. The clinical relevance of these findings is not known, since there have not been reports of adrenal crisis in clinical trials of ICS's in children. However, adrenal crisis has been reported in children treated with excessively high doses of ICS's (Roux et al., 2003).

Recent studies confirm that benefits of ICS, properly prescribed and used, clearly outweigh not only their potential adverse effects but also the risks associated with poorly controlled asthma.

Benefits of oral corticosteroids for asthma include reduction in mucus production, chest tightness, coughing, and wheezing. Other non-asthma related conditions, such as sinus conditions and psoriasis, may also improve due to the anti-inflammatory properties of oral steroids.

Side effects of steroids: Side effects of short-term oral steroids include fluid retention, stomach upset, excessive hunger, and blurred vision. Difficulty concentrating, insomnia, and mood changes can also occur as a result of taking oral corticosteroids. The systemic side-effects of long-term treatment with high doses of ICS's may include cataracts, osteoporosis, easy bruising, and hair loss, Weight gain, an increase in facial hair in women, and muscle weakness. Long term use of oral corticosteroids may also increase the risk of diabetes, high blood pressure, and certain infections. Systemic effects of inhaled glucocorticosteroids are not a problem in adults at doses of ≤ 400 mg budesonide or equivalent daily.

Factors affecting response of ICS's: Three most important factors that appear to have significant impact on the effectiveness of inhaled corticosteroid (ICS) treatment are:

1.) **Patient compliance with inhaled anti-asthma therapy:** The term "Compliance" is defined as the extent to which a patient's behavior matches the prescriber's advice but recently it has mostly been superseded by the term adherence, a similar concept but having fewer negative connotations from physician/patient relationship point of view (Haynes, 1979). Adherence is defined as the extent to which the patient's behavior matches agreed recommendations from the prescriber.

The issue of noncompliance is complicated by different patterns of noncompliance and a variety of measurements of noncompliance. Cochrane GM 1996 identified several patterns of noncompliance, including taking only half of the medications at the prescribed times, taking the medication regularly for a period and stopping, and skipping prescribed doses. Compliance with preventive therapy such as ICSs whose effect is seen over a period of weeks may be less than compliance with drugs that relieve asthma symptoms more rapidly. Patient adherence to medication is influenced by a number of factors relating to how the individual judges the necessity of their treatment relative to their concerns. These factors can be categorized as follows:

1. Treatment factors:
   - Dosing schedule too frequent
   - cost / non-availability of medicine
   - Complexity or inconvenience of treatment regimen
   - Need to use proper inhaler technique
   - Discomfort of drug administration (eg, bad taste, dry throat, hoarseness, fungal infections)
   - Physician's Inertia / Attitude/ lack of communication
   - Proper education about the disease not given by physician
2. Behavioral factors
   - Belief that medication is not really needed (esp. Controller medicine (ICS)
   - Belief that medication would not work
   - Poor perception of the impact of the disease (symptoms, experience, expectations & interpretation of illness)
   - Fear of adverse effects or dependence/ negative orientation to medicines
   - Steroid phobia
   - Forgetting to take medication
   - Volitional non-adherence: voluntarily not taking medication
   - Non-volitional non-adherence: from failure to take medication properly (e.g. ICS± LABA)
3. Contextual issues: Past experiences, Cultural issues/ Social beliefs/ Poor pt /View of others/ Practical difficulties

It is important to keep the medication regimen as simple as possible, prioritize recommendations, educate the patient regarding disease management, and individualized the dosing and schedule of ICS as per patient's requirment.

2.) Inhalation technique. The effectiveness of inhaler therapy depends not only on compliance, but also on the inhaler technique. Various types of inhaler devices are available including trubohaler, discus etc however they can be broadly categorized based on the form of drugs used as dry powder inhalers (DPI) and Metered Dose inhalers (MDI). Although both types of inhalers are equally effective but While prescribing ICS to patient due consideration should be given to the age of the patient, comorbid conditions, coordination between the hands & mouth & the educational level of patient, otherwise the inhaled ICS will get deposited in the oropharynx & produce local side effects(such as change in voice, Oropharyngeal candidiasis). Use of Spacer with MDI can largely reduce the deposition of the ICS in throat & hence avoid local side effects of the steroids.

3.) **Impact of inhalation technique and device on drug deposition in the lungs:** For ICSs, the efficacy depends on the topical activity of the drug that reaches the target area, whereas the adverse events depend both on oral deposition and systemic activity. Systemic activity of the drug depends on the amount of the drug absorbed either through the GI tract or through the lungs, as well as on the first-pass metabolism for drug absorbed through the GI tract.

The amount of drug delivered to the lungs depends on the inhalation technique,(Dolovich, 1981, Jackson & Lipworth , 1995) as well as on the type of inhaler used and the fine particle size (respirable particle diameter between 1- 4 µm) of the drug. **Table -3** shows the Estimates of the Lung to Systemic Bioavailability Ratios for different types of ICS's.

Product	% Dose Deposited in the Lungs	% Dose Reaching the Systemic Circulation after Absorption from the Gastrointestinal Tract	Lung/Systemic Bioavailability Ratio
BDP via CFC propellant	5.5	14.7	0.27
BDP (non-CFC propellant)	56.1	5.5	0.92
Budesonide via MDI	15	7.7	0.66
Budesonide via DPI	30	5.3	0.85

BDP-beclomethasone dipropionate. CFC-chlorofluorocarbon. MDI-metered-dose inhaler, DPI- dry powder inhaler.

Table 3. Estimates of the Lung to Systemic Bioavailability Ratios for Inhaled Corticosteroids

Recent Recommendations about the delivery device for ICS from American College of Chest Physicians/American College of Asthma, Allergy, and Immunology states that:

1. For the treatment of asthma in the outpatient setting, both the MDI with a spacer/holding chamber and the DPI are appropriate devices for the delivery of ICS's.
2. For outpatient asthma therapy, the selection of an appropriate aerosol delivery device for ICS's includes the patient's ability to use the device correctly, the preferences of the patient for the device, the availability of the drug/device combination, the compatibility between the drug and delivery device, the lack of time or skills to properly instruct the patient in the use of the device or monitor the appropriate use, the cost of therapy, and the potential for reimbursement(Dolovich, 2005). **Table -4** summarizes the advantages & disadvantages of all the devices available for the delivery of ICS's

Type	Advantages	Disadvantages
Small-volume jet nebulizer (Respiratory solution, Respules, nebules)	Patient coordination not required Effective with tidal breathing High dose possible Dose modification possible Can be used with supplemental oxygen Can deliver combination therapies if compatible	Lack of portability Pressurized gas source required Lengthy treatment time Device cleaning required Contamination possible Not all medication available in solution form Does not aerosolize suspensions well Device preparation required Performance variability Expensive when compressor added
Ultrasonic nebulizer	Patient coordination not required High dose possible Dose modification possible Small dead volume small and portable Faster delivery than jet nebulizer No drug loss during exhalation (breath actuated devices)	Expensive Need for electric power source Contamination possible Not all medication available Device preparation required before treatment Does not nebulize suspensions well Possible drug degradation airway irritation with some drugs
Pressurized MDI (CFC/ HFA as propellant) accuhaler, Evohalers	Portable and compact Treatment time is short No drug preparation required No contamination of contents Dose-dose reproducibility high Some can be used with breath actuated mouthpiece	Coordination of breathing and device actuation needed High pharyngeal deposition Upper limit to unit dose content Remaining doses difficult to determine Potential for abuse Not all medications available
Holding chamber, reverse flow spacer, or spacer (Zerostat, Zerostat-v **spacer**)	Reduces need for coordination Reduces pharyngeal deposition	Inhalation can be more complex for some patients Can reduce dose available if not used properly More expensive/Less portable Integral actuator devices may alter aerosol properties compared to native actuator
DPI (Turbohaler, Diskus, Rotahaler, Handihaler, aerolizer)	Breath-actuated Less coordination required No Propellant required Small and portable Short treatment time Dose counters	Requires moderate to high inspiratory flow Can result in high pharyngeal deposition Not all medications available

CFC-Cloro-fluor-Carbon, HFA- hydro-fluoro-alkane, MDI- Metered dose inhaler, DPI- Dry Powder inhaler

Table 4. Advantages and Disadvantages of Aerosol-Generating Device or System

In short, effective asthma treatment requires a combination of pharmacology and psychology. Effective prescribing needs to take account of patients' beliefs, expectations, and adherence behavior.

Goal of Asthma Management: According to Global Initiative for Asthma (**GINA 2010**) Guidelines issued by the National Heart Lung & Blood institute, the goals for successful management of asthma are to:

- Achieve and maintain control of symptoms
- Maintain normal activity level including exercise
- Maintain pulmonary functions as close to normal as possible
- Prevent asthma exacerbations
- Avoid side effects from asthma medications
- Avoid asthma mortality

Therefore, for successful management of asthma and optimum control of asthma , patients should always be assessed to know their status of asthma control , Following classification of asthma by level of control is more relevant and **useful** (Figure 2).

Characteristic	Controlled (All of the following)	Partly Controlled (Any measure present in any week)	Uncontrolled
Daytime symptoms	None (twice or less/week)	More than twice/week	Three or more features of partly controlled asthma present in any week
Limitations of activities	None	Any	
Nocturnal symptoms/ awakening	None	Any	
Need for reliever/ rescue treatment	None (twice or less/week)	More than twice/week	
Lung function (PEF or FEV$_1$)‡	Normal	< 80% predicted or personal best (if known)	
Exacerbations	None	One or more/year*	One in any week†

Adopted from Global Initiative for Asthma (GINA 2010) Guidelines
* Any exacerbation should prompt review of maintenance treatment to ensure that it is adequate.
† By definition, an exacerbation in any week makes that an uncontrolled asthma week.
‡ Lung function testing is not reliable for children 5 years and younger.

Figure 2. Classification of asthma by level of control

To reach this goal, four interrelated components of therapy are required:

Component 1: Develop patient/doctor partnership: In order to help in the effective management of asthma so that the asthmatic patient can learn how to: avoid risk factors, take medications correctly, understand the difference between "controller" and "reliever" medications, monitor their status using symptoms and, if relevant Peak expiratory Flow (PEF) recognize signs that asthma is worsening and take action, seek medical help as appropriate.

Component 2: Identify and Reduce Exposure to Risk Factors: To improve control of asthma and reduce medication needs, despite physical activity is a common cause of asthma symptoms however patients should not avoid exercise. Common strategies for avoiding allergens and pollutants include the followings; Stay away from tobacco smoke, patients and parents should not smoke, avoid drugs, foods, and additives if they are known to cause symptoms, reduce or, preferably, avoid exposure to occupational sensitizers.

Component 3: Assess, Treat, and Monitor Asthma: Each patient is assigned to one of five treatment "steps" based on the frequency and severity of symptoms, PFT values and the exacerbations. At each treatment step, asthma education, environmental control & vaccination are important component of asthma control. Rescue medication should be provided for quick relief of symptoms as needed. As the severity of disease increases, from Steps 2- 5, patients should be given one or more regular controller medications (*ICS*) in order to keep asthma under control & to avoid the morbidity & mortality related with asthma and to prevent the long term consequences of the disease. Regular use of ICS has *demonstrated* high efficiency in reducing asthma symptoms, reducing frequency & severity of exacerbations, reducing mortality, improving quality of life, improving lung function, decreasing airway hyper-responsiveness & controlling airway inflammation.

Component 4: Managing asthma exacerbations: Exacerbations of asthma are characterized by episodes of progressive increase in shortness of breath, cough, wheezing or chest tightness, or some combination of these symptoms. Mamgement of asthma exacerbation requires close objective monitoring (both clinical and using PEF), repetitive administration of rapid-acting inhaled bronchodilators, early introduction of systemic glucocorticosteroids and oxygen supplementation. It is very important to use systemic steroids early in case of exacerbation in order to control the underlying inflammation earliest possible. GINA guidelines have simplified the recognition of severity of acute exacerbation of asthma and management in acute care setting base on the severity of symptoms & response to treatment (For details: www.ginasthma.org)

Stepwise approach for asthma Management: GINA guidelines have simplified the management of asthma at all stages in stepwise manner starting from rescue medicines to regular controller medicine. (**Figure 3**)

4. Glucocorticoid resistance

Although glucocorticoids are highly effective in the control of chronic inflammation or immune dysregulation occurring in asthma pts however a small proportion of patients displays persistent immune activation and airway inflammation and fail to respond despite high doses of oral corticosteroids imposing a big challenge for the physicians. (Barnes, 1995, 1995, Sze⁻er, 1997). This group of patients has been classified as "steroid-resistant"

Step 1	Step 2	Step 3	Step 4	Step 5
Asthma education / Environmental control				

Step 1	Step 2	Step 3	Step 4	Step 5
		Asthma education Environmental control		
As needed rapid-acting β₂-agonist	As needed rapid-acting β₂-agonist			
Controller options	Select one	Select one	Add one or more	Add one or both
	Low-dose inhaled ICS*	Low-dose ICS plus long-acting β₂-agonist	Medium-or high-dose ICS plus long-acting β₂-agonist	Oral glucocorticosteroid (lowest dose)
	Leukotriene modifier **	Medium-or high-dose ICS	Leukotriene modifier	Anti-IgE treatment
		Low-dose ICS plus leukotriene modifier	Sustained release theophylline	
		Low-dose ICS plus sustained release theophylline		

* ICS=inhaled glucocorticosteroids
** =Receptor antagonist or synthesis inhibitors

Adopted from Global Initiative for Asthma (GINA 2010) Guidelines

Figure 3. Stepwise approach for asthma Management

Steroid resistant asthma: American Thoracic Society (ATS) defined Steroid resistant patients as characterized by a pre-bronchodilator Force expiratory volume in 1 sec (FEV1) of less than 70% predicted with a maintained bronchodilator response. Steroid resistance is defined by administering a course of oral prednisone e.g. 40 mg/d (divided doses) for 7 days or preferably 2 wk, and observing the effect on morning pre-bronchodilator FEV1 (Lee, 1996). If the FEV1 fails to increase by 15% (and 200 ml), the patient is considered steroid resistant (Sally et al., 2000). These patients show the typical diurnal variability in peak expiratory flow and bronchodilatation with inhaled B-2 agonists. This type of trial can also assess the possibility of poor adherence to the maintenance regimen.

Patients with steroid resistance can be grouped into two broad categories,

Type 1 steroid resistance: is either immune-mediated or acquired as the result of environmental triggers or lifestyle. Clinically, such patients will develop steroid side effects, including adrenal gland suppression, osteoporosis, and cushingoid features from pharmacologic doses of systemic steroids. This is because there is only one (glucocorticoid resistant) GR gene and these patients have steroid resistance only at the level of their immune/inflammatory cells (i.e., T cells). The rest of the tissues in their body remain sensitive to the deleterious effects of systemic steroids.

Type 2 steroid resistances: is rare but involves a generalized primary cortisol resistance that affects all tissues and is likely associated with a mutation in the GR gene or genes that modulate GR function. This form is not associated with the development of steroid's side effects or suppression of morning cortisol levels (**Table 5**). It is analogous to genetically inherited familial cortisol resistance. When patients present with a history of no side effects after high doses of prednisone, it is critical to confirm that they are taking the oral prednisone by checking their morning serum cortisol after a course of therapy under strict supervision. Such individuals need alternative approaches to control their pulmonary inflammation.

Features	Type 1 steroid resistances	Type 2 steroid resistances
AM cortisol levels	Suppressed	No
Cushingoid side effects	Yes	No
Cause	Cytokine induced(May be genetic), Allergy, Microbes	Genetic
GCR ligand and DNA binding affinity	Reduced	Normal
GCR numbers	Normal or High	Low
Reversibility of GCR defect	Yes	No

Table 5. Summarizes difference in both Types of steroid resistance

It is imperative to exclude confounding factors when trying to make the diagnosis of steroid-resistant asthma in a patient. These factors include non-adherence with asthma medication, inadequate inhalation technique, incorrect diagnosis, unrecognized concomitant diagnoses, and ongoing exposure to environmental allergens, abnormal corticosteroid pharmacokinetics, and psychosocial disturbances. Low dose methotrexate, cyclosporine, Intravenous immunoglobulin, leukotriene antagonists, such as zafirlukast and montelukast and Nedocromil sodium has been used in steroid resistant patients with varying success rates and with associated side effects.

5. Clinical features of glucocorticoid-resistant asthma

Glucocorticoid resistance in asthma was first described in six patients with asthma who did not respond clinically to high doses of systemic glucocorticoids and in whom there was also a reduced eosinopenic response (Schwartz et al .,1968). Larger groups of patients with chronic asthma who were glucocorticoid resistant were subsequently identified (Carmichael et al ., 1981). These patients were not Addisonian and did not suffer from the abnormalities in sex hormones described in familial glucocorticoid resistance (see below). Plasma cortisol and adrenal suppression in response to exogenous cortisol is normal (Lane et al., 1996). Complete glucocorticoid resistance in asthma is very rare, but reduced responsiveness is more common, so that oral glucocorticoids are needed to control asthma adequately (steroid-dependent asthma).

Mechanisms of glucocorticoid resistance: There may be several mechanisms for resistance to the effects of glucocorticoids. Although a family history of asthma is more common in patients with GCR than GCS asthma, little is known about its inheritance. It is possible that a certain proportion of the population has glucocorticoid resistance which only becomes manifest when they develop a severe immunological or immune disease that requires glucocorticoid therapy. Resistance to the inflammatory and immune effects of glucocorticoids should be distinguished from the rare familial glucocorticoid resistance, where there is an abnormality of glucocorticoid binding to GR.

Glucocorticoid resistance may be *primary* (inherited or acquired of unknown cause) or *secondary due to* reduced glucocorticoid responsiveness (glucocorticoids themselves, cytokines, b-adrenergic agonists).

Primary glucocorticoid resistance: There are several possible mechanisms for a reduced anti-inflammatory response to glucocorticoids.

a. Pharmacokinetic abnormalities.
b. Antibodies to lipocortin-1.
c. Cellular abnormalities.
d. Abnormality in GR function.
e. Interaction between GR and transcription factors.

Secondary glucocorticoid resistance: various probable mechanisms include:

a. Down-regulation of GR.
b. Effects of cytokines.
c. Effect of B2 agonists.

6. Factors contributing to corticosteroid resistance

A variety of factors known to contribute to immune activation and pulmonary disease have been found to alter corticosteroid responsiveness (**Table 6**).

Clinical allergy and allergen exposure
Infection
Smoking
Obesity
Stress
Ethnicity
Low vitamin D level

Table 6. Factors Contributing to Corticosteroid Insensitivity

6.1. Allergen exposure

Allergen exposure in vivo reduces GR binding affinity in PBMCs from atopic asthmatics. In vitro treatment with cat allergen of peripheral blood mononuclear cell (PBMC) from cat-allergic asthmatics was also observed to reduce GR binding affinity and T-cell proliferation induced by allergens compared with control antigens. The induction of these GR binding abnormalities was found to be IL-2 and IL-4 dependent.

6.2. Infection

Infection is a common trigger for pulmonary disease. An analysis of the T-cell repertoire in patients whose asthma was poorly controlled (FEV_1 <75% predicted despite use of high-dose corticosteroids) revealed that their T cells were activated by a microbial superantigen. To determine whether microbial super antigens could alter corticosteroid sensitivity, the capacity of corticosteroids to inhibit the activation of T cells from normal subjects with super antigens as compared with the mitogen, phytohemagglutinin, was studied. While corticosteroids caused a 99% inhibition of phytohemagglutinin-induced PBMC proliferation, there was only 19% inhibition of super antigen-induced T-cell proliferation. The mechanism by which super antigens induce corticosteroid resistance of human T cells is via activation of the Mitogen-Activated protein Kinase Kinase/Extracellular signal-Regulated Kinase (MEKK-ERK) pathway (Li et al., 2004, Goleva et al., 2004). Viruses can also alter response in corticosteroids. In particular, rhinovirus has been reported to reduce GR nuclear translocation and thereby reduce corticosteroid response.

6.3. Neutrophilia

The nature of the inflammatory infiltrate will also determine whether the particular pulmonary disease being treated is likely to resolve with corticosteroid therapy. Pulmonary diseases associated with infiltration of neutrophils are likely to be Steroid resistant. To determine the potential mechanism of corticosteroid resistance in neutrophils, Strickland et al.,2001 examined relative amounts of GRα and GRβ in freshly isolated neutrophils and observed increased GRβ, but not GRα, protein and mRNA expression in neutrophils at baseline and after IL-8 exposure (Strickland et al. 2001). High constitutive expression of GR-β by neutrophils may provide a mechanism by which these cells escape corticosteroid-induced cell death.

6.4. Other factors contributing to steroid resistance

Other factors contributing to steroid resistance include smoking, stress, obesity, ethnicity, and vitamin D deficiency. In smokers, oxidative stress results in reduced levels of histone deacetylase-2 (Barnes, Adcock, 2009). Stress may induce steroid resistance via multiple mechanisms, including the chronic elevation of the stress hormone, cortisol, which downregulates expression of the GR (Haczku , Panettieri, 2010). The association of steroid resistance with obesity may be related to the systemic inflammation found in this condition, leading to chronic elevation of TNF and mitogen-activated protein kinase (MAPK) activation that causes GR dysfunction (Sutherland et al., 2008) Black patients with asthma have also been found to have reduced steroid responsiveness compared with white asthmatics (Federico, 2005), although the reason for this is not known, but it could be due to a combination of genetic and environmental factors.

Several recent studies on asthmatics have now shown that low vitamin D levels are associated with increased corticosteroid requirements, and there is a potential role for vitamin D in the enhancement of corticosteroid response (Sutherland et al., 2010)

7. Management of corticosteroid resistance

The management of steroid resistant (SR) asthma poses a significant challenge to the clinician. Identification of the SR patient early in the course of illness is important to prevent tissue remodeling and irreversible changes in lung pathology. Definitions of clinical response to steroid therapy will be dictated by the pulmonary disease being treated and time frame for improvement of clinical disease before unacceptable steroid side effects occur. In the case of asthma, clinical studies have suggested that favorable response to inhaled steroids is associated with high levels of exhaled nitric oxide, high bronchodilator response, and a low FEV_1/FVC ratio prior to treatment (Barnes,2008)

A systematic, stepwise approach is important for a successful outcome (Leung and Bloom, 2003). **Table 7** lists factors to be considered in the evaluation of patients with a history of steroid resistance.

Correct diagnosis
Comorbid conditions- rhinosinusitis, congestive heart failure, COPD, Gastro Esophageal reflex
Drug adherence
Drug delivery
Drug interactions causing enhanced metabolism of steroids
Alternative anti-inflammatory therapies

Table 7. Considerations in Treating Steroid Resistance

Step 1.   Complete Evaluation including history, physical examination, pulmonary function testing, and appropriate laboratory tests to confirm the diagnosis and rule out concomitant medical disorders such as vocal cord dysfunction, Gastroesophageal reflux/aspiration, chronic rhinosinusitis, allergic bronchopulmonary aspergillosis, heart failure, COPD & broncholitis etc.(**Figure 4**)

Step 2.   Try to find out psychological & social factors including adherence to therapy and take corrective measures for them.

Step 3.   Observe the inhalational technique of patient, reeducate, reinforce about the proper technique especially in patients requiring high doses of ICS for severe persistent asthma. Spacer devices should be used to maximize ICS dose delivery and reduce adverse effects.

Step 4.   Strict environmental control at home, in school, and at work including finding the source of allergens & eliminating the same because persistent allergen exposure will increase the symptoms of asthma & reduces steroid responsiveness.

Step 5.   Search for concomitant bacterial/ mycobacterial/ fungal infection of the tracheobronchial tree especially in patients taking high doses of ICS or chronic oral steroids. Chronic colonization with *Mycoplasma pneumoniae* or *Chlamydia pneumoniae*, can trigger airway inflammation in chronic asthmatics and thus poor responsiveness to steroids.

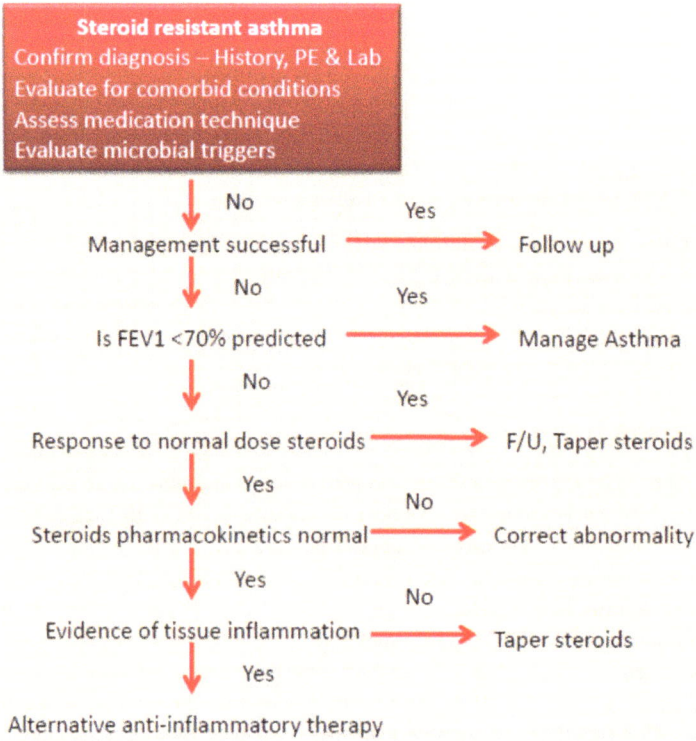

Figure 4. Flow diagram to manage steroid resistant asthma

Step 6. Search for factors affecting lifestyle and steroid responsiveness. Patients with Vitamin D deficiency have increased steroid requirements. Other cofactors, including obesity, smoking, no or little exposure to sunlight and pigmented skin are well known to lower vitamin D levels.

Step 7. Combination therapy can be used to maximize clinical response. Inhaled long-acting β_2-agonists (LABA) have been found to enhance Glucocorticoid receptor (GR) nuclear translocation and reduced corticosteroid requirements. Consider addition of other steroid-sparing drugs such as leukotriene modifiers, anticholinergic drugs, nidocromil sodium(Marin, 1996) and theophylline.

Step 8. In very difficult case, studies to identify systemic steroid pharmacokinetics and receptors to assess the basis for corticosteroid resistance to determine whether there is incomplete corticosteroid absorption, failure to convert corticosteroids to an active form, or rapid elimination of steroids (frequently as a result of interactions with other medications). Patients with poor absorption of prednisone usually respond well to oral liquid steroid preparations. In patients with rapid corticosteroid elimination, a split dosing regimen (morning & afternoon) is suggested.

Step 9. Consider Steroid sparing anti-inflammatory therapies that would enhance corticosteroid action including cyclosporine (Alexander et al., 1992), IV Immunoglobulin (Mazer , 1991), methotrexate (Mullarkey et al. 1998, Erzurum et al., 1991), mycophenolate mofetil, azathioprine, Macrolides, trolendamycin and gold, depending on the severity of asthma and the potential of significant side effects. Omalizumab (recombinant anti IgE antibody) is useful in patients with primarily allergic asthma & with severe persistent allergic rhinitis.

Further Studies are needed to determine whether cytokine antagonism—TNF-α, IL-2, IL-4, or IL-13—could restore steroid responsiveness because such cytokines have been found to induce steroid resistance. Vitamin D has recently been demonstrated to induce IL-10-producing regulatory T cells (Xystrakis et al., 2006) and enhance steroid action, and may therefore be steroid sparing(Zhang et al., 2010)

8. Novel steroids

Steroids, either systemic or inhaled, are exquisitely active and effective in asthma, but their mechanism of action is broad, and concern for toxicity—even with topical steroids—has limited their wider use. A variety of approaches are being pursued to maximize local activity within the airways and at the same time to minimize systemic absorption and toxicity. One approach is development of on-site-activated steroids such as ciclesonide, which is a nonhalogenated ICS prodrug that requires endogenous cleavage by esterases for activity. Soft steroids are also being developed; these have improved local, topical selectivity and have much less steroid effect outside the target area. They may be inactivated by esterases or other enzymes (for example a lactone–glucocorticosteroid conjugate).

Dissociated glucocorticoids: The recognition that most of the anti-inflammatory effects of glucocorticoids are mediated by repression of transcription factors (transrepression), whereas the endocrine and metabolic effects of steroids are likely to be mediated via glucocorticoid response element binding (transactivation) has led to a search for novel corticosteroids that selectively transrepress, thus reducing the potential risk of systemic side effects. These dissociated steroids which favor monomeric glucocorticoid receptor complexes (i.e., they produce transrepression) and avoid dimerization or transactivation, which is undesirable in asthma would make the treatment of asthma more effective without the current fear of steroid's side effects. Agents from each of these categories are undergoing clinical trials.

Steroid sparing : The combination of long acting beta agonist (LABA) with inhaled corticosteroid (ICS) is used frequently in asthma and a benefit from adding LABA to ICS has been described. One review compared reduced dose (mean 60% reduction in inhaled steroid) ICS/LABA combination to either a fixed moderate/high dose ICS or a reduced/tapering ICS dose. In adults with asthma, who use moderate to high maintenance doses of ICS, the addition of LABA has an ICS-sparing effect. LABA permit a reduction of 37% (253 mcg BDP) in subjects on minimum maintenance ICS and up to 60% (300 mcg FP) in subjects on maintenance ICS without deterioration in asthma control. They are most effective when combined with ICS, and this combination therapy is the preferred treatment when a medium dose of ICS alone fails to achieve control of asthma (Gibson, 2005). The addition of a LABA to a daily regimen of ICS improves symptom scores, decreases nocturnal symptoms, improves lung function, decreases the use of relief medication, reduces the number of exacerbations and achieves clinical control of asthma in more patients, more rapidly, and at a lower dose of ICS, than ICS given alone(Greening,1994, Pauwel, 1997).

Certain case reports have documented tiotropium as a useful steroid sparing agent however future clinical trials are warranted that explore the use of tiotropium as a potential 'steroid-sparing agent' in severe refractory asthma (Kapoor, 2009).

9. Immunomodulator therapy as steroid sparing

Methotrexate: Methotrexate may have a small steroid sparing effect in adults with asthma who are dependent on oral corticosteroids. However, the overall reduction in daily steroid use is probably not large enough to reduce steroid-induced adverse effects. This small potential to reduce the impact of steroid side-effects is probably insufficient to offset the adverse effects of methotrexate (Davies, 1998)

Azathioprine : Currently there is a clear lack of evidence to support the use of azathioprine in the treatment of chronic asthma as a steroid sparing-agent. Large, long-term studies with pre-defined steroid reducing protocols are required before recommendations for clinical practice can be made (Dean, 2004)

Cyclosporine: The improvement in asthma with cyclosporin are small and of questionable clinical significance. Given the side effects of cyclosporin, the evidence available does not recommend routine use of this drug in the treatment of oral corticosteroid dependent asthma (Evans, 2001)

Chloroquine : There is insufficient evidence to support the use of chloroquine as an oral steroid-sparing agent in chronic asthma. Further trials should optimise oral steroid dosage before addition of the steroid-sparing agent (Dewey, 2003)

Troleandomycin : There is insufficient evidence to support the use of troleandomycin in the treatment of steroid dependent asthma.(Evans ,2001)

Gold: Gold has limited clinically significanct benefits as steroid sparing agent & given the side effects of gold and necessity for monitoring the use of gold as a steroid sparing agent in asthma cannot be recommended.(Evans , 2001)

10. Conclusion

Inhaled Corticosteroids are the most effective first line of therapeutic intervention to control the primary immunologic mechanism of the disease and to avoid the devastating consequences of this disease with resultant cost- effectiveness and risk benefits analysis leading to best control of asthma. As far as steroids are concerned, there is over fear of its side effects in the patients as well as physicians which has to be removed. It should be make clear that steroids are friends of asthma pts if optimally used but if overused it may turned out to be foe, hence emphasis should be given on the optimized and appropriate use of steroids based on the asthma severity, Hence physicians should try to use the both edges of this **"double edged sword"** for the benefit of patients.

In addition to pharmacological intervention, emphasis should always be given on the patient's education about asthma including its pathogenesis, medications, inhalation technique and strict environmental control on every visit of the patient. Definitively the safety issues of the use of

Steroids in asthma has to be taken in to consideration in order to address the instructions of Hippocrates, **"first do no harm"** in relation to the steroids, however steroids continue to be the most potent and the most effective controller medication for asthma, and their use in the appropriate clinical setting remains invaluable for the control & management of asthma in clinical practice.

Author details

Mahboub Bassam and Vats Mayank
Department of Pulmonology and Allergy & Sleep Medicine , Rashid Hospital, Dubai

11. References

Agertoft L, Pedersen S. (1998). Bone mineral density in children with asthma receiving long-term treatment with inhaled budesonide. *Am J Respir Crit Care Med*; 157(1):178-83.

Agertoft L, Pedersen S. (2000).Effect of long-term treatment with inhaled budesonide on adult height in children with asthma. *N Engl J Med*;343(15):1064-9.

Alexander AG, Barnes NC, Kay AB.(1992). Trial of cyclosporin in corticosteroid dependent chronic severe asthma. *Lancet*,339:324–328.

Barnes PJ, Adcock IM. (1995). Steroid-resistant asthma. Q J Med, 88: 455-468.

Barnes PJ, Greening AP, Crompton GK. (1995). Glucocorticoid resistance in asthma. *Am J Respir Crit Care Med*, 152: 125-140.

Barnes PJ, Adcock IM.(1998) Transcription factors and asthma. *Eur Respir J*;12:221–234.

Barnes PJ. (2008). Emerging pharmacotherapies for COPD. *Chest*, 134(6):1278-1286.

Barnes PJ, Adcock IM. (2009). Glucocorticoid resistance in inflammatory diseases. *Lancet*, 373(9678):1905-1917.

Barreto M. L., Cunha S. S., Alc^antara-Neves N et al., (2006). Risk factors and immunological pathways for asthma and other allergic diseases in children: background and methodology of a longitudinal study in a large urban center in Northeastern Brazil (Salvador-SCAALA study). *BMC Pulmonary Medicine*, vol. 6, article 15.

Bassam M, Vats M, Afzal S, Sharif W, Iqbal MN. (2012). Environmental Exposure and nonadherence with Medicines directly correlate with Exacerbations and Hospitalization for

Asthma: A Population-Based Survey from UAE. ISRN Pulmonology, Volume 2012.

Beato M, Herrlich P, Schutz G. Steroid hormone receptors: many actors in search of a plot. *Cell* 1995;83:851–857.

Bianchi M, Meng C, Ivashkiv BL (2000). Inhibition of IL-2-induced Jak-STAT signaling by glucocorticoids. PNAS, vol. 97, no. 17, pg 9573–9578.
www.pnas.orgycgiydoiy10.1073ypnas.160099797

Braman SS.(2006). The global burden of asthma. *Chest*,130(suppl 1):4S-12S

Carmichael J, Paterson IC, Diaz P, Crompton GK, Kay AB, Grant IWB. (1981) Corticosteroid resistance in chronic asthma. *Br Med J*, 282: 1419-1422.

Cochrane GM. (1996) Compliance and outcomes in patients with asthma. *Drugs*, 52:12–19

Darnell, J.E. (1997). STATs and gene regulation. *Science*. 277:1630–1635.

Davies HRH R, Olson LLG, Gibson PG. (1998). Methotrexate as a steroid sparing agent for asthma in adults. *Cochrane Database of Systematic Reviews*, Issue 3. Art. No.: CD000391

Dean TP, Dewey A, Bara A, Lasserson TJ, Walters EH. (2004)Azathioprine as an oral corticosteroid sparing agent for asthma. *Cochrane Database of Systematic Reviews*, Issue 1. Art. No.: CD003270

Dewey A, Bara A, Lasserson TJ, Walters EH.(2003) Chloroquine as a steroid sparing agent for asthma. *Cochrane Database of Systematic Reviews*, Issue 4. Art. No.: CD003275.

Dolovich M, Ruffin RE, Roberts R, et al. (1981)Optimal delivery of aerosols from metered dose inhalers. *Chest*; 80(suppl): 911–915,

Dolovich MB, Ahrens CR, Hess DR et al . (2005)Device Selection and Outcomes of Aerosol Therapy: Evidence-Based Guidelines : American College of Chest Physicians/American College of Asthma, Allergy, and Immunology *Chest*,127;335-371

Erzurum Sc, Leff JA, et al. (1991). Lack of benefit of methotrexate in severe, steroid dependent

asthma. *Ann Intern Med.*,114:353–360.

Evans DJ, Cullinan P, Geddes DM, Walters EH, Milan SJ, Jones P. (2001)Gold as an oral corticosteroid sparing agent in stable asthma. *Cochrane Database of Systematic Reviews*, Issue 2. Art. No.: CD002985

Evans DJ, Cullinan P, Geddes DM, Walters EH, Milan SJ, Jones P. (2001)Troleandomycin as an oral corticosteroid sparing agent in stable asthma. *Cochrane Database of Systematic Reviews*, Issue 2. Art. No.: CD002987

Evans DJ, Cullinan P, Geddes DM, Walters EH, Milan SJ, Jones P. (2001)Cyclosporin as an oral corticosteroid sparing agent in stable asthma. *Cochrane Database of Systematic Reviews*, Issue 2. Art. No.: CD002993

Federico MJ, Covar RA, Brown EE, Leung DY, Spahn JD. (2005). Racial differences in T-lymphocyte response to glucocorticoids. *Chest*,127(2):571-578.

Gibson P.G. Powell H, Ducharme FM.(2005) Long-acting beta2-agonists as an inhaled corticosteroid-sparing agent for chronic asthma in adults and children. *Cochrane Database of Systematic Reviews*, Issue 4. Art. No.: CD005076

Global Strategy for Asthma Management and Prevention. Global INitiative for Asthma (GINA), 2010. Available from www.ginasthma.org Date last updated, 2010.www.ginasthma.org

Greening AP, Ind PW, Northfield M, Shaw G. (1994)Added salmeterol versus higher-dose corticosteroid in asthma patients with symptoms on existing inhaled corticosteroid. Allen & Hanburys Limited UK Study Group. *Lancet*; 344: 219-224.

Goleva E, Hall CF, Ou LS, Leung DY. (2004)Superantigen-induced corticosteroid resistance of human T cells occurs through activation of the mitogen-activated protein kinase kinase/extracellular signal-regulated kinase (MEK-ERK) pathway. *J Allergy Clin Immunol.*,114(5):1059-1069

Haczku A, Panettieri RA Jr. (2010). Social stress and asthma: the role of corticosteroid insensitivity. *J Allergy Clin Immunol,*125(3):550-558.

Haynes RB, Taylor DW, Sackett DL, eds. (1979) Compliance in health care. Baltimore, MD: Johns Hopkins University Press.

Hopp RJ, Degan JA, Biven RE, Kinberg K, Gallagher GC.(1995) Longitudinal assessment of bone mineral density in children with chronic asthma. *Ann Allergy Asthma Immunol*;75(2):143-8.

Horne R, (2003). *Concordance and Medicines Management in the Respiratory Arena*, Hayward Medical Publications, London, UK.

Ito K, Barnes PJ, Adcock IM.(2000) Glucocorticoid receptor recruitment of histone deacetylase 2 inhibits interleukin-1beta-induced histone H4 acetylation on lysines 8 and 12. *Mol Cell Biol* 20:6891–6903.

Jackson C, Lipworth B. (1995)Optimizing inhaled drug delivery in patients with asthma. *Br J Gen Pract*; 45:683–687)

Kapoor AS, Olsen SR , CO'Hara C , et al. (2009). The efficacy of tiotropium as a steroid-sparing agent in severe asthma. *Can Respir J* Vol 16; No 3.

Karin M. (1998). New twists in gene regulation by glucocorticoid receptor: is DNA binding dispensable? *Cell*;93:487–490.

Kirkham B, Corkill MM, Davison SC, Panayi GS. (1991) Response to glucocorticoid treatment in rheumatoid arthritis: *in vitro* cell mediated immune assays predicts *in vivo* response. *J Rheumatol* 18: 1130-1133.

Lane SJ, Atkinson BA, Swimanathan R, Lee TH. (1996) Hypothalamic pituitary axis in corticosteroid-resistant asthma. *Am J Respir Crit Care Med*, 153: 1510 -14.

Lee TH, Brattsand R, Leung DYM, editors (1996). Corticosteroid action and resistance in asthma. *Am J Respir Cell Mol Biol*; 154(Suppl): S1–S79.

Leung DYM, Martin RJ, Sze¯er SJ, et al. (1995) Dysregulation of interleukin 4, interleukin 5, and interferon c gene expression in steroid-resistant asthma. *J Exp Med*, 181: 33±40.

Leung DY, Bloom JW.(2003). Update on glucocorticoid action and resistance. *J Allergy Clin Immunol.* 111(1):3-22.

Li LB, Goleva E, Hall CF, Ou LS, Leung DY. (2004).Super antigen-induced corticosteroid resistance of human T cells occurs through activation of the mitogen-activated protein kinase kinase/extracellular signal-regulated kinase (MEK-ERK) pathway. *J Allergy Clin Immunol.*;114(5):1059-1069.

Marin JM, Carrizo SJ, Garcia R, Ejea MV.(1996). Effects of nedocromil sodium in steroid-resistant asthma: a randomized controlled trial. *J Allergy Clin Immunol.*; 97:602–610.

Masoli M, Fabian D, Holt S, Beasley R.(2004). Global Initiative for Asthma (GINA) program: the global burden of asthma: executive summary of the GINA Dissemination Committee report. *Allergy,* 59:469-478.

Mazer BD, Gelfand EW. (1991). An open-label study of high-dose intravenous immunoglobulin in severe childhood asthma. *J Allergy Clin Immunol,* 87:976–983.

Mullarkey MF, Blumenstein BA, et al. (1988). Methotrexate in the treatment of corticosteroid-dependent asthma. *N Engl J Med.,*318:603–607.

Murphy, K.M., et al. (2000). Signaling and transcription in T helper development. *Annu. Rev. Immunol.* 18:451–494.

National Institutes of Health, Bethesda: (2006) National Institutes of Health/US Department of Health and Human Services; Inc., c1998. National Heart Lung and Blood Institute. Practical Guide for the Diagnosis and Management of Asthma, April, http://www.nhlbi.nih.gov/health/prof/lung/asthma/ practgde.htm.

Pauwels RA, Lofdahl CG, Postma DS, et al. (1997) Effect of inhaled formoterol and budesonide on exacerbations of asthma. Formoterol and Corticosteroids Establishing Therapy (FACET) International Study Group. N Engl J Med; 337: 1405- 1411.

Pedersen S. (2001)Do inhaled corticosteroids inhibit growth in children? *Am J Respir Crit Care Med*;164(4):521-35.

Rengarajan, J., Szabo, S.J., and Glimcher, L.H. (2000). Transcriptional regulation of Th1/Th2 polarization. *Immunol. Today.* 21:479–483.

Roux C, Kolta S, Desfougeres JL, Minini P, Bidat E. (2003)Long-term safety of fluticasone propionate and nedocromil sodium on bone in children with asthma. *Pediatrics*;111(6 Pt 1): e706-13.

Sally E. W., Fahy JV, Irvin C et al. (2000)Proceedings of the ATS Workshop on Refractory Asthma Current Understanding, Recommendations, and Unanswered Questions. *Am J Respir Crit Care Med* Vol 162. pp 2341–2351,

Schwartz, Lowell FC, Melby JC. (1968) Steroid resistance in bronchial asthma. *Am J Int Med,* 69: 493-499.

Sharek PJ, Bergman DA.(2000) Beclomethasone for asthma in children: effects on linear growth. *Cochrane Database Syst Rev*;2.

Strickland I, Kisich K, Hauk PJ, et al. (2001). High constitutive glucocorticoid receptor beta in human neutrophils enables them to reduce their spontaneous rate of cell death in response to corticosteroids. *J Exp Med.*;193(5):585-593.

Sutherland ER, Goleva E, Strand M, Beuther DA, Leung DY. (2008).Body mass and glucocorticoid response in asthma. *Am J Respir Crit Care Med.*;178(7):682-687.

Sutherland ER, Goleva E, Jackson LP, Stevens AD, Leung DY. (2010)Vitamin D levels, lung function, and steroid response in adult asthma. *Am J Respir Crit Care Med.*;181(7):699-704.

Szefler SJ, Leung DY. (1997) Glucocorticoid-resistant asthma: pathogenesis and clinical implications for management. *Eur Respir J,* 10(7): 1640-47.

Wills-Karp, M. (1999). Immunologic basis of antigen-induced airway hyperresponsiveness. *Annu. Rev. Immunol.* 17:255–281.

Woolcock A , Rubinfeld AR, Seale JP et al. (1989) Thoracic society of Australia and New Zealand. Asthma management plan, 1989. *The Medical Journal of Australia*, vol. 151, no. 11- 12, pp. 650–653,

World Health Organization.(2003). *Adherence to Long-Term Therapies: Evidence for Action*, World Health Organization, Geneva, Switzerland.

Wurster, A.L., Tanaka, T., and Grusby, M.J. 2000. The biology of Stat4 and Stat6. *Oncogene.* 19:2577–2584.

Xystrakis E, Kusumakar S, Boswell S, et al. (2006) Reversing the defective induction of IL-10-secreting regulatory T cells in glucocorticoid-resistant asthma patients. *J Clin Invest.* 116(1):146-155

Zhang Y, Goleva E, Leung DYM. (2010).Vitamin D has corticosteroid sparing effects by enhancing glucocorticoid induced mitogen-activated protein kinase phosphatase-1 [abstract]. *J Allergy Clin Immunol.*;125(2):216

New Formula of Glucocorticoids in Clinical Treatment

Soft Glucocorticoids: Eye-Targeted Chemical Delivery Systems (CDSs) and Retrometabolic Drug Design: A Review

Pritish Chowdhury and Juri Moni Borah

Additional information is available at the end of the chapter

1. Introduction

Steroids play a vital role in human physiology and medicine. Glucocorticoids have dominated the class of anti-inflammatory agents quite successfully over other drugs since their introduction to dermatology more than fifty years ago. Later they have been developed both as topical and systemic anti-inflammatory agents. From studies it has been found that glucocorticoids normally release their anti-inflammatory effects mainly through the modulation of the cytosolic glucocorticoid receptor (GR) at the genomic level [1, 2]. The activated glucocorticoid-GR complex formed *via* binding of glucocorticoid with the GR in the cytoplasm, migrates to the nucleus, where it upregulates the expression of anti-inflammatory proteins and repress the expression of pro-inflammatory proteins. In some recent work, it has been reported that the activated glucocorticoid-GR complex has also been found to initiate nongenomic effects like inhibition of vasodilation, vascular permeability and migration of leukocytes [1, 3]. Glucocorticoids also mediate anti-inflammatory activity through membrane-bound GR-mediated nongenomic effects and also through direct non specific interaction with cellular membranes [3, 4]. Since GR is involved in a plethora of signalling pathways, more than 5000 genes are expressed or suppressed following glucocorticoid exposure [4, 5]. Therefore long term use or high dosages of glucocorticoids could result in adverse drug reactions (ADRs) like increased Intraocular Pressure (IOP) [6, 7] in ocular therapeutics. Glucocorticoids- induced ocular hypertension is of great concern in ophthalmic therapeutics as it can lead to secondary iatrogenic open-angle glaucoma. Glaucoma is a group of eye diseases characterized by progressive optic nerve cupping with visual field loss leading to bilateral blindness. It has been reported that glaucoma is estimated to affect more than 50 million people worldwide as defined by the World Health Organization (WHO) [8].

However, the use of corticosteroids has become more and more restricted and unacceptable because most of these agents are found to be associated with severe side effects, including percutaneous absorption and cutaneous atrophy [9]. Also allergic contact dermatitis is an unexpected adverse effect in most of these corticosteroids. On the other hand because of their high efficacy, their use is inevitable to give them the status of life saving drugs. The severe side effects associated with these glucocorticoids, has led to the pharmaceutical industry to make a productive effort towards the introduction of new generation of topical corticosteroids with specific substituents in their parent molecules to make them safer in comparison to the old generation glucocorticoids [10].

The effectiveness of hydrocortisone was first demonstrated by Sulzberger and Witten during 1950 [11] and soon after the new and more effective fluorinated hydrocortisones were introduced in the market during 1960 [12]. Further R&D works on these glucocorticoids led to introduction of super potent corticosteroids in the 1970s and 1980s. Cornell and Stoughton [13] had proposed a potency rating of these topically applied glucocorticoids in 1984, based primarily on the vasoconstrictor assay or skin-blanching of corticosteroid preparations. Again based upon the consensus of the United States Pharmacopoeia (USP) Dermatology Advisory Panel, a classification of the potency ranking for these glucocorticoids had been done as low, medium, high and very high [14]. New generation of glucocorticoids do not cause much cutaneous atrophy or systemic absorption in human body. Molecular configuration of these new corticosteroids tends to display a rapidly declining concentration gradient in the skin. Many of these new generation glucocorticoids are developed through the concept of prodrugs – a tool for improving physiochemical, biopharmaceutical or pharmacokinetic properties of pharmacologically active agents. Thus prodrugs are bioreversible derivatives of drug molecules that undergo an enzymatic or chemical transformation *in vivo* to release the active parent drug, which could then exert the desired pharmacological effect. These new generation glucocorticoids primarily act in the top layers of the skin where the most important mediators of the inflammatory reactions are [10, 14] found.

As for these new generation glucocorticoids, the action in the deeper layer is considerably diminished making them having less systemic side effects [14]. European and North American based clinical studies have shown that the new generation corticosteroids with their improved risk- benefit ratio are as effective as products currently available in the market [15]. These new generation glucocorticoids are highly effective in treating plethora of disease including psoriasis, allergies, asthma, rheumatoid arthritis and lupus [2-8, 14,15].

Again the application of anti-inflammatory agents in ophthalmic therapeutic is a challenging task because of severe complications arising out of the currently used anti-inflammatory agents. The eye is vulnerable to damage from low level of intraocular inflammation. The blood-aqueous and blood-retinal barriers generally limit penetration of protein and cells from peripheral circulation, while regulatory molecules and cells in the eye actively suppress immunological responses [16]. The fact that ocular inflammatory conditions and surgical trauma induce changes in the blood- aqueous and blood-retinal barriers [16-18], due to which immune cells and mediators of inflammation could enter the eye, resulting in the development of symptoms of ocular inflammation such as redness, pain, swelling and itching [19]. Ocular inflammation is a serious problem, negligence of which may lead to temporary or permanent blindness [20].

Clinical studies suggest that topical glucocorticoids are effective in the management of anterior segment inflammation. They impart a number of potent anti-inflammatory effects [21]. They are found to suppress cellular infiltration, capillary dilution, proliferation of fibroblasts, collagen deposition leading to scar formation; they also stabilize intracellular and extracellular membranes. Glucocorticoids increase the synthesis of lipocortins which block *phospholipase A$_2$* and also inhibit Histamine (**A**) synthesis in mast cells. A critical step in the inflammatory cascade is the inhibition of *phospholipase A$_2$* that inhibits the transformation of Phospholipids (**B**) to Arachidonic acid (**C**). Glucocorticoids are also found to increase the enzyme histaminase and modulate transcription factors present in mast cell nuclei [21, 22]. The formation of cataract is also one of the severe adverse drug reactions (ADRs) associated with glucocorticoids when used for ocular problems.

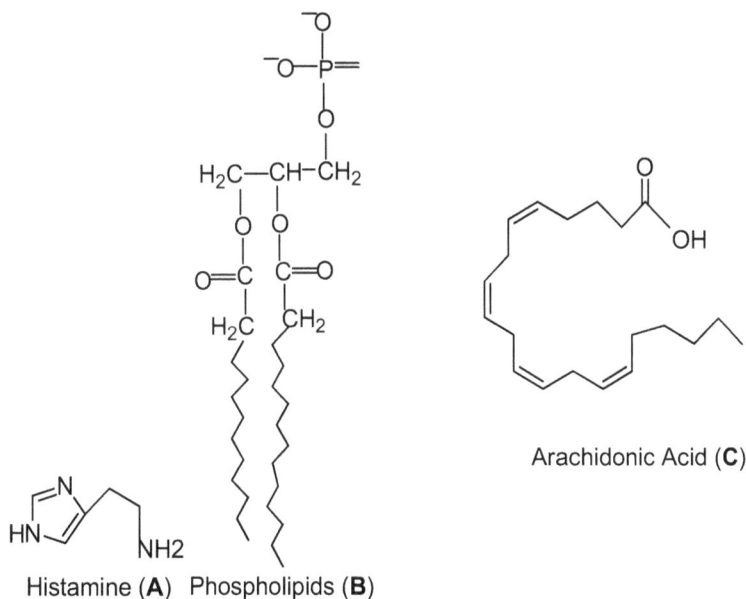

Arachidonic Acid (**C**)

Histamine (**A**) Phospholipids (**B**)

It has been reported by Manabe *et al* [23] that the mechanism of steroid-induced cataract formation is chemically based and possibly not related to the downstream effects of glucocorticoid receptor (GR) activation. At present the most accepted hypothesis of this mechanism is likely to involve non-enzymatic formation of Schiff base intermediates between the steroid C-20 ketone group and nucleophilic groups such as β -amino groups of lysine residues of proteins (**Figure 1**). Schiff base formation is followed by a Heyns rearrangement [23] involving the nearby C-21 hydroxyl group of the glucocorticoid molecule furnishing stable amine-linked adducts. This covalent binding results in the destabilization of the protein structure allowing further oxidation leading to steroid-induced cataract formation [23].

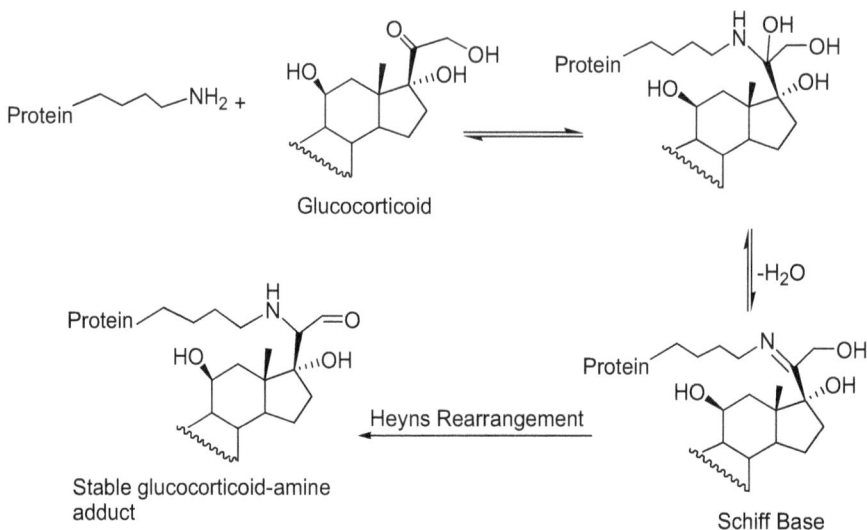

Figure 1. Mechanism of steroid-induced cataract formation due to the synthesis of the stable steroid-amine adduct between the C-20 carbonyl group of glucocorticoids and nucleophilic group such as β-amino groups of lysine residues of proteins via formation Schiff Base

R&D work in understanding the mechanism of action of steroids, both for their anti-inflammatory effects and adverse drug reactions (ADRs) has lead to the development new generation glucocorticoids mainly through prodrug design approach to find use in treating plethora of diseases as mentioned earlier. All these new generation glucocorticoids are not designed for ophthalmic therapeutics. Hence a real breakthrough in the field of ophthalmic therapeutic could be achieved only by specifically designing new drug entities to incorporate the eye targeting possibility into their chemical structure [24,25]. Chemical Delivery Systems (CDSs) and Retrometabolic drug design principles have led to development of a new but unique class of glucocorticoids which are safe and effective in treating a wide variety of ocular inflammatory conditions including giant papillary conjunctivitis, seasonal allergic conjunctivitis, and uveities as well as in the treatment of ocular inflammation and pain following cataract surgery. This new and unique class of glucocorticoids are now known as soft glucocorticoids which are associated with highly minimized ADRs to justify terming them as `soft drugs' [24, 26].

It is pertinent to note that, this important drug design based on Chemical Delivery Systems (CDSs) and Soft drug (SD) approaches integrate the specific pharmacological, metabolic, and targeting requirements for ophthalmic therapeutics. .A number of glucocorticoid soft drugs and soft β -blockers have been developed this way for clinical trials. Their potential is already documented by the results obtained with several soft drugs designed within this framework. Glucocorticoid soft drugs such as Loteprednol Etabonate, and Etiprednol Dicloacetate and β -blockers such as Betaxoxime, and Adaprolol are some of the new chemical entities developed as soft drugs for ocular applications. Besides, many of these soft drugs have already reached the clinical development phase in various ophthalmic areas and one of them Loteprednol Etabonate has already been marketed [24]. Herein we review the important aspects of the development of new generation glucocorticoids through prodrug approach with special reference to the development of the first and second generation glucocorticoid soft drugs by the application chemical delivery systems (CDSs) and retrometabolic drug design approaches towards ophthalmic therapeutics. A few examples of soft ocular β –blockers have also been cited to know more about the retrometabolic drug design approach in depth as have been put forwarded by Bodor and his co-workers (24).

2. New generation glucocorticoids: Prodrugs

As discussed earlier several numbers of new entities of glucocorticoids have been developed during the last two decades. Many of them are already in market for their high efficacy and less systemic side effects. These new generation corticosteroids were developed with modifications made in the basic glucocorticoid molecules, *viz.*, Betamethasone **1** or Dexamethasone **2** extensively used during early stage of glucocorticoids therapy. The main object of synthesizing these modified glucocorticoids was to get better skin penetration, slower enzyme degradation, and greater affinity for cytosol receptors [5].

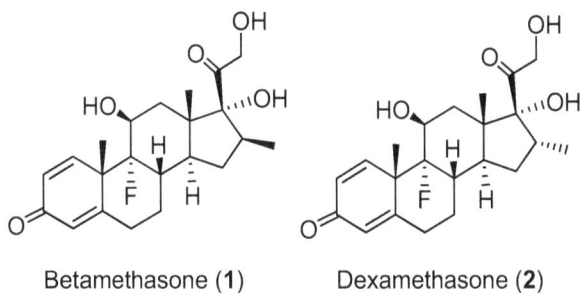

Betamethasone (**1**)   Dexamethasone (**2**)

Even then in some cases it was observed that the changes that increased potency, also led sometimes to more systemic side effects. As per clinical investigations by various workers, these new generation glucocorticoids have been found to act *via* hepatic or extra hepatic biotransformation. These results in lesser systemic side effects and hence are much safer drugs to be used specially by adults and non- erythrodermic patients. However, while systemic side effects are of concern, cutaneous side effects are generally common involving problems such as striae formation, atrophy, purpura, peri-oral dermatitis, steroid rosacea, hypertrichosis and steroid acne [2,6]. Most of the side effects associated even with these new generation glucocorticoids are basically related to the duration and potency of the application, the manner of application, the presence of penetration-enhancing substances and the state of skin barrier. Besides these, the anatomic site and the age of the patient could also adversely influence the side effect profile [2, 6]. In both drug discovery and development, prodrug design approach helped to maximize the amount of an active drug to reach its target through changing the physicochemical, pharmacokinetics or biopharmaceutical properties of the drug. Therefore the term prodrug refers to a pharmacologically inactive compound which is converted to an active drug by metabolic biotransformation which may occur prior, during or after absorption or at specific target sites within the body because of their specific molecular configurations [28-30]. The labile `prodrug' corticosteroids such as 17-Prednicarbate, Alclometasone, Methylprednisolone aceponate, Fluticasone Propionate and Fluocortin butylester are some of these new generation glucocorticoids which are developed through prodrug approach [2,6]. Based on the molecular configuration of these new generation glucocorticoids, they are classified into several categories [**Table1**] [2, 6].

Molecular Configurations	Structures	Names
Asymmetric acetonides		Budesonide (**3**)
C-21-Carboxylesters		Fluocortin butylester (**4**)
		Methylprednisolone aceponate (**5**)
		Alclometasone dipropionate(**6**)
		Beclomethasone (**7**)

		Ciclesonide (8)
C-17 –Prednicarbonates		17-Prednicarbate (9)
Carbothiates		Mometasone furoate (10)
		Fluticasone propionate (11)

Table 1. Classification of new generation glucocorticoids on the basis of their molecular configurations

Chemical stability is another criteria for classification of these new generation corticosteroids. Based on this, most of these newer drugs can be regarded as prodrugs because immediately after application to the system, they undergo metabolization and acyl-exchanges to form the active molecule to fight the ailment in the system. As mentioned earlier, all these glucocorticoids have been developed through prodrugs design approach in order to maximize the amount of an active drug reaching its target through changing the physicochemical, biopharmaceutical or pharmacokinetic properties of drugs. Prodrugs are bioreversible derivatives of drug molecules that undergo an enzymatic or chemical transformation *in vivo* to release the active parent drug, which can then exert the desired pharmacological effect [28-30]. Most of the new generation corticosteroids have been found belonging to the class of molecules having high potency. By introducing various substituents at different positions, changes or modifications were made on the parent hydrocortisone molecules, such as Betamethasone (1) and Dexamethasone (2) in order to get better skin penetration, slower enzymatic degradation and greater affinity for the cytosol receptor for these molecules to reduce or eliminate their systemic side effects [6]. The systemic side effects of these new corticosteroids are reduced due to rapid biotransformation while applying them for treatment of atopic dermatitis. However it is pertinent to note that there are still risks of having potential hypothalamus and pituitary axis (HPA) suppression with some of these new generation glucocorticoids while treating young children and erythrodermic patients. Clinical safety has been demonstrated in most of these newer corticosteroids with restricted duration of treatment up to six weeks [2, 6]. Even then skin atropy and some telangiectasia have been observed in some patients. A large number of reports of contact allergic reactions associated with these new generation glucocorticoids were still of great concern. To explain the increased allergenicity, data from clinical studies and literature were reviewed to define precisely some of the more important groups of cross-reacting molecules [31]. **Table2** represents the various allergy groups of these newer glucocorticoids based on their molecular structures and configurations. Clinical studies have revealed that Tixocortol pivalate (19) has been identified as a good screening agent for the Group A [32]. Budesonide (3) is infact a 1:1 mixture of two diasteriomers (R- and S- isomer). The R-isomer has been found to be a marker for the Group B while the S-isomer for the Group D. Glucocorticoid members of Group C cause minimized contact sensitivity and do not cross react with other groups. As shown in **Table2**, Group D has been divided in two sub-groups D_1 and D_2 based on recent studies [2, 33] with respect to their mode of substitutions.

Group	Molecular configuration	Characteristics of substituent
A	Hydrocortisone (12) type	No substitution in D ring, except a short chain ester on C-17 or C-21 or a thioester on C-21
B	Triamcinolone (13) type	C-16,C-17-*cis*-ketal or –diol structure
C	Betamethasone (1) type	C-16 methyl substitution, no side chain on C-17; possible side chain at C-21.
	Fluocortin Butylester (4)	
D	Hydrocortisone-17α-butyrate(14) type	Long chain ester at C-17 and/or C-21 with or without C-16 methyl substitution.
D_1	Betamethasone Dipropionate(15)	Long chain ester at C-17 and/or C-21 with C-16 methyl substitution; halogen substituent in ring B
	Betamethasone17α-Valerate (16)	
	Clobetasol 17α -Propionate (17)	
	Mometasone Furoate (10)	
	Fluticasone Propionate (11)	
D_2	Hydrocortisone-17α-butyrate(14)	Long chain ester at C-17; possibly a side chain at C-21; no methyl substitution at C-16 and no halogen substituent in ring B.
	Hydrocortisone 17α-Valerate (18)	
	17-Prednicarbate (9)	
	Methylprednisolone Aceponate (5)	

Table 2. Allergy Groups of new generation corticosteroids based on their molecular structures and configurations

To the Group D₁, belong not only the old generation glucocorticoid molecules like Betamethasone dipropionate (**15**), Betamethasone-17α-valerate (**16**) and Clobetasol 17α propionate (**17**) but also new generation corticosteroids such as Mometasone furoate (**10**) and Fluticasone propionate (**11**). These glucocorticoids are found to possess very less systemic side effects and so can be used safely even in case of patients who are allergic to other corticosteroids. To the Group D₂ belong Hydrocortisone-17α- valerate (**18**) and Hydrocortisone - 17α-butyrate (**14**) as well as the labile new generation glucocorticoids like 17-Prednicarbate (**9**) and Methylprednisolone Aceponate (**5**). They are sometimes found to cause allergic reactions.

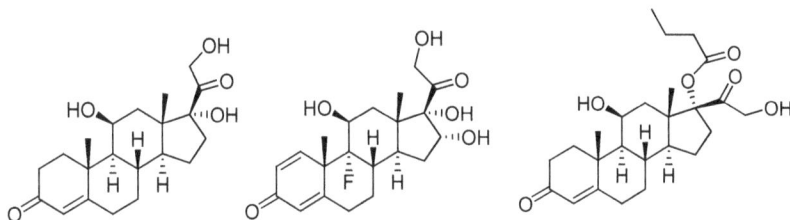

Hydrocortisone (**12**)   Triamcinolone (**13**)   Hydrocortisone-17α-butyrate (**14**)

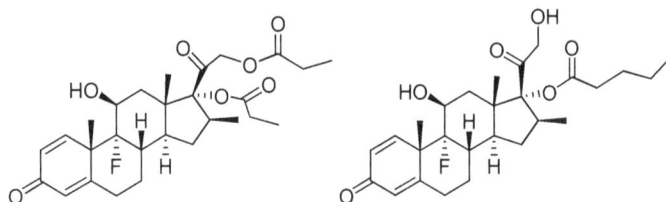

Betamethasone Dipropionate (**15**)   Betamethasone-17α-Valerate (**16**)

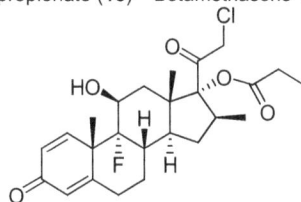

Clobetasol-17α-Propionate (**17**)

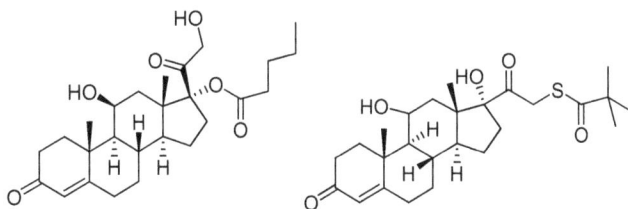

Hydrocortisone-17α-Valerate (**18**)   Tixocortol pivalate (**19**)

S-isomer of Budesonide (**3**) is the marker for this Group D$_2$, but they can cross react with the Group A. **Table 3** illustrates the safety profile, potency , side effects and allergy groups of some of the new generation glucocorticoids along with their manufactures.

Product	Manufacturer	Safety profile	Potency	Side effect	Allergygroup
Budesonide(3)	Astra, Entcort	A Stable asymmetric acetonide undergoing rapid biotransformation in liver with less systemic side effects	High potency	May be problem with contact sensitivity	B
Mometasone Furoate (10)	Schering-Plough, Elocom	A stable chlorinated topical glucocorticoid with low penetration with high biliary excretion, and also low resorption in the circulation with fast biotransformation in the liver resulting in rare local systemic side effect.	High potency	Very rare contact hypersensitivity	D$_1$
Fluocortin butylester(4)	Schering Corp.- Essex, Varlane	Biotransformation into the non- active fluocortolone-21-acid in skin.	Medium potency	Rare contact hyper-sensitivity	C
Alclometasone dipropionate(6)	Schering-Plough, Aclovate, Glaxo- -welcome	A labile prodrug metabolizing to inactive compound	High potency	Occasional Contact hyper-sensitivity	D$_2$
17-Prednicarbate(9)	Hoechst-Roussel,Dermatop Emollient	A labile prodrug glucocorticoid, converting to prednisolone in the skin	High potency	Contact hyper-sensitivity is observed. Also can cross-react with the Group A	D$_2$
Methylprednisolone aceponate(5)	Schering Corp. Essex, Advantan	A labile prodrug. Get transformed into methyl prednisolone in the skin and into nonactive derivatives in the liver	High potency	Contact hyper-sensitivity is not rare	D$_2$

Fluticasone propionate (11)	Cutivate, Glaxo Wellcome	A fluorinated topical glucocorticoid. Readily metabolized in the liver resulting in a locally potent sterid drug with a low HPA inhibitory potency	High potency	Contact hyper-sensitivity is very rare	D1
Beclomethasone(7)	Schwitz Biotech, Havione Farmaciencies, Portugal	A chlorinated topical corticosteroid. Readily metabolized in the liver resulting in a locally potent steroid with a low HPA inhibitory potency	High potency	Contact hyper-sensitivity is very rare	D1
Cyclesonide (8)	Brand Name: Alvesco, Taj Pharmaceuticals Ltd. India	A triamcinolone type Gluco-corticoid with low HPA inhibitory potency	High Potency	Contact hyper-sensitivity is rare	D1

Table 3. Some of the marketed new generation glucocorticoids and their allergy groups:

Continuous efforts are still being still sought after by pharmaceutical companies worldwide to develop and market more and more safer glucocorticoids as anti-inflammatory agents, because clinical investigations on some already marketed newer glucocorticoids have revealed that many of them are still prone to cause allergic reactions and other systemic side effects specially on prolonged use. However, glucocorticoids are still regarded as life saving drugs dominating over the other anti-inflammatory agents for the treatment of a number of diseases including psoriasis, allergies, acute asthma, rheumatoid arthritis and lupus.

Eye–targeted Chemical Delivery Systems (CDSs) and retrometabolic drug design: Soft β-Blockers and Soft Glucocorticoids

Soft corticosteroids or Soft glucocorticoids can be termed as a unique class of new generation glucocorticoids that are designed specifically for ophthalmic therapeutics [24-27]. The new generation glucocorticoids developed by prodrug approach as described earlier have brought revolution in treating a plethora of disease including psoriasis, allergies, asthma, rheumatoid arthritis and lupus because of their minimized systemic side effects. However, these new generation glucocorticoids are still not useful for ophthalmic applications due to their association with adverse drug reactions (ADRs) including elevation of intraocular pressure (IOP) and steroid-induced cataract formation [23] in ophthalmic applications. For the therapeutic treatment of most of ocular problems, topical administration undoubtedly seems preferred mode, because for systemically administered drugs, only a very small fraction of the total dose will reach the eye from the general circulatory system. Even distribution for this fraction to the inside of the eye is further hindered by the blood-retinal barrier (BRB), which is almost as effective as blood-brain barrier (BBB) in restricting the passage of xenobiotics from the blood stream [34]. Therefore despite its apparent accessibility, the eye, in fact, is well protected against the absorption of foreign materials, including drug molecules, by the eyelids, by flow of tears, and also by the permeability barriers imposed by the cornea on one side and the blood-retinal barrier on the other side as mentioned above [24]. Because of this a significant portion of the applied drug is absorbed through nasolacrimal duct and the mucosal membranes of the nasal, oropharyngeal, and gastrointestinal tract to pass to the system. It has been found that no more than 2% of medication introduced topically to the eye is adsorbed [35-37]. Again clinical studies by various workers reveal that the main biological barrier for penetration to the eye is represented by the cornea. The relatively lipophilic corneal epithelium tissue having low porosity and high tortuosity due to tight annular junctions, is the primary barrier for hydrophilic drugs, where as the middle stromal layer consisting mainly of water interspersed with collagen fibrils(major thickness of cornea), is the main barrier for the lipophilic drugs [38-41]. All these facts result not only in a low net eye drug delivery, but also in substantial systemic availability of ophthalmic drugs after

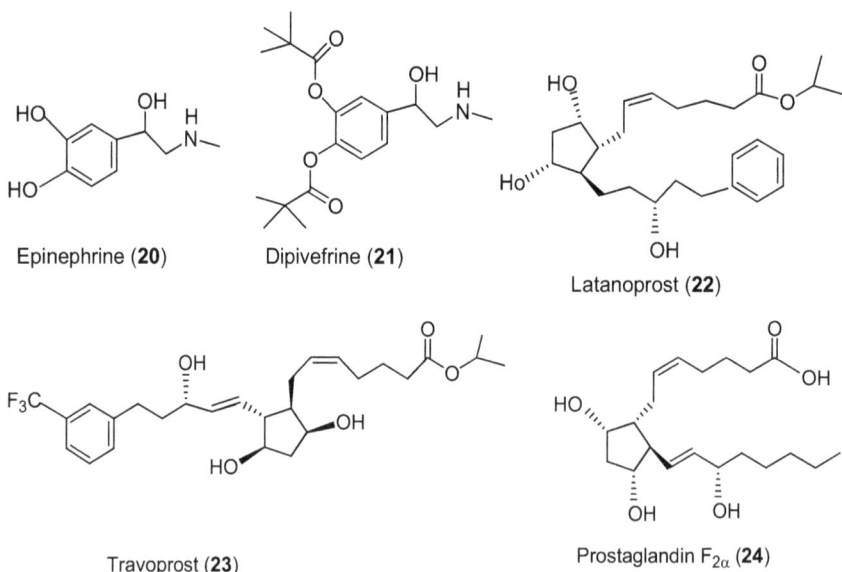

Epinephrine (20)   Dipivefrine (21)

Latanoprost (22)

Travoprost (23)

Prostaglandin $F_{2\alpha}$ (24)

topical administration giving systemic side effects [42]. Moreover as mentioned earlier, existing ophthalmic drugs are actually not developed for ocular applications, they were intended for other therapeutic areas which were later converted to ocular applications following their high efficacy. This further has decreased the likelihood of achieving eye-specific delivery along with reduced systemic side effects. In view of this, various drug design approaches have been tried to eliminate the problems of low ocular delivery and potential for substantial systemic side effects [6, 43]. It has been found that prodrug approach here had some limitations. Prodrugs are pharmacologically not active (or may be weakly active) compounds that results from transient chemical modifications of biologically active species, so that they are metabolically transformed into effective drugs following administration [28-30, 44-47]. Compared with the original structures, prodrug structures incorporate chemical modifications to get improvement in some deficient physiological properties, such as membrane permeability or water solubility or to overcome some other problems like rapid elimination, bad taste, a formulation difficulty etc. After administration, the prodrug because of its improved characteristics, is more systemically or locally available than the parent drug. However the prodrug must undergo chemical or biochemical conversion to the active form before exerting its biological effect. Some of the marketed ophthalmic prodrugs include Dipivefrine (**21**)-the dipivalate ester prodrug of epinephrine (**20**), latanoprost (**22**) and travoprost (**23**) -isopropyl ester prodrugs that are prostaglandin $F_{2\alpha}$ (**24**) analogs [24].

Retrometabolic Drug Design:

Because of the adverse drug reactions (ADRs) associated even with the new generation glucocorticoids in ocular treatment, the real breakthrough in the area of ophthalmic therapeutics could be achieved only by specifically designing new drugs with their ophthalmic applications in mind, so that the possibility of eye targeting with reduced systemic side effects is already incorporated in their chemical structures. In an effort to minimize ADRs and other complicacies associated with glucocorticoids, Bodor and his colleagues for the first time have developed the concept of retrometabolic drug design for ophthalmic therapeutics to introduce a new and unique class of glucocorticoids now known as soft corticosteroids or soft glucocorticoids that helped in developing glucocorticoid soft drugs for ophthalmic use [24, 48-50]. Soft β-blockers are also falling in this soft drug category. The concept of soft drugs has been originated from the pioneer work of Prof. N Bodor and his co-workers at the Center for Drug Discovery, University of Florida, Health Science Center, Gainesville, FL 32610-0497, USA [24, 48-50]. The possibility of developing these soft drugs has been extensively studied along the lines of retro- metabolic drug design for two important classes of ophthalmic drugs, β- blockers and glucocorticoids [24]. The underlying principle of retrometabolic drug design involves synthesizing analogs of lead molecules or reference molecules, starting from one of the known inactive metabolites of that lead compound. The inactive metabolite is then converted to an isosteric or isoelectronic analog with structural modifications designed for a rapid and predictable metabolism back to the original inactive metabolite after exerting the desired therapeutic effect at the site (**Figure 2**) [24, 26]. These analogs or soft drugs were predicted to have therapeutic potential similar to that of the lead compound, but because of the structural modifications provided by the design, any active drug remaining after attainment of the therapeutic effect would be metabolically deactivated, thus reducing adverse drug reactions (ADRs) [24, 26, 48-51]. According to Prof Bodor, in developing soft drugs the goal is not to avoid metabolism but rather to control and direct it. Inclusion of a metabolically sensitive moiety into the parent drug molecule can make possible the design and prediction of the major metabolic pathway preventing the formation of undesired toxic, active, or high-energy intermediates. It is desired that, If possible, inactivation should take place as the result of a single, low- energy and high- capacity step that gives the inactive species subject to rapid elimination. Most critical metabolic pathways in a biological system are mediated by *oxygenases*, a consequence of the fact that the normal reaction of an organism to a foreign material is to burn it up as food [52]. However *oxygenases* exhibit not only interspecies, but also inter individual and are subject to inhibition and induction (24) and because the rates of hepatic *mono-oxygenases* reactions are at least two orders of magnitude lower than the slowest of the other enzymatic reactions [53,54], it is usually desirable to avoid oxidative pathways as well as these slow, easily saturable *oxidase*s. In view of this, the design of soft drugs must be based on moieties activated by hydrolytic enzymes. Rapid metabolism could be more reliably performed by these ubiquitously distributed *esterases*. Bodor et al (26) suggested that it is desirable not to rely exclusively on metabolism by organs such as kidney or liver to have an additional advantage because blood flow and enzyme activities in these organs can be fatally damaged in critically ill patients. However, the increase in the therapeutic index can only be achieved if the drug is stable enough to reach its receptor site to deliver the desired effect, and any free drug remaining thereafter should be metabolized to minimize ADRs [24].

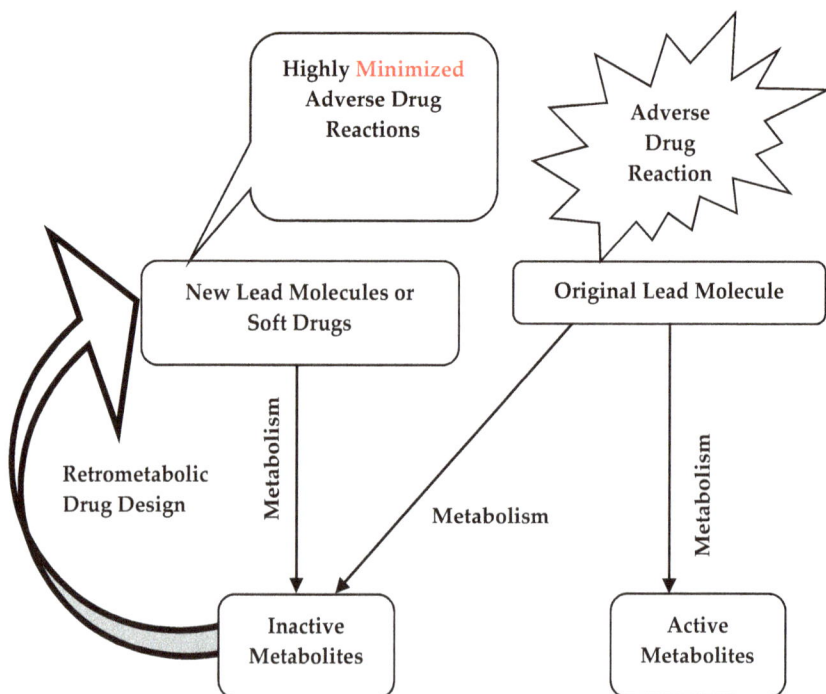

Figure 2. Retrometabolic drug design approach: Synthesis of new lead molecules (Soft drugs) based on an inactive metabolite of an original lead molecule

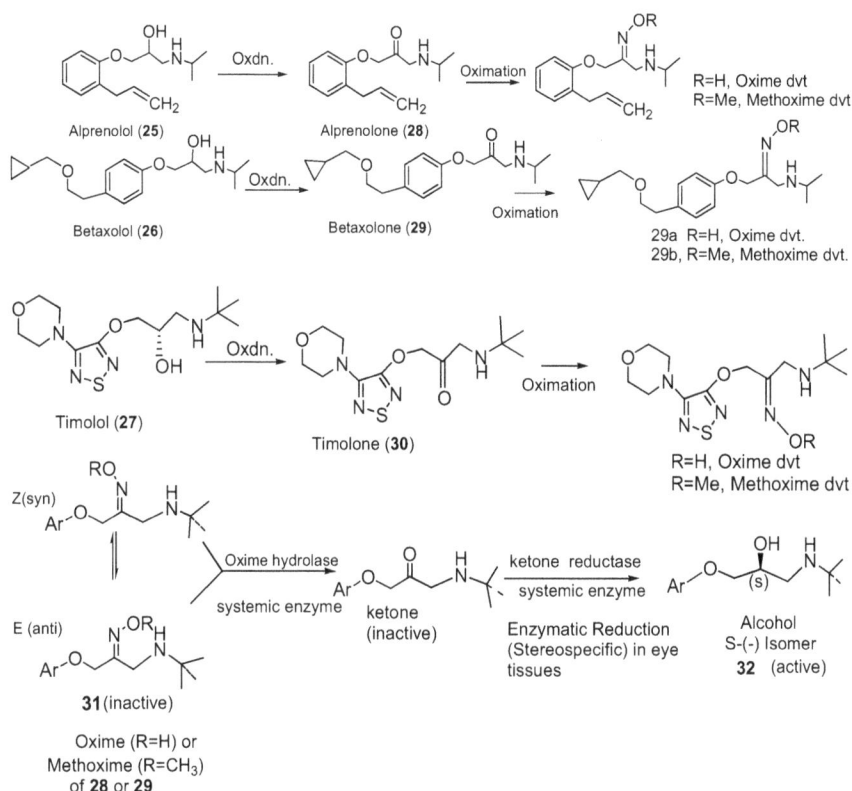

Figure 3. Site- and Stereospecific delivery of β-adrenergic antagonists to the eye through sequential activation of their oximes and alkyl oximes.

Soft- β-Blockers:

As because soft drug design is a general concept, topically applied soft drugs that show local activity with reduced systemic side effects could become potential therapeutics for any ocular diseases [24]. During the last three decades, Bodor and his colleagues have applied retrometabolic drug design to a variety of therapeutic agents such as β- blockers, antimicrobials, analgesics, and acetyl *cholinesterase* (ACE) inhibitors and were successful in developing retrometabolically designed compounds with market potential. As for example, in addition to the oxime or methoxime β -blocker analogs, the development of soft β - blockers could represent another possible route toward improved and safer antiglaucoma agents [54-62]. Several oxime and methoxime analogs of known β -Adrenergic blockers such as Alprenolol (25), Betaxolol (26)l, Timolol (27) etc. were synthesized from their respective ketone derivatives, *viz.*, Alprenolone (28), Betaxolone (29), Timolone (30) and studied clinically [54-62]. They are potential drugs which have been developed applying general retrometabolic drug design principle and can be recognized as site-specific enzymatic chemical delivery systems (CDSs) [54-62]. In these compounds, a β -amino oxime or alkyloxime function replaces the corresponding β -amino alcohol pharmacore part of the original molecules (**Figure 3**). These oxime or alkyloxime derivatives (**31**) are found to exist in Z (syn) or E (anti) configuration. They are hydrolyzed within the eye by enzymes located in the iris-cillary body and subsequently again by reductive enzymes present there producing only the active S- (-) stereoisomeric alcohol (**32**) of the corresponding β-blockers [54]. For aryl β -amino alcohol-type β -adrenergic agonists and antagonists, most of the activity has been known to be

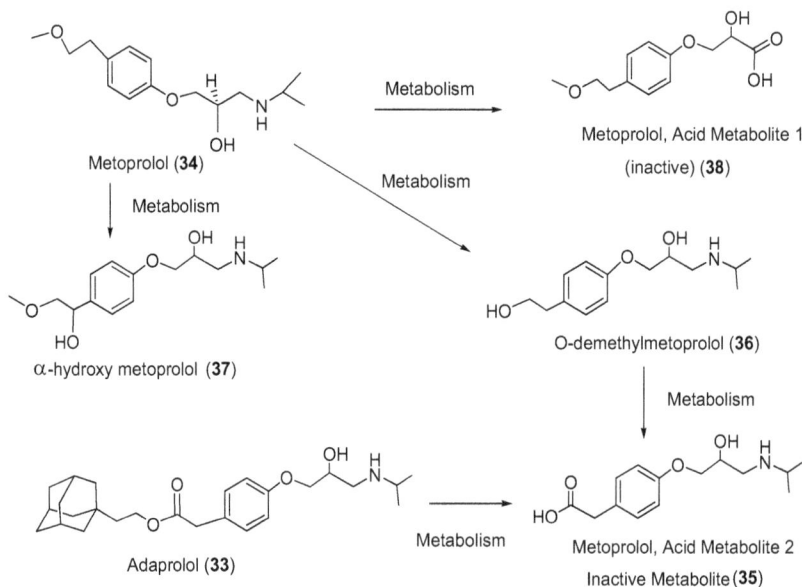

Figure 4. Inactive Metabolite-based Soft Drug Design: Comparison of the structure and metabolism of the soft β -blocker Adaprolol (23) with that of the traditional β -blocker Metoprolol(24).

present with the S- (-) stereoisomer [63-65], possibly because this isomer allows better interaction of all three important functionalities (aromatic, amino and β -hydroxyl moieties) with the β -adrenoceptor. In fact these oxime and alkyloxime derivatives have been found to exhibit significant intraocular pressure (IOP) lowering activity, but even their intravenous administration did not produce the active β -blocker metabolically; as a result they are void of any cardiovascular activity, which has been found to be a major drawback of classical antiglaucoma agents [26].

According to Bodor and his team [24], the oxime-type CDS approach clearly demonstrates the site- specific or site-enhanced drug delivery through sequential, multi-step enzymatic and/or chemical transformations through a targetor moiety that is converted into a biologically active function by enzymatic reactions which take place primarily at the site of action as a result of differential distribution of some enzymes found in the eye [24].

Again as Prof. Bodor and his team suggest [24,26], soft drugs (SDs) represent a different, conceptually opposite targeting concept; whereas eye-targeting CDSs, represented here by the above discussed oxime analogs, are inactive compounds designed to achieve the targeted effects *via* a multi-step activation process by enzymes found at their intended site of action. However soft drugs represented by β-blockers or glucocorticoids are active compounds designed to achieve the targeted effects *via* a single-step inactivation process involving enzymes found ubiquitously in the systemic circulation. Because in this class, inactive metabolite based soft drugs can be achieved introducing the hydrolytically sensitive functionality at a flexible pharmacophore region, there is considerable freedom for structural modifications. As a result, transport and metabolism properties are easier to control. From the various soft β-blockers developed along these lines by Bodor and Buchwald [24], Adaprolol (**33**), an adamantane ethyl ester was selected as a potential candidate for a new topical antiglaucoma agent [24]. The metabolism of the well-known β - blocker Metoprolol (**34**) has been compared with that of the soft β -blocker Adaprolol which has been designed starting from one of Metoprolol`s inactive acid metabolite (**35**), *viz.,* phenyl acetic acid (**Figure 4**). Its other metabolites include α-hydroxymetoprolol (**36**) and O-Dimethylmetoprolol (**37**) both of which are active. Another inactive metabolite includes the acid derivative **38**. Adaprolol was chosen because of the fact that if membrane transport (lipophilicity) and relative stability are important for pharmacological activity as they are needed to achieve right corneal permeability, then the ester goup should be relatively lipophilic and should provide ester stability [66-70]. In clinical trials Adaprolol (**33**) indeed produced prolonged and significant IOP-reduction while hydrolyzed relatively fast [67, 68]. Therefore, it was possible to separate local activity from undesired systemic cardiovascular or pulmonary activity, a characteristic highly desirable in development of antiglaucoma therapy [24]. Adaprolol (**33**) could be now a potent antiglaucoma soft β -blocker to replace the traditional β -blocker Metoprolol (**34**). Further clinical studies confirmed that Adaprolol is not only effective in reducing intraocular pressure (IOP) but also has a safer cardiovascular profile than Timolol (**27**) because unlike Timolol, Adaprolol did not reduce the systolic blood pressure [24].

Glucocorticoid Soft Drugs: Ophthalmic Therapeutics

Along the line of soft β-blockers, development of soft anti-inflammatory glucocorticoids represents a promising and successful ophthalmic drug design area initiated by Bodor and his colleagues [24,26]. Inflammation in the eye could result from surgery, injury, infection, conjunctivitis, or uvitis-conditions that can cause severe discomfort even leading to loss of vision. As mentioned earlier, topical glucocorticoids represent an important class of molecules to treat ocular inflammations and allergies as they are the most effective anti-inflammatory compounds offering the broadest range of treatment. However a number of contradictions limit their usefulness severely [12]. In addition to the general systemic side effects or adverse drug reactions (ADRs) associated with these glucocorticoids, they also cause several ocular complications such as IOP-elevation resulting steroid- induced glaucoma, induction of cataract formation and other secondary complications [12, 71]. In this context design of soft anti-inflammatory glucocorticoids has been one of the most active and productive fields of soft drug design. Ophthalmic use of glucocorticoids usually causes increased intraocular pressure (IOP) as a result of increased resistance to aqueous humour outflow. The design of soft anti-inflammatory glucocorticoids has been one of the most important and most successful areas of Soft Drug design. Although the soft nature of such drugs are mainly associated with fast hydrolytic degradation, in fact it is not necessarily be so as Bodor and his co-workers suggested [24].Too much rapid hydrolysis may in fact result in weak activity. The desired increase of therapeutic index can be obtained only if the drug is sufficiently stable to reach the receptor sites at the target organ to produce the desired effect, but the free, non-protein-bound drug undergoes facile hydrolysis to avoid undesired systemic side effects. Therefore to develop a soft drug and hence separating successfully the desired local activity from systemic toxicity, an adequate balance between intrinsic activity, solubility/lipophilicity, tissue distribution, protein binding and rate of metabolic deactivation have to be achieved. In the case of slow, sustained release to the general circulatory system from delivery site, even a relatively slow hydrolysis could result in a very low, almost steady-state systemic concentration [24]. Based on these concepts of eye-targeting chemical delivery systems (CDSs) and retrometabolic drug design approaches, Bodor and his group was successful in developing glucocorticoid soft drugs for ophthalmic therapeutics having potential market value.

First Generation Cortienic Acid (39)-based Glucocorticoid Soft Drugs: Loteprednol Etabonate (41) and its Analogs (42):

Synthesis of Dug molecules and Structure-Activity Studies:

As already mentioned, Bodor and his colleagues [24, 26] have applied retrometabolic drug design approach to a variety of therapeutic agents such as β- blockers, antimicrobials, analgesics, and acetyl cholinesterase (ACE) inhibitors and were successful in developing retrometabolically designed molecules reaching towards market application. They had designed a number of analogs starting with Δ^1-cortienic acid (40), the primary metabolite of prednisolone that lacks corticosteroid activity [25]. Hydrocortisone can undergo a variety of oxidative and reductive metabolic conversions [72] by local *esterases* within the system. Thus oxidation of its dihydroxyacetone side chain leads to the formation of cortienic acid *via* 21-dehydrocortisol (21-aldehyde) and cortisolic acid (21-acid) [**Figure 5**]. Cortienic acid (39) is an ideal lead molecule for the inactive metabolite soft drug (SD) approaches because it is lack of corticosteroid activity and therefore is major metabolite excreted in human urine. To get the new lead compounds, the pharmacophore moieties of the 17α-hydroxyl and 17β-carboxy substituents of the lead compound had to be restored by suitable isosteric/isoelectronic substitution containing esters or other types of functions that could restore the anti-inflammatory potency of the original corticosteroid while at the same time incorporating hydrolytic features to ensure metabolism. Other structural considerations included the presence or absence of double bond at C-1 position, presence of 6 α or 9 α fluorine, and 16 α & 16 β –methyl group (**Figure 6**). More than hundred possible drug molecules were synthesized and tested in pre-clinical anti-inflammatory models [5]. Structure-activity studies by Bodor and his group [24] of these molecules have confirmed that the best substituent for maximal therapeutic activity included a haloester at 17β– position and a carbonate or ether moiety at 17α– position. Incorporation of 17 α carbonates or ether was preferred over 17α– esters to increase stability and to prevent potential formation of mixed anhydrides by reaction of a 17α ester with a 17β acid functionality and subsequent potential for lens protein binding leading to steroid- induced cataract formation.

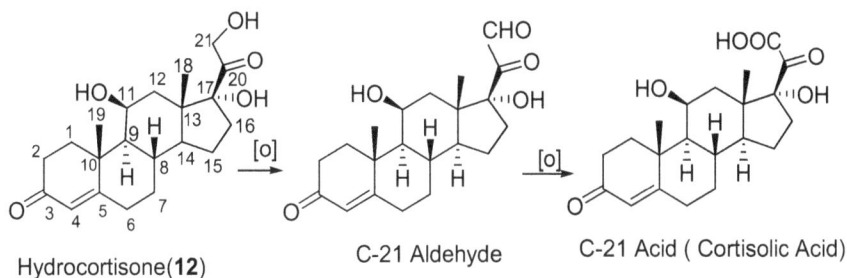

Hydrocortisone(**12**)   C-21 Aldehyde   C-21 Acid (Cortisolic Acid)

Figure 5. Oxidative metabolism of hydrocortisone by local esterases into C-21 Aldehyde and C-21 Acid (Cortisolic Acid)

Therefore in addition to the C-20 ketone functionality of prednisolone being replaced to eliminate the possibility of Schiff base intermediates, other chemical features associated with cataracterogenesis were also eliminated by the proposed design. The carbonates were expected to be less reactive than the corresponding esters due to the lower electrophilicity of the carbonyl carbon [24].

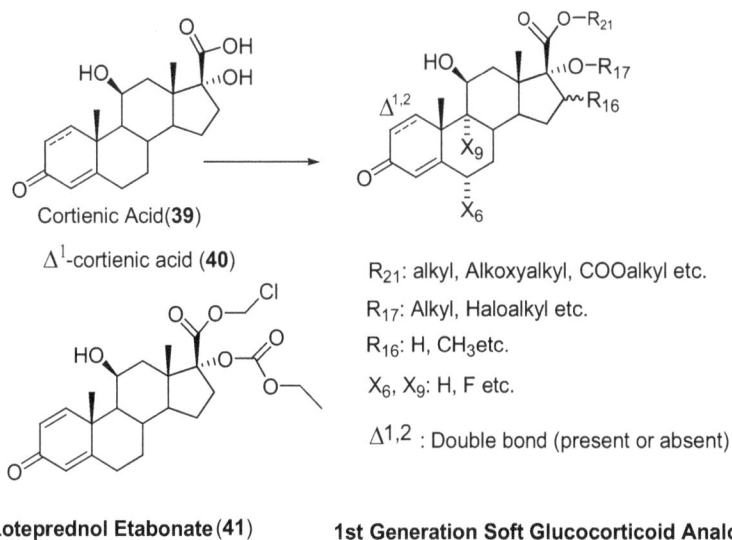

Cortienic Acid(**39**)

Δ^1-cortienic acid (**40**)

R_{21}: alkyl, Alkoxyalkyl, COOalkyl etc.

R_{17}: Alkyl, Haloalkyl etc.

R_{16}: H, CH_3etc.

X_6, X_9: H, F etc.

$\Delta^{1,2}$: Double bond (present or absent)

Loteprednol Etabonate (**41**)   **1st Generation Soft Glucocorticoid Analogs (42)**

Figure 6. Design of 1st Generation Cortienic acid-based Glucocorticoid Soft Drugs (**42**) with their Glucocorticoid Soft Drug representative Loteprednol Etabonate (LE)(**41**)

Loteprednol Etabonate (LE) namely chloromethyl- 17α-[(ethoxycarbonyl) oxy]-11β-hydroxy-3-oxoandrosta-1, 4-diene-17 β -carboxylate (**41**), was the most promising drug candidate among the various cortienic acid-based derivatives synthesized by Bodor and his group (**Figure 6**)]. In Loteprednol Elaborate (**41**), a metabolically labile ester function occupies 17 β - position, while a stable carbonate group occupies 17α-position. The ester is hydrolyzed to an inactive carboxylic acid, Δ^1-cortienic acid etabonate (**43**), and then into Δ^1-cortienic acid (**40**) in biological systems after exerting the desired therapeutic effect, thereby minimizing the likelihood of toxicity [**Figure 7**]. As a result of the predictable conversion of Loteprednol Etabonate into an inactive metabolite in the eye following topical administration, this glucocorticoid has a low propensity for undesirable toxicity while possessing increased anti-inflammatory activity. In fact Loteprednol Etabonate (**41**) has been found to be 1.5 times more potent than the parent anti-inflammatory agent dexamethasone [24].

Loteprednol Etabonate (41) and its Clinical Investigations in Ophthalmic Therapeutics:

Clinical study confirmed that Loteprednol Etabonate and some of the other soft glucocorticoids synthesized, provided a significant improvement of the therapeutic index, determined as the ratio between the anti-inflammatory activity and the thymus evolution activity [24]. In addition, binding studies using rat lung cytosolic corticosteroid receptors exhibited that the receptor binding affinity of LE and some of its analogs even exceeded that of the most potent glucocorticoids known[24]. Loteprednol Etabonate (**41**) is the one of the first-generation cortienic acid-based glucocorticoid soft drugs to get approved by Food and Drug Administration (FDA), USA for use in all inflammatory and allergy-related ophthalmic disorders, including inflammation after cataract surgery, uveitis, allergic conjunctivitis, and giant papillary conjunctivitis (GPC) [73-76]. Clinical tests on LE (**41**) by various groups of workers suggest it to be a potent glucocorticoid soft drug for ocular therapeutics. LE has also been selected for development as a potent glucocorticoid soft drug based on various considerations including the therapeutic index, availability, synthesis, and `softness' (the rate and easiness of metabolic deactivation). LE is now the active ingredient of a number of ophthalmic preparations available in the market (*Lotemax, Alrex, Zylet etc.*) [73, 74, 76].

Loteprednol Etabonate (**41**) has been found to be highly lipophilic which is 10 times greater than that of Dexamethasone (**2**), a characteristic that could increase its efficacy by enhancing penetration through biological membranes [24,26]. Competitive binding studies with rat lung type II GRs confirmed that binding affinity of LE was more than 4 times that of Dexamerhasone [77]. A vasoconstriction test in humans used to assess the bioavailability exhibited that LE could produce a blanching response similar to that of Betamethasone 17α-valerate (**16**) to confirm its good penetration properties and strong potency [11]. Bodor and his group, have reported the therapeutic index of LE having more than 20-fold better than that of other glucocorticoids including Hydrocortisone 17α-butyrate (**14**), Betamethasone 17α-valerate (**16**) and Clobetasol 17α-propionate (**17**) based on their cotton pellet glaucoma test and thymolysis potency [9]. LE (**41**) has been rightly selected on the basis of considerations including Therapeutic Index (TI) which is the ratio between the median toxic dose (TD$_{50}$) and the median effective dose (ED$_{50}$), availability, synthesis and the rate and easiness of metabolic deactivation (Softness)[24]. In traditional glucocorticoids such as Hydrocortisone 17α-butyrate (14), Betamethasone 17α-valerate (16) and Clobetasol 17α-propionate (17), efficacy and toxicity are closely correlated (r^2 =0.996) applying the relationship between the anti- inflammatory and thymus involution activities [24] determined in the cotton pellet granuloma test (**Figure 8**). In these glucocorticoids, the reported results [24] have shown that TI have been found to be almost similar regardless of their intrinsic activities; however glucocorticoid soft drug Loteprednol Etabonate (41) owing to its softness and improved toxicity profile, provides a significant improvement(24) (**Table 4**).

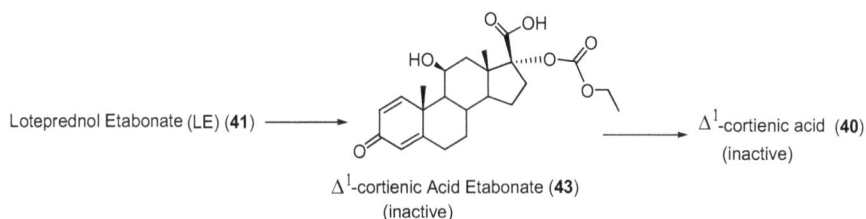

Loteprednol Etabonate (LE) (41) ⟶ ⟶ Δ^1-cortienic acid (40)
(inactive)

Δ^1-cortienic Acid Etabonate (43)
(inactive)

Figure 7. Metabolism of Loteprednol Etabonate (41) to Δ^1-Cortienic acid etabonate (43) and then to Δ^1-Cortienic acid(40).

Loteprednol Etabonate (LE) is predictably metabolized by local *esterases* into its inactive metabolite Δ^1-cortienic acid (40) which has been confirmed through animal studies [20]. Clinical studies by Druzgala *et al* [78] have confirmed that the highest concentration of LE was found in cornea, followed by the iris/ciliary body and aqueous humour. The cornea also showed the highest ratio of metabolite to Loteprednol Etabonate (41), indicating that the cornea was the prime site of metabolism, while aqueous humour concentrations of LE were nearly 100-fold lower. This finding suggested that Loteprednol Etabonate may exert a decreased IOP effect as compared to other glucocorticoids [78]. Further a comparison of the IOP-elevating activity of Loteprednol Etabonate with that of Dexamethasone (2) in rabbits confirmed a lack of IOP effect with LE [79, 80]. LE was found to have a terminal half- life (t1/2) of 2.8 hrs in dogs following intravenous administration [81]. Further when absorbed systemically, LE was found to be metabolized to Δ^1-cortienic acid etabonate (43) and then to Δ^1-cortienic acid (40) (**Figure 7**) and have been found to be eliminated rapidly through the bile and urine [26, 81, 82]. So far numerous preclinical tests were carried out on Loteprednol Etabonate (41) including more recent ones by Comstock and DeCory [20, 83]. Most of these clinical studies have confirmed that Loteprednol Etabonate achieves the required balance between the solubility/lipophilicity, ocular tissue distribution, receptor binding, and subsequent rate of metabolic deactivation as have been outlined by Bodor when he conceptualized for the first time the retrometabolic drug design.

Since the design of this glucocorticoid soft drug LE by Bodor and his group, various ophthalmic suspension formulation of LE *viz.*, a 0.2% suspension, a 0.5% suspension and a combination suspension of LE 0.5% plus tobramycin 0.3%, have been developed and clinically tested in various ocular inflammatory conditions and postoperative ocular inflammation.

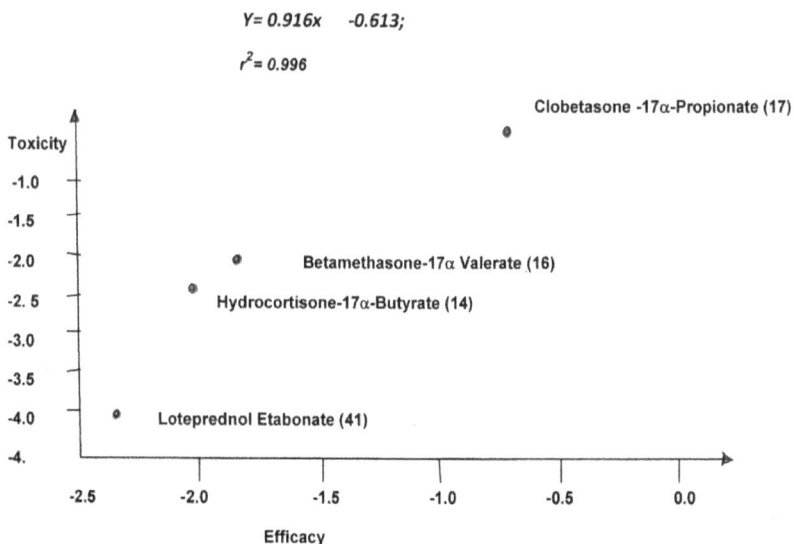

Figure 8. Literature reported [24] graph showing the relationship between the Efficacy [log $1/ED_{50}$ (μg/pellet)] and Toxicity [log $1/TD_{50}$ (μg/pellet) of Hydrocortisone-17 α-Butyrate (14: 0.1%), Betamethasone-17 α-Valerate (16: 0.12%), Clobetasone-17 α-Propionate (17: 0.1%) and Loteprednol Etabonate (41: 0.1%). Relative TI being computed with Betamethasone-17 α-Valerate (16) as reference.

Glucocorticoids	Therapeutic Index (TI) TD_{50}/ED_{50}	Relative Therapeutic Index (Rel TI) TI/TI_{BMV}
Loteprednol Etabonate (41)	56.2	22.5
Clobetasone-17α-Propionate (17)	3.8	1.5
Hydrocortisone-17 α -Butyrate (14)	3.1	1.3
Betamethasone-17 α -Valerate (BMV: 16)	2.5	1.0

Table 4. Literature reported Therapeutic Index (TI) and Relative Therapeutic Index (Rel. TI) of some glucocorticoids and Loteprednol Etabonate (**41**). Relative Therapeutic Index was computed with Betamethasone-17α -Valerate (BMV)(**16**) as the reference.

Ocular diseases against which LE formulations were clinically tested included Giant Papillary Conjunctivitis, Prophylaxis of Seasonal Allergic Conjunctivitis, Seasonal Allergic Conjunctivitis, Anterior Uveitis, Blepharokerato Conjunctivitis, and Keratoconjunctivitis sicca etc. All these studies confirmed the clinical anti-inflammatory potency of LE and lack of significant IOP after its use [20]. Again two identical placebo-controlled trials examined the safety and efficacy of LE in treating post operative inflammation following cataract surgery with intraocular lens implantation [92]. Ilyas et al [93] have studied the long term safety of LE 0.2% by conducting a retrospective review of more than 350 seasonal and perennial conjunctivitis patients who used LE 0.2% on a daily basis for extended periods of time. The results showed the absence of significant ADRs as there were no reports of posterior subcapsular opacification with quite insignificant IOP in most of the patients. In fact there was no observation of IOP elevation greater than 4mm Hg over base line at any period of time.

Besides, safety and efficacy of LE ophthalmic ointment 0.5% in the treatment of inflammation and pain following cataract surgery was studied in two randomized, multicentre, double-masked, parallel group, vehicle-controlled studies [20]. A very fewer LE ointment-treated patients needed rescue medication and most of them did not showed any ocular adverse event. Clinical trials on gel formulation of LE in treatment of ocular inflammation and pain after cataract surgery have been taken up more recently [20]. It is because of the high lipophilic nature of LE, gel formulation could provide improved product homogeneity over a suspension formulation to enhance its more consistent clinical response.

LE has been designed by Bodor and his group with a C-20 ester rather than a C-20 ketone and so LE is unable to form covalent adduct with lens protein, the main reason behind steroid-induced cataract formation as discussed earlier. Global market research indicates that an estimated more than 20 million LE units have been distributed globally. Clinical studies suggest the rapid metabolism of LE into inactive metabolites in conjunction with the lack of C-20 carbonyl functionality have resulted in LE – to become a unique glucocorticoid soft drug with significantly less, if any, potential for promoting steroid-induced cataract formation.[20]. LE has now been proved as a safe and effective treatment for contact lens-associated GPC, seasonal allergic conjunctivitis, postoperative inflammation or uveitis. Retrospective study established that even long time (>1 year) use of LE caused no reported adverse effects. .

Synthesis of the Side Chain of Loteprednol Etabonate (41) directly from 20-Oxopregnane (44) to furnish an Analog (45) of LE:

Based on promising results from animal studies, further clinical trials on Loteprednol Etabonate (41) are also going on for a safer treatment of gastrointestinal inflammation and other diseases such as asthma, rhinitis, and dermatological problems [76,82,84-86]. Success story of this retrometabolically designed glucocorticoid soft drug Loteprednol Etabonate has drawn attention to pharmaceutical industries as well as people working in steroid field worldwide. The authors of this chapter [87], recently, have reported a facile synthesis of the side chain of this potent ocular glucocorticoid soft drug, starting directly from 20-oxopregnanes, *viz.*, 3β-acetoxy-pregn-5(6),16(17)-diene-20-one (16- dehydropregnenolone acetate i.e. 16-DPA) (44)- a potent steroid drug intermediate, utilizing their recently developed metal mediated halogenation technique as a key reaction [88,89] to furnish the final product –an analog (45) of Loteprednol Etabonate (41) with the requisite side chain [**Scheme 1**].

The present methodology paves a useful and productive way to construct the side chain of this important glucocorticoid soft drug directly from 20-oxopregnanes *via* its C-21 functionalization in much simpler and easier way with their newly developed metal mediated halogenation technique, which avoids application of harsh and tedious reaction conditions associated with this conversion [90, 91].

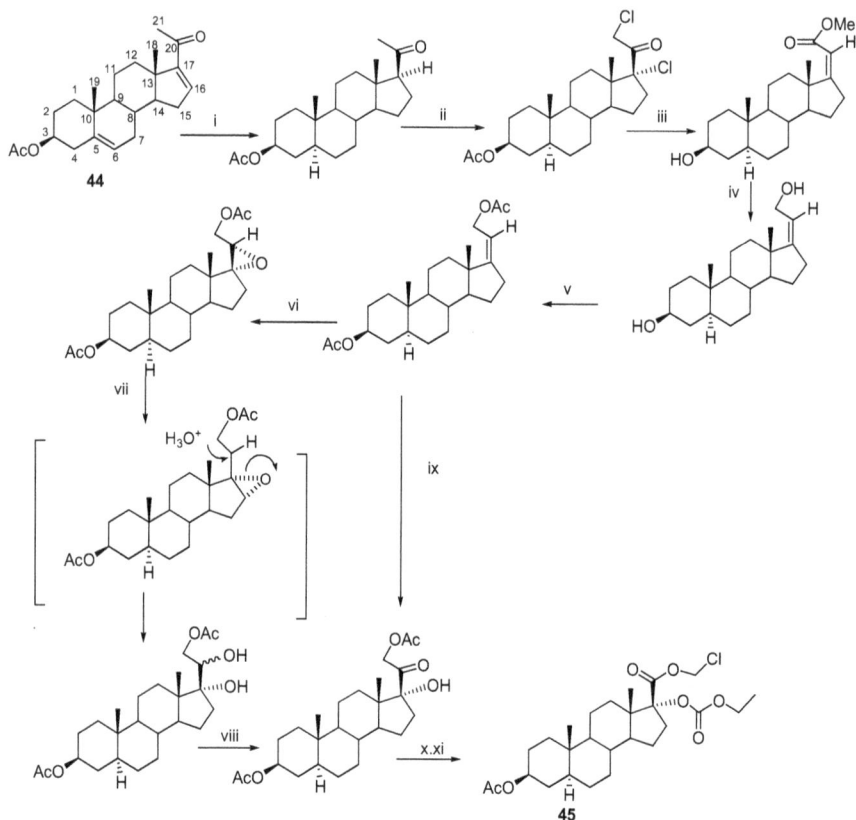

Scheme 1. Reagents and conditions: (i) H_2,Pd-C, 95% (ii) MnO_2-TMSCl/AcCl-AcOH, 81% (iii) 3% KOH, MeOH-H_2O, 75% (iv) LiAlH$_4$,THF, 88% (v) CAN, AcOH, 75% (vi) m-CPBA, CHCl$_3$, 62% (vii) H_2SO_4,acetone-H_2O, 48% (viii) Jones reagent, 57% (ix) OsO_4 – H_2O_2, rt., 50% (x) NaIO$_4$, Ethyl chloroformate, 70% xi) Chloromethyl iodide, 75% .

Second –generation Cortienic Acid (39)-based Glucocorticoid soft drugs: Etiprednol dicloacetate (46) and its Analogs (47):

Synthesis of Drug molecules and Structure-Activity Studies:

Based on their retrometabolic drug design approach, Nicholas Bodor [94] have more recently introduced another new class of soft glucocorticoids with 17α-dicloroester substituent. These are now known as the second generation soft glucocorticoids (**Figure 9**). This is said to be a unique design as no known glucocorticoid has been found to contain a halogen substituent at the 17α position. Nevertheless, the pharmacophore portions of these second- generation cortienic acid-based soft glucocorticoids, having the halogen atoms at 17α position, can be positioned so as to provide excellent overlap with those of the traditional glucocorticoids [24, 95]. It has been conceived the idea that dichlorinated substituents seem required for activity and sufficiently soft nature. Molecular configuration suggests that with dicholrinated substituents, one of the chlorine atom would necessarily point in the direction needed for pharmacophore overlap, whereas with monochlorinated substituents, steric hindrance might force the lone chlorine atom to point away from this desired direction. Secondly experimentally it has been found that as compared with the unsubstituted ester, dichloro substituents could cause ~20 fold increase in the second-order rate constant k_{cat}/K_M of enzymatic hydrolysis in acetate esters, on the other hand monochloro

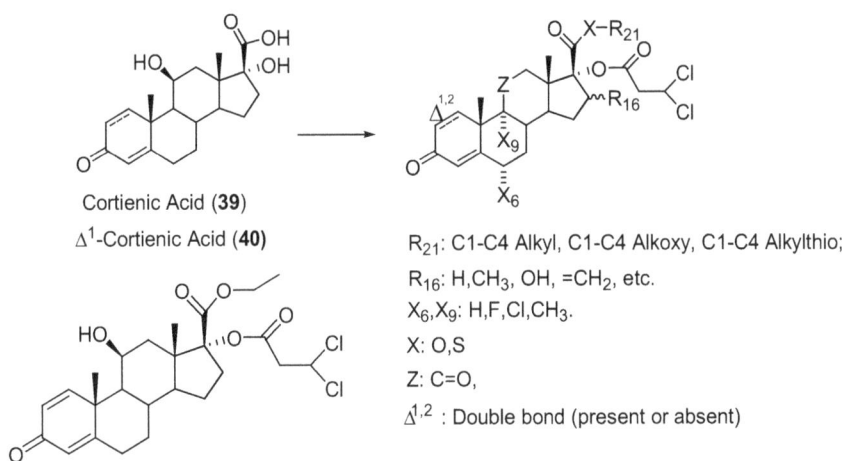

Cortienic Acid (**39**)
Δ^1-Cortienic Acid (**40**)

R_{21}: C1-C4 Alkyl, C1-C4 Alkoxy, C1-C4 Alkylthio;
R_{16}: H,CH$_3$, OH, =CH$_2$, etc.
X_6,X_9: H,F,Cl,CH$_3$.
X: O,S
Z: C=O,
$\Delta^{1,2}$: Double bond (present or absent)

Etiprednol Dicloacetate(**46**)   **2nd Generation Soft Glucorticoid Analogs** (**47**)

Figure 9. Design of 2nd Generation Cortienic Acid-based Soft Glucocorticoids Soft Drugs (**47**) and their Glucocorticoid Soft Drug representative Etiprednol Dicloacetate (ED)(**46**)

substituent did not cause any change [96]. Unlike first generation soft glucocorticoids, in the second generation of this soft steroid series, hydrolysis primarily cleaves the 17α- ester group and not the 17β-ester group. The corresponding metabolites are also not active. From large no of compounds synthesized in this series, Etiprednol Dicloacetate (ED) (**46**) had been selected for development as a potent ocular glucocorticoid soft drug [24].

Etiprednol Dicloacetate (46) and its Clinical Investigations in Ophthalmic Therapeutics:

In animal and in human clinical trials, in accordance with its soft nature, Etiprednol Dicloacetate (**46**) was found to have low systemic toxicity [94, 97-99]. Etiprednol Dicloacetate had also shown better receptor binding capacity than Loteprednol Etabonate and was found to be more effective than Budesonide (**3**) in various asthma models [24]. Further No Observable Adverse Effect Level (NOAEL) of ED after oral administration for 28 days was found to be 2mg/kg in rats and dogs, and about 40 times higher than that of Budesonide [97].

The comparison of the transrepressing and transactivating activity of Etiprednol Dicolacetate (46) and Budesonide(3) were done by measuring their inhibition in interleukin(IL)-1β production of a simulated human monocyte cell line and by evaluating glucocorticoid-induced increase in the activity of tyrosine-amino-transferase (TAT) of a rat hepatoma cell line respectively [99] and the measured activities were expressed relative to Dexamethasone (2) From the results it was found that ED (46) possesses less transactivating activity with a preserved transrepressing acivity, and hence ED is to be called as a dissociated glucocorticoid. Dissociation of transactivating (carbohydrate metabolism altering) and transrepressing (anti-inflammatory) activity found in Etiprednol Dicloacetate(ED) is a fruitful advantage in subsequent help in separating the most beneficial anti-inflammatory activity from the undesired side effects or adverse drug reactions (ADRs).A comparison of transrepression (anti-inflammatory effect) and transactivation (carbohydrate metabolism altering) effects of dexamethasone (2), used as 100% reference, Budesonide (3) and Etiprenol Dicloacette (46) determined on an average of two experiments for concentrations of 10 $^{-7}$ (98) is depicted in **Figure 10** [24]. Hence this productive effort in developing dissociated glucocorticoids can be termed as one of the novel and sought after mechanistic approaches towards the development of newer glucocorticoid soft drugs [24, 100,101].

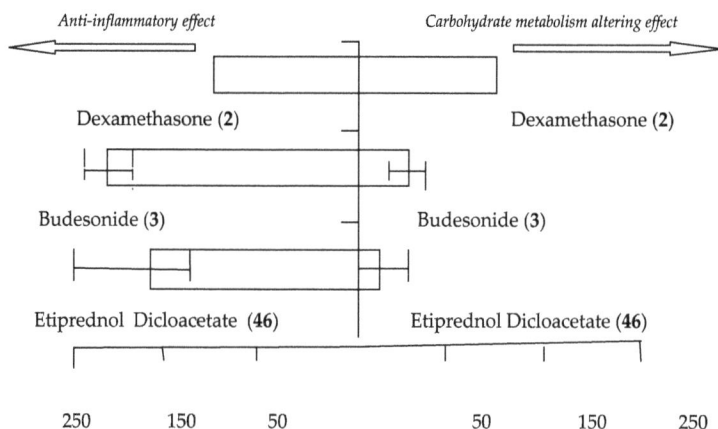

Figure 10. Literature reported [24] tentative comparison of transrepression (anti-inflammatory effect) and transactivation (carbohydrate metabolism altering) effects of dexamethasone (2)(used as 100% reference), Budesonide (3) and Etiprednol Dicloacetate (46)

3. Conclusion

Since the introduction of glucocorticoids in drug industry more than a half century ago, new series of glucocorticoids have been introduced for site specificity as well as for minimizing systemic side effects. At the initial stage, several new generation glucocorticoids were developed using prodrug design approach involving changes or modifications made in glucocorticoid molecules introducing specific substituents at various specific positions of the basic glucocorticoid skeletons to obtain better skin penetration, slower enzyme degradation and greater affinity for the cytosol receptor. The term prodrug refers to a pharmacologically inactive molecule that is converted to an active drug by metabolic biotransformations that may occur prior, during or after adsorption or at specific target sites within the body. This approach has given several potent new generation glucocorticoids such as Budesonide (**3**), 17-Prednicarbate (**9**), Fluticasone propionate (**11**), Methyl prednisolone aceponate (**5**), Beclomethasone (**7**) etc towards successful treatment of plethora of diseases including psoriasis, allergies, asthma, rheumatoid arthritis and lupus, with significantly minimized systemic side effects. However, all these old and new generation glucocorticoids are effective in reducing anterior segment inflammation only and not suitable for ophthalmic therapeutics as they are found to be associated with Adverse Drug Reactions (ADRs) including elevation of Intraocular Pressure (IOP) and steroid-induced cataract formation in case of ophthalmic therapeutics as they were not designed for ocular treatment. Successful eye-specific therapeutic agents can only be achieved by suitable drug-design approaches which thoroughly can integrate the specific pharmacological, metabolic, and targeting requirements of ophthalmic drugs. Chemical Delivery Systems (CDSs) and Retrometabolic Soft Drug Design approaches initiated by Prof.Nicholas Bodor and his group at the Center for Drug Discovery, University of Florida, Health Science Center, USA, are found to be quite successful with a major break through for this purpose providing flexible and generally applicable solutions. Their potential is indeed well illustrated by the results obtained with a number of soft β-blockers and glucocorticoid soft drugs designed within this framework towards ophthalmic therapeutics. Soft β-blockers, *viz.*, Betaxoxime (**29a**), Adaprolol (**33**) and Glucocorticoid Soft drugs *viz.*,, Loteprednol Etabonate (**41**) and Etiprednol Dicloacetate (**46**) are some of the soft drugs developed by this retrometabolic drug design approach which have already reached the clinical development phase in various ophthalmic areas and one of them Loteprednol Etabonate (LE) is already being in the market as a promising glucocorticoid soft drug in ophthalmic therapeutics. Not only that, based on clinical results from animal studies, LE now also finds place in safer treatment of gastrointestinal inflammations and other diseases such as asthma, rhinitis and dermatological problems. Moreover dissociation of transactivating and transrepressing activity found in the second generation glucocorticoid soft drug, viz., Etiprednol Dicloacetate (ED) could open up a novel and promising mechanistic pathways towards the development of more and more potent glucocorticoid soft drugs in future.

Author details

Pritish Chowdhury and Juri Moni Borah
Natural Products Chemistry Division CSIR- North East Institute of Science & Technology, Jorhat, India

Acknowledgement

We sincerely thank Prof Nicholas Bodor, Executive Director, Center for Drug Discovery, University of Florida, USA for his helpful suggestions. Department of Biotechnology (DBT), New Delhi, India is thankfully acknowledged for financial support. Thanks are also due to Ms Ashma Begum, PhD scholar, for her help in preparing the manuscript.

4. References

[1] Rhen T, Cidlowski JA (2005) Antiinflammatory Action of Glucocorticoids – New Mechanisms for Old Drugs. n..engl j. Med. 353: 1711-23.

[2] Newton R (2000) Molecular Mechanisms of Glucocorticoid Action: What is Important? thorax. 55: 603-613.

[3] Stahn C, Buttgereit F (2008) Genomic and Nongenomic Effects of Glucocorticoids. nat.clin.pract.rheumatol. 4: 525-533.

[4] Stahn C, Lowenberg M, Hommes DW, Buttgereit F (2007) Molecular Mechanisms of Glucocorticoid Action and Selective Glucocorticoid Receptor Agonists. mol.cell.endocrinol. 275: 71-78.

[5] Cidlowski JA, (2009) Glucocorticoids and their Action in Cells. retina.29: S21-23.

[6] Schake H, Docke WD, Asadullah K (2002) Mechanisms involved in the Side Effects of Glucocorticoids. pharmacol.ther. 96: 23-43.

[7] McGhee CN, Dean S, Danesh-Meyer H (2002) Locally Administered Ocular Corticosteroids: Benefits and Risks. drug safety 25: 33-55.

[8] Quigley H (2002) How Common is Glaucoma World-wide? int.glaucoma rev.[serial online]; Available at:
http://www.glaucoma.com/Meetings/3-3/worldwide.php.Accessed August 16,2005.

[9] Fisher DA (1995) Adverse Effects of Topical Corticosteroid Use. west j med. 162:123-126.

[10] Degreef H (1999) New Corticosteroids. In: Maddin S editor. skin therapy letter vol.4 No.6.

[11] a) Sulzberger M B, Witten V H (1952) The effect of topically applied compound F in selected dermatoses j. invest. dermatol. 19: 101-102. b) Sulzberger M B, Witten V H, Smith C C (1953) Hydrocortisone (Compound F) acetate ointment in dermatological therapy. j.a.m.a., 151: 468- c) Sulzberger M B, Witten V H (1954) Hydrocortisone ointment in dermatological therapy. m. clin. north America, 38: 321-

[12] Diassi PA, Fried J, Palmere RM, Sabo EF (1961) Fluorinated Steroids I Synthesis of 2@-Fluorohydrocortisone j.Am.chem.soc. 83: 4249-4256.

[13] a) Cornell RC, Stoughton RB (1985) Correlation of the vasoconstrictive assay and clinical activity in psoriasis (sôrī`əsĭs), occasionally acute but usually chronic and recurrent inflammation of the skin. The exact cause is unknown, but the disease appears to be an inherited, possibly autoimmune disorder that causes the arch dermatol. 121: 63-67.

b) Stoughton RB (1992) Vasoconstrictor n. Assay--Specific Applications. In: Maibach HI, Surber C,editors. Topical Corticosteroids. New York: Karger. Pp.42-53. 1. causing constriction of blood vessels. 2. a nerve or agent that does th[14] Degreef H, Dooms-Goossens, A (1993) The New Corticosteroids: are they Effective and Safe? dermatol.clin.11: 155-160.

[15] Hadzija BW, Ambrose WW (1996) Comparison of Cosmetic and Physicochemical Properties of Six Topical Corticosteroid Creams. cutis. 57: S13-18.

[16] Stein-Streilein J, Streilein JW (2002) Anterior Chamber Associated Immune Deviation (ACAID): Regulation, Biological Relevance and Implications for Therapy. int. rev. immunol. 21: 123-152.

[17] Lapalus P, Moulin G, Bayer V, Fredj-Reygrobellet D, Elena PP (1986) Effects of a New Anti-allergic Agent : Magnesium Salt of N-Acetyl-Aspartyl-Glutamic Acid on Experimental Allergic Inflammation of the Rabbit Eye. curr. eye res. 5: 517-522.

[18] Ferguson VM, Spalton DJ (1991) Recovery of the Blood-Aqueous Barrier after Cataract Surgery. br. j. ophthalmol. 75: 106-110.

[19] Abelson MB, Schaefer K (1993) Conjunctivitis of Allergic Origin: Immunologic Mechanisms and Current Approaches to Therapy. surv. ophthalmol. 38: S115-132.

[20] Chambless SL, Trocme S (2004) Development in Ocular Surgery. curr. opin.allergy clin. 4: 431-434.

[21] Comstock TL, Paterno MR, Singh A, Erb T, Davis E (2011) Safety and Efficacy of Loteprednol etabonate Ophthalmic Ointment 0.5% for theTreatment of Inflammation and Pain following Cataract Surgery. clin ophthalmol. 5: 177–186.

[22] Pavesio CE, DeCory HH (2008) Treatment of Ocular Inflammatory Conditions with Loteprednol etabonate. br. j. .ophthalmol. 92 :455–459.

[23] Manabe S, Bucala R, Cerami A (1984) Nonenzymatic Addition of Glucocorticoids to Lens Proteins in Steroid-Induced Cataracts. j. clin. invest. 74: 1803-1810.

[24] Bodor N, Buchwald P (2005) Ophthalmic Drug Design Based on the Metabolic Activity of The Eye: Soft Drugs and Chemical Delivery Systems. The AAPS Journal 7: Article 79.

[25] Bodor N, Shek E, Higuchi T (1976) Improved Delivery Through Biological Membranes.1. Synthesis and Properties of 1-Methyl-1,6-Dihydropyridine-2-Carbaldoxime, A Prodrug of N-Methylpyridium-2-Carbalddoxime Chloride. j. med. chem. 19: 102-107..

[26] Bodor N, Buchwald P (2000) Soft Drug Design: General Principle and Recent Applications. med. res. rev. 20: 58-101.

[27] Bodor N, Loftsson T, Wu WM (1992) Metabolism, Distribution and Transdermal Permeation of a Soft Corticosteroid, Loteprednol etabonate pharm.res. 9: 1275-1278.

[28] Hu L (August, 2004) The Prodrug Approach to better Targeting. www.currentdrugdiscovery.com.

[29] Mueller CE (2009) Prodrug Approaches for Enhancing the Bioavailability of Drugs with Low Solubility. 6: 2071-2075.

[30] Verma A, Verma B, Prajapati SK, Tripathy K (2009) Prodrug as a Chemical Delivery System: A Review. 2: 100-102.

[31] Coopman S, Degreef H, Dooms-Goossens A (1989) Identifications of Cross Reaction Patterns in Allergic Contact Dermatitis from Topical Corticosteroids. br. j. dermatol.121: 27-34.

[32] Larochelle P, Du Souich P, Bolte E, Lelorier J, Goyer R (1983). Tixocortol pivalate, a corticosteroid with no systemic glucocorticoid effect after oral, intrarectal, and intranasal application. *clin. pharmaco. therap.* 33: 343–350

[33] Goossens A, Matura M (1999) Corticosteroids in Occupational Skin Diseases, 3rd Edition by Adams R. WB Saunders Co. Philadelphia, USA.

[34] Stewart PA, Tuor UI (1994) Blood-Eye Barriers in the Rat: Correlation of Ultrastructure with Function. j. comp. neurol. 340: 566-576.

[35] Schoenwald RD (1990) Ocular Drug Delivery: Pharmacokinetic Considerations. clin pharmacokinet . 18 : 255 - 269.

[36]. Mitra AK, Mikkelson TJ (1988) Mechanism of Transcorneal Permeation of Pilocarpine. j. pharm sci . 7: 771 - 775.

[37] Davies NM (2000) Biopharmaceutical Considerations in Topical Ocular Drug Delivery. clin exp pharmacol physiol . 27 : 558 - 562 .

[38] Schoenwald RD (1990) Ocular Drug Delivery: Pharmacokinetic Considerations. clin pharmacokinet . 18: 255 - 269.

[39] Grass GM, Robinson JR (1988) Mechanism of Corneal Penetration. *In vivo* and *in vitro* kinetics. j. pharm sci . 7: 3 - 14.

[40] Prausnitz MR, Noonan JS (1998) Permeability of Cornea, Sclera, and Conjunctiva: A Literature Analysis for Drug delivery to the eye. j pharm sci . 87: 1479 - 1488.

[41] Edwards A, Prausnitz MR (2001) Predicted Permeability of the Cornea to Topical Drugs. pharm res . 18: 1497 - 1508 .

[42] Lee VH, Robinson JR (1986) Topical Ocular Drug Delivery: Recent Developments and Future Challenges. j ocul pharmacol . 2 : 67 - 108 .

[43] Sasaki H, Yamamura K, Mukai T (1999) Enhancement of Ocular Drug Penetration. crit rev ther drug carrier syst 16 : 85 -- 146 .

[44] Bundgaard H (1985) ed. Design of Prodrugs . Amsterdam,The Netherlands : Elsevier Science .

[45] Bodor N, Kaminski JJ (1987) Prodrugs and Site-Specifi c Chemical Delivery Systems. *annu rep med chem* . 22 : 303 - 313 .

[46] Wermuth CG, Gaignault J-C, Marchandeau C (1996) Designing Prodrugs and Bioprecursors I: Carrier Prodrugs. In: Wermuth CG, ed. The Practice of Medicinal Chemistry. London, UK: Academic Press. pp 671- 696.

[47] Ettmayer P, Amidon GL , Clement B Testa B (2004) Lessons learned from Marketed and Investigational Prodrugs. j med chem . 47: 2393 – 2404.

[48] Bodor N (1994) Drug Targeting and Retrometabolic Drug Design Approaches. *adv drug deliv rev* 14 : 157 - 166 .

[49] Bodor N, Buchwald P (1997) Drug targeting *via* Retrometabolic Approaches. Pharmacol ther . 76 : 1 - 27 .

[50] Bodor N, Buchwald P (2003) Retrometabolism-Based Drug Design and Targeting. In: Abraham DJ, ed. Drug Discovery and Drug Development. Burger's Medicinal Chemistry and Drug Discovery. Vol 2. 6th ed.New York, John Wiley and Sons. pp 533-608.

[51] Bodor N (1996) Designing Safer Ophthalmic Drugs: In: Trends in Medicinal Chemistry: Proceedings of the Xth International Symposium on Medicinal Chemistry. Amsterdam, The Netherlands. Elsevier : pp 145- 164.

[52] Albert A (1985) Selective Toxicity: The Physico-Chemical Basis of Therapy. London, UK, Chapman and Hall.

[53] El-Koussi A, Bodor N (1989) Formation of Propanolol in the Iris-Ciliary Body from its Propranolol Ketoxime Precursor - A Potential Antiglaucoma Drug. *int j pharm* . 53 : 189 - 194 .

[54] Bodor N, Prokai L (1990) Site- and Stereospecific Ocular Drug Delivery by Sequential Enzymatic Bioactivation p*harm res* . 7 : 723 - 725 .

[55] Bodor N, El-Koussi A Improved Delivery through Biological Membranes. LVI. Pharmacological Evaluation of Alprenoxime - A New Potential Antiglaucoma Agent. *pharm res* . 8 : 1389 - 1395 .

[56] Simay A, Prokai L, Bodor N (1989) Oxidation of Aryloxy-β-Amino Alcohols with Activated Dimethylsulfoxide: A Novel C-N Oxidation facilitated by Neighboring Group Effect. Tetrahedron 45 : 4091 - 4102 .

[57] Simay A, Bodor N (1992) Site- and Stereospecific Drug Delivery to the Eye. In: Sarel S, Mechoulam R, Agranat I, eds. Trends in Medicinal Chemistry '90 .Oxford, UK : Blackwell Scientific Publications. pp 361- 368 .

[58] Bodor N (1995) Retrometabolic Drug Design Concepts in Ophthalmic Targetspecific Dug Delivery. adv drug deliv rev 16 : 21 - 38 .

[59] Polgar P, Bodor N (1995) Minimal Cardiac Electrophysiological Activity of Alprenoxime, A Site-Activated Ocular β -Blocker, in Dogs. life sci .56 : 1207 - 1213 .

[60] Prokai L, Wu W-M, Somogyi G, Bodor N (19950 Ocular Delivery of the β -Adrenergic Antagonist Aprenolol by Sequential Bioactivation of its Methoxime Analog. j. med. chem . 38: 2018 - 2020 .

[61] Bodor N, Farag HH, Somogyi G, Wu W-M, Barros MDC, Prokai L (1997) Ocular-Specific Delivery of Timolol by Sequential Bioactivation of its Oxime and Methoxime Analogs. *J ocul pharmacol* . 13: 389 - 403.

[62] Farag HH, Wu W-M, Barros MDC, Somogyi G, Prokai L, Bodor N (1997) Ocular-Specific Chemical Delivery System of Betaxolol for Safe Local Treatment of Glaucoma. *drug des discov* .15: 117 – 130.

[63] Nathanson JA (1988) Stereospecificity of Beta Adrenergic Antagonists: R-Enantiomers show Increased Selectivity for beta-2 receptors in ciliary process. *j pharmacol exp ther* .245 : 94 - 101 .

[64] Mehvar R, Brocks DR (2001) Stereospecifi c Pharmacokinetics and Pharmacodynamics of β-Adrenergic Blockers in Humans. *j pharm pharm sci* . 4: 185 - 200.

[65] Sharif NA, Xu SX, Crider JY, McLaughlin M, Davis TL (2001) Levobetaxolol (Betaxon) and Other β -adrenergic Antagonists: Preclinical Pharmacology, IOP-Lowering Activity and Sites of Action in Human Eyes. *j ocul pharmacol ther* .17: 305 – 317.

[66] Bodor N, Oshiro Y, Loftsson T, Katovich M, Caldwell W (1984) Soft Drugs. 6. The Application of the Inactive Metabolite Approach for Design of Soft β -Blockers. *pharm res.* 1 : 120 - 125 .

[67] Bodor N, El-Koussi A, Kano M, Khalifa MM (1988) Soft Drugs. 7. β -Blockers for Systemic and Ophthalmic Use. *j med chem* . 31 : 1651 - 1656 .

[68] Bodor N, El-Koussi A (1988) Novel 'Soft' β -Blockers as Potential Safe Antiglaucoma Agents. *curr eye res* . 7 : 369 - 374 .

[69] Polgar P, Bodor N (1991) Cardiac Electrophysiologic Effects of Adaprolol maleate, A New β -Blocker, in Closed Chest Dogs. *life sci* . 48: 1519 - 1528.

[70] Bodor N, El-Koussi A, Zuobi K , Kovacs P (1996) Synthesis and Pharmacological Activity of Adaprolol Enantiomers: A New Soft Drug for Treating Glaucoma. *j ocul pharmacol ther* . 12 : 115 - 122 .

[71] Buchman AL (2001) Side Effects of Corticosteroid Therapy. j clin gastroenterol 33: 289-294.

[72] Monder C, Bradlow HL (1980) Cortoic Acids: Explorations at the Frontier of Corticosteroid Metabolism. *Recent Prog Horm Res* . 36: 345 - 400.

[73] Noble S, Goa KL (1998) Loteprednol etabonate: Clinical Potential in the Management of Ocular Infl ammation. *bio drugs* .10 : 329 - 339 .

[74] Howes JF (2000) Loteprednol Etabonate: A Review of Ophthalmic Clinical Studies. *pharmazie* . 55: 178 - 183.

[75] Bartlett JD, Howes JR, Ghormley NR, Amos JF, Laibovitz, R, Horwitz B (1993) Safety and Efficacy of of Loteprednol Etabonate for Treatment of Papillae in Contact Lens Associated Giantpapillary Conjunctivitis. curr. eye. res. 12: 313-321.

[76] Bodor N, Buchwald P (2002) Design and Development of a Soft Corticosteroid, Loteprednol Etabonate. In: Schleimer RP, O'Byrne PM, Szefl er SJ, Brattsand R, eds. Inhaled Steroids in Asthma. Optimizing Effects in the Airways. New York, NY: Marcel Dekker. pp 541- 564.

[77] Druzgala P, Hochhaus G, Bodor N (1991) Soft Drugs – 10. Blanching Activity and Receptor Binding Affinity of aNew Type of Glucocorticoid: Loteprednol etabonate. j steroid biochem mol biol 2: 115-125.

[78] Druzgala P, Wu WM, Bodor N (1991) Ocular Absorption and Distribution of Loteprednol Etabonate, A Soft Steroid in Rabbit Eyes. curr. eye. res. 10: 933-937.

[79] Bodor N, Wu W-M (1992) A Comparison of Intraocular Pressure Elevating Activity of Loteprednol Etabonate and Dexamethasone in Rabbits. *curr eye res* .11 : 525 - 530 .

[80] Novack GD, Howes J, Crockett RS (1998) Sherwood MB . Change in Intraocular Pressure During Long-Term Use of Loteprednol Etabonate. *j glaucoma* . 7: 266 – 269.

[81] Hochhaus G, Chen LS, Ratka A, Druzgala P, Howes J, Bodor N, Derendorf H (1992) Pharmacokinetic Characterization and Tissue Distribution of the New Glucocorticoid Soft Drug Loteprednol Etabonate in Rats and Dogs. j pharm sci. 81: 1210-1215.

[82] Bodor N, Wu W-M, Murakami T , Engel S (1995) Soft drugs. 19. Pharmacokinetics, Metabolism and Excretion of a Novel Soft Corticosteroid, Loteprednol Etabonate, in Rats. pharm res 12 : 875 - 879 .

[83] Comstock TL, Usner DW (2010) Effect of Loteprednol Etabonate Ophthalmic Suspension 0.5% on Postoperative Pain and Discomfort : Presented at the American Society of Cataract and Surgery Meeting.

[84] Bodor N, Murakami T, Wu W-M(1995) Soft Drugs. 18. Oral and Rectal Delivery of Loteprednol Etabonate, A Novel Soft Corticosteroid, in Rats -for Safer Treatment of Gastrointestinal Infl ammation. pharm res 12 : 869 - 874 .

[85] Szelenyi I, Hermann R, Petzold U, Pahl A, Hochhaus G (2004) Possibilities in Improvement of Glucocorticoid Treatments in Asthma with Special Reference to Loteprednol Etabonate. pharmazie . 59: 409 - 411 .

[86] Szelenyi I, Hochhaus G, Heer S (2000) Loteprednol Etabonate: A Soft Steroid for the Treatment of Allergic Diseases of the Airways. drugs today (Barc) . 36 : 313 - 320 .

[87] Chowdhury P, Borah J.M, Goswami P, Das A.M (2011) steroids, 76: 497–501.

[88] Borah P, Ahmed M, Chowdhury P (1 998) j chem res (M) 1173–1180.

[89] Borah P, Ahmed M, Chowdhury P (1998) j chem res (S) 236–237.

[90] Djerassi C (1963) In: Steroid Reactions (An outline for Organic Chemistry). San Francisco: Holden-Day, USA.

[91] Wuts PGM, Cabaj JE, Meisto KD (1993) synth commun 23: 2199–2211.

[92]Stewart R, Horwitz B, Howes J, Novack GD, Hart K (1998) Double-Masked, Placebo-controlled Evaluation of Loteprednol Etabonate 0.5% for postoperative Inflammation. Loteprednol Etabonate Post-Operative Inflammation Study Group 1. j. cataract. refract. surg. 24: 1480 — 1489.

[93] Ilyas H, Slonim CB, Braswell GR, Favetta JR, Schulman M (2004) Long-term Safety of Loteprednol Etabonate 0.2% in the treatment of Seasonal and Perennial Allergic Conjunctivitis. eye contact lens 30: 10-13.

[94] Bodor N (1999) Inventor. Androstene Derivatives. US patent 5 981 517.

[95] Buchwald P, Bodor N (2004) Soft Glucocorticoid Design: Structural Elements and Physicochemical Parameters Determining Receptor-Binding Affi nity. p harmazie . 59: 396 - 404.

[96] Barton P, Laws AP, Page MI (1994) Structure-Activity Relationships in the esterase-Catalysed Hydrolysis and Transesterifi cation of esters and lactones. j chem. soc, perkin trans 2 . pp 2021 - 2029.

[97] Miklós A , Magyar Z, Kiss É (2002) 28-Day Oral Toxicity Study with Soft Corticosteroid BNP- 166 in Rats and Dogs, followed by a 14-Day Recovery Period. pharmazie 57 : 142 - 146 .

[98] Kurucz I, Tóth S, Németh K (2003) Potency and Specificity of the Pharmacological Action of a New, Antiasthmatic, Topically Administered Soft steroid, Etiprednol Dicloacetate (BNP-166). *j pharmacol exp ther* .307 : 83 – 92.

[99] Kurucz I, Németh K , Mészáros S *et al* (2004) Anti-infl ammatory Effect and Soft Properties of Etiprednol Dicloacetate (BNP-166) A New, Antiasthmatic Steroid. *pharmazie* . 59 : 412 – 416.

[100] Jaffuel D, Demoly P, Gougat C (2000) Transcriptional Potencies of Inhaled Glucocorticoids. *am j respir crit care med* . 162: 57 – 63.

[101] Bhalay G, Sandham DA (2002) Recent Advances in Corticosteroids for the Treatment of Asthma. *curr opin investig drugs* . 3: 1149 - 1156.

Chapter 13

Corticosteroids for Skin Delivery: Challenges and New Formulation Opportunities

Taner Senyigit and Ozgen Ozer

Additional information is available at the end of the chapter

1. Introduction

Currently, corticosteroids are the most widely used class of anti-inflammatory drugs. The introduction of topical hydrocortisone in the early 1950s provided great advantages over previously available therapies and initiated a new era for dermatological therapy. Their clinical effectiveness in the treatment of dermatological disorders is related to their vasoconstrictive, anti-inflammatory, immunosuppressive and anti-proliferative effects. Despite their benefit in the therapy of inflammatory diseases, topical corticosteroids (TC) are associated number of side effects that limit their use. Most TC are absorbed in quantities that can produce both systemic and topical side effects [1-2]. Table 1 shows the currently used TC in various dermatological disorders according to the British classification system [3]. In general, mild and moderate TC are used for long-term treatments while the potent and very potent products especially preferred for shorter regimes.

Over the years, research has focused on strategies to optimize the potency of steroids while minimizing adverse effects due to drug absorption across the skin. In other words, research focus no longer been on the synthesis of more potent derivatives but on safer one. Several attempts have been made to increase the safety of TC treatment, including new application schedules, special vehicles and new synthesized agents [4]. However, "ideal" TC have not yet been synthesized. They should be able to permeate the stratum corneum (SC) and reach adequate concentrations in the epidermis without reaching high systemic concentrations.

One of the approaches to reduce the adverse effects of TC is to enhance their permeability so as to reduce the topically applied dose [5]. Several approaches have been attempted, such as iontophoresis, electroporation or the application of eutectic mixtures [6,7]. However, the use of chemical penetration enhancers is the most widely used approach to increase skin delivery [8].

POTENCY	DOSE % (w/w)	TC
Mild		Hydrocortisone
	1	Hydrocortisone acetate
	0.25	Methylprednisolone
	0.05	Alclometasone dipropionate
	0.01-0.1	Dexamethasone
	0.0025	Fluocinolone acetonide
	0.75	Fluocortyn butyl ester
	0.5	Prednisolone
Moderate	0.05	Clobetasone butyrate
	0.02	Triamcinolone acetonide
	0.005	Fluocinolone acetonide
Potent	0.05	Betamethasone dipropionate
	0.1	Betamethasone valerate
	0.025	Fluocinolone acetonide
	0.1	Hydrocortisone butyrate
	0.05	Halometasone monohydrate
	0.1	Diflucortolone valerate
Very potent	0.1	Halcinonide
	0.05	Clobetasol propionate

Table 1. The currently used TC in various dermatological disorders [3]

TC are formulated in a variety of conventional vehicles, including ointments, creams, lotions and gels. In addition to conventional formulations several innovative systems such as nanoparticles, liposomes, microemulsions, foams and patches have been evaluated for different dermatological conditions. Colloidal drug carrier systems, such as liposomes and nanoparticles, could target TC to the viable epidermis, where the inflammatory reactions take place. In particular, liposomal preparations showed a strong affinity for the SC. Patents filed on topical nanoparticulate formulations also claimed the importance of colloidal drug carrier systems for this type of applications [9-12].

This chapter will review major innovations and advances in TC formulations based on the published articles and patent applications. The main factors influencing the effectiveness and bioavailability of TC will be also briefly discussed before emphasizing formulation alternatives.

2. Skin structure

The skin, in Latin called cutis, is considered the largest organ of the body, accounting more than 10% of the body mass and having an average surface of approximately 2 m^2. The thickness of the skin is highly variable (average thickness of 1.5 mm), depending of several factors as the anatomic location, age and sex. The functions of the skin have been classified as protective, homeostatic, or sensorial. To maintain its characteristics, this organ is in a continual renewing process [13].

Anatomically, the skin consists on 3 basic layers: epidermis, dermis and subcutaneous tissues. Depending on the region considered, the epidermis is made of 4-5 sublayers that, from bottom to top, are: stratum basale, stratum spinosum, stratum granulosum, stratum lucidum (present only in palm and soles) and SC or horny layer. In addition to these structures, there are also several associated appendages: hair follicles, sweat glands, apocrine glands, and nails [14].

The most important skin function is permeability barrier function. The outermost layer of the epidermis, the SC, with its peculiar structure, plays an important role in permeability barrier function [15]. Due to its barrier properties, the skin membrane is equally capable at limiting the molecular transport from and into the body. Overcoming this barrier function will be the purpose of skin drug delivery.

3. Clinical limitations and side effects of TC

TC are successfully used in the treatment of several common cutaneous diseases but their major limitation is still their side effect potential. The most common side-effects occur locally in the areas of skin treated with the steroid. Probably the most well known is thinning of the skin (atrophy), which sometimes results in permanent stretch marks (striae). Fine blood vessels may swell and become prominent under the skin surface (telangiectasia), again a permanent change. In addition, there may be a temporary loss of pigment in the areas of skin treated; this may be more noticeable in dark-skinned people. Sometimes the skin may become allergic to the steroid, making the eczema appear to get worse. The skin may also bruise more easily and become more susceptible to infection.

The occurrence and severity of the side effects are depend on the duration of use, dosage, dosing regime and spesific drug used, along with individual patient variability. However, the highest risk factor seems to be prolonged use [16-18]. The concentration of corticosteroid in systemic circulation and risk of sytemic side effects are increased by prolonged therapy with TC. Systemic side-effects of TC, such as pituitary–adrenal axis suppression, should be taken into account when treating children. Children have a higher ratio of total body surface area to body weight (about 2.5- to 3-fold that of adults) and adrenal suppression may cause growth retardation.

The principle systemic side effects associated with TC are bodyweight gain, Cushing's syndrome, electrolyte imbalance, hypertension, diabetes mellitus, pseudoprimary aldosteronisim, growth retardation, osteoporosis peptic ulser and gastritis. In addition, TC are mostly capable of causing local side effects. One particularly important local side effect is epidermal thinning or atrophy [19]. This effect is characterized with the reduction in cell size and number of cell layers in epidermis. Other local side effects related to TC treatment are steroid acne, rosacea, perioral dermatitis, corticoid acne, allergic contact dermatitis, hypopigmentation, glaucoma, cataracts, worsening of cutaneous infections and hypertrichosis [2]. Table 2 represents the possible local and systemic side effects of TC which are organized in subsections for tissue-organ level.

TISSUE - ORGAN	SIDE EFFECTS
Cardiovascular system	Hypertension
Endocrin system	Adrenal insufficiency, Cushing's syndrome, diabetes mellitus, bodyweight gain, pseudoprimary aldosteronism
Eye	Glaucoma, cataract
Immune system	Increased risk of infection, re-activation of latent viruses
Gastrointestinal	Peptic ulser, gastritis
Central nervous system	Behavioural changes, loss of memory/cognition
Skeleton and muscle	Growth retardation, osteoporosis
Skin	Atrophy, striae, allergic contact dermatitis, delayed wound healing, steroid acne, perioral dermatitis, rosacea, erythema, teleangiectasia, hypertrichosis, hypopigmentation

Table 2. The possible local and systemic side effects of TC

4. Classification of TC

TC are classified in two different ways by American and British National Formulary classification systems [20-21]. The American classification system includes seven potency groups while the British National Formulary contains four groups. In the former system, the potency of a product is defined by the corticosteroid, its concentration and the nature of the vehicle. On the other hand, The British classification system is irrespective of the topical vehicle used. According to the American classification sytem, it is important to note that the greater in potency for TC result in the greater therapeutic efficacy and side effects. Therefore, low-potency formulations should be used for long term treatments by physicians while the more potent products should be chosen for short periods and sites such as palms and soles, where low potency TC are ineffective [1,2].

5. Formulations of TC

It is well known that, besides the active molecule, the potency of each topical formulation can be influenced by vehicle characteristics. Vehicles should allow adequate release of the active compound, spread easily and be aesthetically pleasant [21]. Some important rules should be considered when choosing a vehicle; the solubility, release rate and stability of the therapeutic agent in the vehicle, the ability of the vehicle to hydrate the SC, the physical and chemical interactions of the vehicle with the skin and active molecule and also the phase, localization and extent of disease [22].

TC are formulated in a variety of conventional vehicles, including ointments, creams, lotions and gels. As mentioned previously, the character of the vehicle system defines the potency of topical preparations and its selection is crucial for product performance.

Ointments are semi-solid preparations intended for application to skin or mucous membranes. There are four types of ointment bases; hydrocarbon bases, absorption bases, emulsion bases and water-soluble bases. The potential of the absorption is affected by choice of the bases. Hence, appropriate selection of the base is important for the efficacy of the dermal therapy [23].

Ointment formulations are generally more effective than creams containing the same drug and they are especially preferred for infiltrated, lichenified lesions. In a comparative study, the absorption of clobetasol propionate from ointment and cream formulations was evaluated and it was reported that a greater amount of clobetasol propionate was absorbed from the ointment [24]. Ointments including well-known and new synthesized TC were formulated and they were still first-option for treatment of dermatological diseases. However, the greasy nature and hardness of the removal from the skin due to their lack of water-washability is their disadvantages.

Mobile dispersions intended for topical application are generally described as lotions and semi-solid systems as creams. Although, creams are usually emulsions of the oil-in-water type (aqueous creams) or water-in-oil type (oily creams), lotions are mostly oil-in-water emulsions [25]. Regarding to the phase of disease, lotions and creams are generally recommended in acute and subacute dermatoses. Good compliance is obtained by prescribing creams and lotions which are easily applied by patients rather than ointments in case of large extensional dermatoses. Sequeira et al. [26] filed a patent application which provided a corticosteroid lotion formulation exhibiting high vasoconstrictor and excellent anti-inflammatory activities in steroid responsive dermatoses. The addition of propylene glycol to a hydro-alcoholic lotion base exhibited and significantly higher vasoconstrictor activity than the corresponding lotion without propylene glycol.

Gels are semi-solid systems with dispersions of small or large molecules in an aqueose vehicle with a gelling agent. The gel formulations are suitable for topical delivery of drugs for treatment of diseases due to lack of irritating components. Pharmaceutical gel formulations for topical drug delivery include drug and gelling agent [27]. Gels based on carbopol, cellulose derivatives and chitosan are commonly used in the pharmaceutical and cosmetic industries [28, 29].

Recently, new hydrogel formulation intended for cosmetic use was introduced as a novel formulation of steroids for the treatment of atopic dermatitis. The formulation was prepared with carbopol-based polymer that contained 0.05% (w/w) of micronized desonide which is a well-known synthetic corticosteroid. This formulation was easily applied for atopic dermatitis patients aged 3 months. A wide variety of studies have been performed to validate the safety and efficacy of this product and these studies supported very favourable safety, tolerability and efficacy profile [30, 31].

Senyigit et al. [32] investigated the effect of vehicles (chitosan and sodium-deoxycholate gel) on the skin accumulation and permeation of two topical corticosteroids: clobetasol propionate and mometasone furoate. Commercial cream formulations containing the same amount of drug were also used for comparison. It was reported that sodium-deoxycholate gel formulation dramatically improved the amount of drug in the skin although chitosan gel produced the same skin accumulation as commercial creams for both active agents. In addition, all of these gel formulations did not induce the permeation.

For conventional formulations it can be stated that the effectiveness of the active agent is directly related to the composition of the formulation. In general, the potency of the corticosteroids in the formulations could be listed in order such as; ointments> gels> creams> lotions. This generalization was supported with a patent filed by McCadden [33]. The brief summary about conventional TC formulations including pharmaceutical characteristics, clinical usage, benefits and disadvantages were given in Table 3.

Formulation type	Pharmaceutical characteristics	Clinical usage	Benefits	Disadvantages
Ointment	Semi-solid preparations containing different types of ointment bases	Infiltrated, lichenified lesions	Occlusive property on the skin for inducing skin hydration at the skin-ointment interface	Greasy nature and hardness of the removal from the skin due to their lack of water-washability
Cream	Oil-in-water (aqueous creams) or water-in-oil (oily creams) type of emulsion	Acute and subacute dermatoses	Easy application and good patient compliance	Difficulty of spreadability and soiling linen and clothing during treatment for oily creams
Lotion	Generally oil-in-water emulsions	Acute and subacute dermatoses	Easy application and good patient compliance	Not suitable for use on dry skin
Gel	Dispersions formulated with a gelling agent	Suitable for all types of skin diseases	Easy application, easy to attach to the skin, good patient compliance and lack of irritating components	-

Table 3. The summary about conventional TC formulations

The activity of a TC formulation can be enhanced by adding a chemical penetration enhancer which may result in an increase of drug delivery into skin. Chemical penetration enhancers have been reviewed by several researchers and the authors underline the difficulty to select rationally a penetration enhancer for a specific permeant [34-36]. Recent studies showed that terpenes appear to be promising penetration enhancers for pharmaceutical formulations with favourable properties such as low cutaneous irritancy and possess good toxicological profile [32, 37].

Recently, it has been a great interest in developing new drug carriers for TC that may contribute to reduction of side effects. Therefore, in addition to previously mentioned conventional formulations several innovative systems such as nanoparticles, liposomes, microemulsions, foams and patches have been developed for TC.

Liposomes, microemulsions, solid lipid and polymeric nanoparticles have been proposed to increase percutaneous absorption of therapeutic agents while mitigating the damage to the skin barrier function [38,39]. Besides, the drug targeting to the skin or even to its substructures could be realized by micro- and nanoparticulate systems [40,41]. These drug carrier systems could target glucocorticoids to the viable epidermis, where the inflammatory reactions take place [9]. In particular, liposomal preparations showed strong affinity for the SC [42].

The loading of therapeutic agents into nanoparticles and administration to the skin using a simple vehicle offer many advantages over other traditional topical formulations, including enhanced formulation aesthetics, protection of unstable active agents against degradation, targeting of active agents to the skin layers and prolonged active agent release [43]. As a consequence of their proposed advantages in dermal/transdermal formulations two most common types of particles have been produced: Lipid nanoparticles and polymeric nanoparticles. The uses of lipid and polymeric nanoparticles for pharmaceutical formulations applied to skin have been reviewed by several authors [40, 44-46]. Most of the data reported on TC was obtained using lipid nanoparticles of differing lipid compositions.

The inclusion of prednicarbate into solid lipid nanoparticles (SLN) of various composition appeared to increase the penetration of the drug into human skin by 30% as compared to cream, permeation of reconstructed epidermis increased even 3-fold [47]. In a subsequent report SLN were shown to induce prednicarbate targeting in the epidermal layer in excised human skin and reconstructed epidermis [9]. Epidermal targeting was evidenced also for prednisolone, the diester prednicarbate and the monoester betamethasone 17-valerate included in solid lipid nanoparticles [48]. The authors hypothesized specific interactions of the drug-carrier complex and the skin surface, possible by the lipid nature and nanosize of the carrier. On the other hand, using the appropriate lipid combination, the skin retention of betamethasone 17 valerate was increased when SLN was used as a vehicle compared to a conventional formulations [49], both using intact skin as well as barrier impaired [50].

Clobetasol propionate was included in SLN as well [51]. SLN containing cream registered significant improvement in therapeutic response (1.9 fold inflammation, 1.2 fold itching) in terms of percent reduction in degree of inflammation and itching against marketed cream.

de Vringer disclosed a stable aqueous suspension of SLNs, comprising at least one lipid and preferably also at least one emulsifier for topical application to the body. According to this invention steroidal anti-inflammatory compound such as hydrocortisone, hydrocortisone-17α-butyrate, budesonide or TA, anti-proliferatives, anti-psoriatics, anti-eczema agents and dithranol could be succesfully incorporated into the suspension of SLNs. It was stated that a combination of two or more topically effective medicaments could also be used [52]. Senyigit et al. [53] prepared lecithin/chitosan nanoparticles containing clobetasol propionate and found a preferential retention in the epidermis while no permeation across the skin was observed. In vivo studies including transepidermal water loss measurements, anti-inflammatory effect and histological evaluation of the formulations on wistar albino rats were also performed and the results were promising (Data not published).

Liposomes are lipid vesicles prepared with phospholipids which have been shown to facilitate transport of drugs into and across skin [54]. Recently, many reports have been published on percutaneous enhancing property of liposomes for both hydrophilic and lipophilic compounds [55]. Liposomes do not only enhance the drug penetration into the skin by showing slow release, but also decrease the clearence of drug by minimizing its absorption into the systemic circulation [56]. Hence, the liposomes can improve the therapeutic effectiveness of TC while reducing systemic side effects. However, many stability problems are reported for liposomes.

Mezei et al. [57, 58] applied triamcinolone acetonide (TA) in liposomes and compared it with TA in Dermabase®. In this study, four- to five fold higher TA concentrations in the epidermis and dermis, with lower systemic drug levels were observed when the drug was delivered from liposomal lotion in comparison with conventional formulations of the same drug concentration.

Lasch and Wohlrab [59, 60] studied the skin distribution of cortisol and hydrocortison after application in a cream and liposomes. As a result, improved concentration-time profile was observed in skin layers by liposomes for both drugs.

Korting et al. [61] compared the efficacy of betamethasone dipropionate encapsulated in liposomes and cream. The liposomes were prepared with egg lecithine and incorporated in a polyacrylate gel. The in vivo studies were carried out in patients with atopic eczema and psoriasis vulgaris. It was concluded that, betamethasone encapsulated in liposomes improved the antiinflammatory action, but not the antiproliferative effect.

Fresta et al. [62] prepared skin-lipid liposome formulations of different corticosteroids (hydrocortisone, betamethasone valerate and TA). They indicated that skin lipid liposomes showed a 6 and 1.3 fold higher blanching effect than control formulations of ointment and the phospholipid-based liposomes, respectively. Skin-lipid liposomes also produced a reduction in drug levels in the blood and urine. Consequently, this liposome formulation was proposed for improving the pharmacological effectiveness and reducing the systemic absorption of TC.

In order to overcome the stability problem of liposomes, new attempts have been maden and new drug carrier systems have been developed by adding some functional chemicals into the liposome structure. These systems are niosomes, transfersomes and ethosomes.

Niosomes, non-ionic surfactant vesicules, are widely studied as an alternative to liposomes for topical and transdermal drug delivery. Niosomes alleviate the disadvantages associated with liposomes, such as chemical instability, variable purity of phospholipids and high cost. In addition, they have the potential for controlled and targeted drug delivery to the skin [63-65]. Deformable liposomes (Transfersomes®) are the first generation of elastic vesicles introduced by Cevc [66]. They consist of phospholipids and an edge activator. An edge activator is often a single chain surfactant that destabilizes lipid bilayers of the vesicles and increases deformability of the bilayers [67-68].

Cevc et al. [69] investigated the regio-specificity potential of transfersomes which included different corticosteroids (hydrocortisone, dexamethasone and TA). They demonstrated that transfersomes ameliorate the targetability of all tested corticosteroids into the viable skin. They also suggested that the introduction of transfersomal corticosteroids creates new opportunities for the well controlled topical medication.

In another study performed by Fesq et al. [70], the efficacy of transfersomes was compared with commercially available cream and ointment formulations of TA in humans. According to the results of this study, 10-fold lower dose of TA in transfersome was found bioequivalent to conventional formulations as measured by erythema suppression. Ultrasonic measurements also revealed significantly reduced atrophogenic potential of transfersomes in comparison to commercial formulations.

Ethosome is another novel lipid carrier showing enhanced skin delivery and recently developed by Touitou. The ethosomal system is composed of phospholipid, ethanol and water. The use of high ethanol content was decribed for ethosomes although liposomal formulations containing up to 10% ethanol [71, 72].

Microemulsions are thermodynamically stable, transparent, isotropic, low-viscosity colloidal dispersions consisting of microdomains of oil and/or water stabilized by an interfacial film of alternating surfactant and cosurfactant molecules [73]. Microemulsions are effective formulations for the dermal and transdermal delivery of particularly lipophilic compounds like TC because of their solubilizing properties and also their components may act as penetration enhancers [74, 75].

Wiedersberg et al. [76] studied the dermato-pharmacokinetic properties of betamethasone valerate from two different formulations either in the reference vehicle consisting of medium chain triglycerides or in the microemulsion. The results showed that microemulsion significantly increased the extent of drug delivery into the SC.

In another study, the penetration behaviour of hydrocortisone from the microemulsion system and a commercialy available cream formulation containing the same amount of hydrocortisone (0.5%) was investigated. *Ex vivo* penetration studies on human breast skin were carried out and the drug contents in the different skin layers were measured. With regard to the cream, the results showed that, a higher percentage of hydrocortisone was found in the epidermis and dermis. This result pointed out the skin targeting effect achieved by microemulsion formulation [77, 78].

Formulation type	Pharmaceutical characteristics	Benefits	Disadvantages
Nanoparticles	Solid lipid nanoparticles include solid or the mixture of solid and fluid lipids Polymeric nanoparticles contain non-biodegradable and biodegradable polymers	Enhanced formulation aesthetics, protection of unstable active agents against degredation, targeting of active agents to the skin layers and prolonged active agent release	Mechanism of interaction between nanoparticles - skin structures and in vivo toxicity issues are need to be clarified
Liposomes	Lipid vesicles prepared with phospholipids	Percutaneous absorption enhancing property, slow release and decrease the clearence of drug by minimizing its absorption into the systemic circulation	Stability problems
Niosomes	Non-ionic surfactant vesicules	Alleviate the disadvantages associated with liposomes, such as chemical instability, variable purity of phospholipids and high cost. Controlled and targeted drug delivery to the skin.	Less effective drug delivery in comparison to liposomes
Transfersomes	Consist of phospholipids and an edge activator	Improved therapeutic risk-benefit ratio,due to better targeting and longer drug presence in the skin	-
Ethosomes	Composed of phospholipid, ethanol and water.	Improved dermal/transdermal delivery of lipophilic or hydrophilic molecules	The mechanism of action is not clear

Formulation type	Pharmaceutical characteristics	Benefits	Disadvantages
Microemulsions	Thermodynamically stable, transparent, isotropic, low-viscosity colloidal dispersions consisting of microdomains of oil and/or water stabilized by an interfacial film of alternating surfactant and cosurfactant molecules	Ease of manufacturing and high loading capacity. Effective formulations for the dermal and transdermal delivery of particularly lipophilic compounds.	-
Patches	Drug delivery systems intended for skin application	Provides the administration of effective and known drug amount to the skin and the occlusive effect	Skin irritation
Foams	Incorporate active agents, solvents, co-solvents, surfactants and propellants in a sealed canister under pressure	More convenient topical drug delivery with easy application and spreadability characteristics in comparision to other topical dosage forms	-

Table 4. The summary about innovative TC formulations

Patches are other innovative drug delivery systems intended for skin application in view of achieving local or systemic effect. The patch provides the administration of effective and known drug amount to the skin [79].

The occlusive effect of Actiderm® (hydrocolloid dermatological patch) has been studied on the percutaneous penetration of several drugs including corticosteroids. It was found to be effective in controlling and sustaining the localized delivery of the steroid into the skin and enhancing the healing of dermatological disorders [80, 81].

Ladenheim et al. [82] investigated the effect of occlusion on *in vitro* TA penetration using hydrocolloid containing patches by measuring transepidermal water loss. They found that the diffusion rate of TA was increased 3-4 fold when applied occluded patch in comparison with unoccluded. Same research group was also evaluated the occlusive properties of a range of hydrocolloid patches containing TA on the drug penetration *in vivo* using visual assessment and the graded multiple-measuremet procedure. They concluded that these patch formulations showed great potential for localized prolonged delivery of drugs to the skin, which would be desirable for the topical use of other corticosteroids [83].

More recently, novel foam formulations of TC have been developed and proposed as alternative therapy to conventional formulations. They offer more convenient topical drug delivery with easy application and spreadability characteristics in comparision to other topical dosage forms [84, 85].

A novel foam formulation with enhanced BMV bioavailability has been shown to be superior in efficacy when compared with a lotion in the treatment of disease, without an concomitant increase in toxicity [86]. Another study has been performed comparing the ability of a foam formulation to release the active ingredient (betamethasone benzoate) with ointment, gel, and cream formulations. It was found that the release of betamethasone benzoate from the foam formulation better than the release from the cream [87].

The thermolabile and low-residue foam formulations of corticosteroids (betamethasone valerate and clobetasol propionate) are available in USA market. These foam formulations are associated with better patient compliance and improvements in quality of life [88, 89]. Table 4 summarizes the new drug carrier formulations of TC.

6. Conclusion

Current therapy of dermatological disorders with conventional dosage forms including TC is insufficient due to the low absorption rate and the risk of side effects. Therefore, it is necessary to synthesize the new topical corticosteroid molecules with adequate anti-inflammatory activity and minimal side effects. Fluticasone propionate, mometasone furoate and prednicarbate are very promising molecules showed lower side effects and better tolerability as a member of new generation TC. Also, improved dermal absorption of established TC may be obtained by new designed vehicle system as an alternative to conventional formulation. Recently, lipid and polymeric based carriers such as liposomes, niosomes, transfersomes, ethosomes, microemulsions and nanoparticles have been studied intensively and the potential of these carrier systems have also been described. Another alternative approach for TC treatment is a combined therapy which is more effective than in case of drug alone. The combined use of TC and synthetic vitamin D analogues such as calcipotriol would be promising for the treatment of inflammatory skin diseases. I

In conclusion, due to the difficulty of synthesizing new steroid molecules, developing the novel alternative drug carrier systems which improve the risk-benefit ratio of TC would be more beneficial in topical corticosteroid treatment. Besides, more in vivo study is required to validate the ability of new formulations in enhancing topical delivery of corticosteroids.

Author details

Taner Senyigit and Ozgen Ozer

Ege University, Faculty of Pharmacy, Department of Pharmaceutical Technology, Bornova, Izmir, Turkey

7. References

[1] Wiedersberg S, Leopold CS, Guy RH (2008) Bioavailability and Bioequivalence of Topical Glucocorticoids. Eur. j. pharm. biopharm. 68:453–466.

[2] Brazzini B, Pimpinelli N. (2002) New and Established Topical Corticosteroids in Dermatology. Am. j. clin. dermatol. 3:47-58.

[3] British National Formulary (2004) London: British Medical Association and the Royal Pharmaceutical Society of Great Britain.

[4] Schackert C, Korting HC, Schafer-Korting M (2000) Qualitative and Quantitative Assessment of the Benefit-Risk Ratio of Medium Potency Topical Corticosteroids In Vitro and In Vivo Characterisation of Drugs with an Increased Benefit-Risk Ratio. BioDrugs. 13:267-277.

[5] Fang JY, Fang CL, Sung KC, Chen HY. (1999) Effect of Low Frequency Ultrasound on the In Vitro Percutaneous Absorption of Clobetasol 17-Propionate. Int. j. pharm. 191:33-42.

[6] Banga AK, Bose S, Ghosh TK (1999) Iontophoresis and Electroporation: Comparisons and Contrasts. Int. j. pharm. 179:1-19.

[7] Kaplun-Frischoff Y, Touitou E (1997) Testesterone Skin Permeation Enhancement by Menthol Through Formation of Eutectic with Drug and Interaction with Skin Lipids. J. pharm. sci. 86:1394-1399.

[8] Moster K, Kriwet K, Naik A, Kalia YN, Guy RH (2001) Passive Skin Penetration Enhancement and Its Quantification In Vitro. Eur. j. pharm. biopharm. 52:103-112.

[9] Santos-Maia C, Mehnert W, Schaller M, Korting HC, Gysler A, Haberland A, Schafer-Korting M (2002) Drug Targeting by Solid Lipid Nanoparticles for Dermal Use. J. drug target. 10:489-495.

[10] Schaller M, Preidel H, Januschke E, Korting HC (1999) Light and Electron Microscopic Findings in a Model of Human Cutaneous Candidosis Cased on Reconstructed Human Epidermis Following the Topical Application of Different Econazole Formulations. J. drug target. 6:361-372.

[11] Beumer R, Chen C, Gutzwiller H, Maillan PE, Nowotny M, Schlegel B, Vollhardt J (2008) Topical compositions comprising nanoparticles of an isoflavone. US Patent Application 20080311209.

[12] Dmowski P, Dipiano GT (2008) Topical Administration of Danazol, US Patent Application, 20080153789, (2008).

[13] Walters KA, Roberts MS (2002) The Structure and Function of Skin. In: Walters KA, editor Dermatological and Transdermal Formulations: Drugs and the Pharmaceutical Sciences New York: Marcel Dekker Inc., pp. 1-39.

[14] Menon GK (2002) New Insight into Skin Structure: Stratching the Surface. Adv. drug del. rev. 54:S3-S17.

[15] Elias P (1983) Epidermal Lipids, Barrier Function and Desquamation. J. invest. Dermatol. 80:44-49.

[16] Schoepe S, Schacke H, May E, Asadullah K (2006) Glucocorticoid Therapy-Induced Skin Atrophy. Exp. dermatol. 15:406-420.

[17] Schacke H (2002) Mechanisms Involved in the Side Effects of Glucocorticoids. Pharmacol. ther. 96:23–43.

[18] Adcock IM (2004) Corticosteroids: Limitations and Future Prospects for Treatment of Severe Inflammatory Disease. Drug dev. tech. 1:321-328.

[19] Korting HC, Kerscher MJ, Schafer-Korting M (1992) Topical Glucocorticoids with Improved Benefit/Risk Ratio: Do They Exist? J. am. acad. dermatol. 27:87–92.

[20] P.O. National Psoriasis Foundation, Steroids (1998) www.psoriasis.org.

[21] Buhse L, Kolinski R, Westenberger B (2005) Topical Drug Classification. Int. j. pharm. 295:101-112.

[22] Fang JY, Leu YL, Wang YY, Tsai YH (2002) In Vitro Topical Application and In Vivo Pharmacodynamic Evaluation of Nonivamide Hydrogels Using Wistar Rat as an Animal Model. Eur. j. pharm. sci. 15:417-423.

[23] Singh SK, Naini V. (2007) Dosage Forms: Non-parenterals. In: Swarbrick J. editor. Encyclopedia of Pharmaceutical Technology. New York: Informa Healthcare, pp. 988-1000.

[24] Harding SM, Sohail S, Busse MJ (1985) Percutaneous Absorption of Clobetasol Propionate from Novel Ointment and Cream Formulations. Clin. exp. dermatol. 10:13-21.

[25] Eccleston GM (1997) Functions of Mixed Emulsifiers and Emulsifying Waxes in Dermatological Lotions and Creams. Colloid surface physicochem. eng. aspect. 123-124:169-182.

[26] Sequeira JA, Munayyer FJ, Galeos R (1988) US4775529.

[27] Beaurline JM, Roddy PJ, Tomai MA (1998) WO1998024436.

[28] Patel NA, Patel NJ, Patel RP (2009) Formulation and Evaluation of Curcumin Gel for Topical Application. Pharm. dev. tech. 14:80-89.

[29] Ozer O, Ozcan I, Cetin EO (2006) Evaluation of In Vitro Release and Skin Irritation of Benzoyl Peroxide-Containing Products. J. drug del. sci. tech. 16:449-454.

[30] Hebert A, Cook-Bolden F, Ford R, Gotz V (2008) Early Relief of Atopic Dermatitis Symptoms with a Novel Hydrogel Formulation of Desonide 0.05% in Pediatric Subjects. J. am. acad. dermatol. AB51:614.

[31] Kerney DL, Ford R, Gotz V. (2009) Patient Assessment of Desonide Hydrogel for the Treatment of Mild to Moderate Atopic Dermatitis. J. am. acad. derm. 60:AB69.

[32] Senyigit T, Padula C, Ozer O, Santi P (2009) Different Approaches for Improving Skin Accumulation of Topical Corticosteroids. Int. j. pharm. 380:155-160.

[33] McCadden, ME (2005) US6890544.

[34] Williams AC, Barry BW (2004) Penetration Enhancers. Adv. drug. deliv. rev. 56:603-618.

[35] Thong HY, Zhai H, Maibach HI (2007) Percutaneous Penetration Enhancers: An Overview. Skin pharmacol. physiol. 20:272-282.

[36] Asbill CS, Michniak BB (2000) Percutaneous Penetration Enhancers: Local Versus Transdermal Activity. PSTT 3:36-41.

[37] El-Kattan AF, Asbill CS, Michniak BB (2000) The Effects of Terpene Enhancer Lipophilicity on the Percutaneous Permeation of Hydrocortisone Formulated in HPMC Gel Systems. Int. j. pharm. 198:179-189.

[38] Shim J, Kang HS, Park W, Han S, Kim J, Chang I (2004) Transdermal Delivery of Minoxidil with Block Copolymer Nanoparticles. J. Control. release 97:477–484.

[39] Alvarez-Roman R, Naik A, Kalia YN, Guy RH, Fessi H (2004) Skin Penetration and Distribution of Polymeric Nanoparticles. J. control. release 99:53–62.

[40] Schafer-Korting M, Mehnert W, Korting HC (2007) Lipid Nanoparticles for Improved Topical Application of Drugs for Skin Diseases. Adv. drug deliv. rev. 59:427–443.

[41] Alvarez-Roman R, Naik A, Kalia YN, Guy RH, Fessi H (2004) Enhancement of Topical Delivery from Biodegradable Nanoparticles. Pharm. Res. 21:1818–1825.

[42] Schaller M, Preidel H, Januschke E, Korting HC (1999) Light and Electron Microscopic Findings in a Model of Human Cutaneous Candidosis Based on Reconstructed Human Epidermis Following the Topical Application of Different Econazole Formulations. J. drug target. 6:361–372.

[43] Zhao Y, Brown MB, Jones SA (2010) Pharmaceutical Foams: Are They Answer to the Dilemma of Topical Nanoparticles? Nanomedicine 6:227-236.

[44] Prow TW, Grice JE, Lin LL, Faye R, Butler M, Becker W, Wurm EMT, Yoong C, Robertson TA, Soyer HP, Roberts MS (2011) Nanoparticles and Microparticles for Skin Drug Delivery. Adv. drug deliv. rev. 63:470-491.

[45] Muller RH, Radtke M, Wissing SA (2002) Solid Lipid Nanoparticles (SLN) and Nanostructured Lipid Carriers (NLC) in Cosmetic and Dermatological Preparations. Adv. drug deliv. rev. 54:131-155.

[46] Muller RH, Petersen RD, Hommoss A, Pardeike J (2007) Nanostructured Lipid Carriers in Cosmetic Dermal Products. Adv. drug deliv. rev. 59:522-530.

[47] Maia CS, Mehnert W, Schafer-Korting M (2000) Solid Lipid Nanoparticles as Drug Carriers for Topical Glucocorticoids. Int. j. pharm. 196:165-167.

[48] Schlupp P (2011) Drug Release and Skin Penetration from Solid Lipid Nanoparticles and a Base Cream: a Systematic Approach from a Comparison of Three Glucocorticoids. Skin pharmacol. physiol. 24:199-209.

[49] Zhang J, Smith E (2011) Percutaneous Permeation of Betamethasone 17-Valerate Incorporated in Lipid Nanoparticles. J. pharm. sci. 100:896-903.

[50] Jensen LB, Petersson K, Nielsen HM (2011) In Vitro Penetration Properties of Solid Lipid Nanoparticles in Intact and Barrier-Impaired Skin. Eur. j. pharm. biopharm. :79(1):68-75.

[51] Kalariya M (2005) Clobetasol Propionate Solid Lipid Nanoparticles Cream for Effective Treatment of Eczema: Formulation and Clinical Implications. Indian j. exp. biol. 43:233-240.

[52] de Vringer T (1997) US5667800.

[53] Senyigit T, Sonvico F, Barbieri S, Ozer O, Santi P, Colombo P (2010) Lecithin/Chitosan Nanoparticles of Clobetasol-17-Propionate Capable of Accumulation in Pig Skin. J. control. release 142:368-373.

[54] Schreier H, Bouwstra J (1994) Liposomes and Niosomes as Topical Drug Carriers: Dermal and Transdermal Drug Delivery. J. control. release 30:1-15.

[55] Lopez-Pinto JM, Gonzalez-Rodriguez ML, Rabasco AM (2005) Effect of Cholesterol and Ethanol on Dermal Delivery from DPPC Liposomes. Int. j. pharm. 298:1-12.

[56] Manosroi A, Kongkaneramit L, Manosroi J (2004) Stability and Transdermal Absorption of Topical Amphotericin B Liposome Formulations. Int. j. Pharm. 270:279-286.

[57] Mezei M, Gulasekharam V (1980) Liposomes: A Selective Drug Delivery System for the Topical Route of Administration. Life sci. 26:1473-1477.

[58] Mezei M, Gulasekharam V (1982) Liposomes: A Selective Drug Delivery System for the Topical Route for Administration: Gel Dosage Form. J. pharm. Pharmacol. 34: 473-474.

[59] Lasch J, Wohlrab W (1986) Liposome-Bound Cortisol: A New Approach to Cutaneous Therapy. Biomed. biochim. acta 45:1295-1299.

[60] Wohlrab W, Lasch J (1987) Penetration Kinetics of Liposomal Hydrocortisone in Human Skin. Dermatologica 174: 18-22.

[61] Korting HC, Zienicki H, Schafer-Korting M, Braun-Falco O (1990) Liposome Encapsulation Improves Efficacy of Betamethasone Dipropionate in Atopic Eczema but not in Psoriasis Vulgaris. Eur. j. clin. pharmacol. 39:349-351.

[62] Fresta M, Puglisi G (1997) Corticosteroid Dermal Delivery with Skin-Lipid Liposomes. J. control. release 44:141-151.

[63] Williams AC (2003) Physical and Technological Modulation of Topical and Transdermal Drug Delivery. In: Transdermal and Topical Drug Delivery London: Pharmaceutical Press, pp. 123-167.

[64] Uchegbu IF, Vyas SP (1998) Non-Ionic Surfactant Based Vesicles (Niosomes) in Drug Delivery. Int. j. pharm. 172: 33-70.

[65] Sinico C, Fadda AM (2009) Vesicular Carriers for Dermal Drug Delivery. Expert opin. drug deliv. 6:813-825.

[66] Cevc G, Blume G (1992) Lipid Vesicles Penetrate into Intact Skin Owing to the Transdermal Osmotic Gradients and hydration force. Biochim. biophys. acta 1104:226–232.

[67] Cevc G (1996) Transfersomes, Liposomes and Other Lipid Suspensions on the Skin: Permeation Enhancement, Vesicle Penetration, and Transdermal Drug Delivery. Crit. rev. ther. drug carrier syst. 13(3/4): 257–388.

[68] Cevc G, Blume G, Schatzlein A, Gebauer D, Paul A. (1996) The Skin: A Pathway for Systemic Treatment with Patches and Lipid-based Agent Carriers. Adv. drug deliv. rev. 18(3):349–378.

[69] Cevc G, Blume G, Schatzlein A. (1997) Transfersomes-mediated Transepidermal Delivery Improves the Regio-Specifity and Biological Activity of Corticosteroids In Vivo. J. Control. release 45(3):211-226.

[70] Fesq H, Lehmann J, Kontny A, Erdmann I, Theiling K, Rother M, Ring J, Cevc G, Abeck D. (2003) Improved Risk-benefit Ratio for Topical Triamcinolone Acetonide in Transfersome® in Comparison with Equipotent Cream and Ointment: a Randomized Controlled Trial. British j. dermatol. 149(3):611-619.

[71] Touitou E, Alkabes M, Dayan N. (1997) Ethosomes: Novel Lipid Vesicular System for Enhanced Delivery. Pharm res. S14:305–306.

[72] Touitou E, Dayan N, Bergelson L, Godin B, Eliaz M. (2000) Ethosomes—Novel Vesicular Carriers for Enhanced Delivery: Characterization and Skin Penetration Properties. J. control. release 65(3):403–418.

[73] Date AA, Naik B, Nagarsenker MS. (2006) Novel Drug Delivery Systems: Potential in Improving Topical Delivery of Antiacne Agents. Skin pharmacol. physiol. 19(1):2–16.

[74] Kreilgaard M. (2002) Influence of Microemulsions on Cutaneous Drug Delivery. Adv. drug deliv. rev. 54(S1):77–98.

[75] Santos P, Watkinson AC, Hadgraft J, Lane ME. (2008) Application of Microemulsions in Dermal and Transdermal Drug Delivery. Skin pharmacol. physiol. 21(5):246–259.

[76] Wiedersberg S, Leopold CS, Guy RH. Dermatopharmacokinetics of betamethasone 17-valerate: Influence of formulation viscosity and skin surface cleaning procedure. Eur J Pharm Biopharm 2009; 71(2): 362–366.

[77] Krause SA, Wohlrab WA, Neubert RHH. (1998) Release of Hydrocortisone from a Microemulsion and Penetration into Human Skin. The First european graduate student meeting, Frankfurt, Germany.

[78] Jahn K, Krause A, Martin J, Neubert RHH. (2002) Colloidal Drug Carrier Systems. In: Bronaugh RL, Maibach HI. editors. Topical Absorption of Dermatological Products. New York: Marcel Dekker pp. 483-493.

[79] Padula C, Nicoli S, Santi P. (2009) Innovative formulations for the delivery of levothyroxine to the skin. Int. j. pharm. 372(1/2):12-16.

[80] Queen D, Martin GP, Marriott C, Fairbrother JE. (1988) Assessment of the Potential of a New Hydrocolloid Dermatological Patch (Actiderm) in the Treatment of Steroid Responsive Dermatoses. Int. j. pharm. 44:25-30.

[81] Juhlin L. (1989) Treatment of Psoriasis and Other Dermatoses with a Single Application of a Corticosteroid Left Under a Hydrocolloid Occlusive Dressing for One Week. Acta dermatol. venereol. 69(4):355-357.

[82] Ladenheim D, Martin GP, Marriott C, Holligsbee DA, Brown MB. (1996) An In-vitro Study of the Effect of Hydrocolloid Patch Occlusion on the Penetration of Triamcinolone Acetonide Through Skin In Man. J. pharm. pharmacol. 48(8):806-811.

[83] Martin GP, Ladenheim D, Marriott C, Hollingsbee DA, Brown MB. (2000) The Influence of Hydrocolloid Patch Composition on the Bioavailability of Triamcinolone Acetonide In Humans. Drug dev. ind. pharm. 26(1):35-43.

[84] Purdon CH, Haigh JM, Surber C, Smith EW. (2003) Foam Drug Delivery In Dermatology: Beyond the Scalp. Am. j. drug deliv. 1(1):71-75.

[85] Tamarkin D, Friedman D, Shemer A. (2006) Emollient Foam In Topical Drug Delivery. Expert opin. drug deliv. 3(6):799-807.

[86] Feldman SR, Sangha N, Setaluri V. (2000) Topical Corticosteroids In Foam Vehicle Offers Comparable Coverage Compared with Traditional Vehicles. J. am. acad. dermatol. 42(6):1017-1020.

[87] Woodford R, Barry BW. (1977) Bioavailability and Activity of Topical Corticosteroids from a Novel Drug Delivery System: the Aerosol Quick Break Foam. J. pharm. sci. 66(1):99-103.

[88] Stein L. (2005) Clinical Studies of a New Vehicle Formulation for Topical Corticosteroids in the Treatment of Psoriasis. J. am. acad. dermatol. 53(S1):39-49.

[89] Franz TJ, Parsell DA, Halualani RM, Hannigan JF, Kalbach JP, Harkonen WS. (1999) Betamethasone Valerate Foam 0.12%: A Novel Vehicle with Enhanced Delivery and Efficacy. Int. j. dermatol. 38(8):628–632.

Permissions

The contributors of this book come from diverse backgrounds, making this book a truly international effort. This book will bring forth new frontiers with its revolutionizing research information and detailed analysis of the nascent developments around the world.

We would like to thank Dr. Xiaoxiao Qian, for lending her expertise to make the book truly unique. She has played a crucial role in the development of this book. Without her invaluable contribution this book wouldn't have been possible. She has made vital efforts to compile up to date information on the varied aspects of this subject to make this book a valuable addition to the collection of many professionals and students.

This book was conceptualized with the vision of imparting up-to-date information and advanced data in this field. To ensure the same, a matchless editorial board was set up. Every individual on the board went through rigorous rounds of assessment to prove their worth. After which they invested a large part of their time researching and compiling the most relevant data for our readers. Conferences and sessions were held from time to time between the editorial board and the contributing authors to present the data in the most comprehensible form. The editorial team has worked tirelessly to provide valuable and valid information to help people across the globe.

Every chapter published in this book has been scrutinized by our experts. Their significance has been extensively debated. The topics covered herein carry significant findings which will fuel the growth of the discipline. They may even be implemented as practical applications or may be referred to as a beginning point for another development. Chapters in this book were first published by InTech; hereby published with permission under the Creative Commons Attribution License or equivalent.

The editorial board has been involved in producing this book since its inception. They have spent rigorous hours researching and exploring the diverse topics which have resulted in the successful publishing of this book. They have passed on their knowledge of decades through this book. To expedite this challenging task, the publisher supported the team at every step. A small team of assistant editors was also appointed to further simplify the editing procedure and attain best results for the readers.

Our editorial team has been hand-picked from every corner of the world. Their multi-ethnicity adds dynamic inputs to the discussions which result in innovative outcomes. These outcomes are then further discussed with the researchers and contributors who give their valuable feedback and opinion regarding the same. The feedback is then collaborated with the researches and they are edited in a comprehensive manner to aid the understanding of the subject.

Apart from the editorial board, the designing team has also invested a significant amount of their time in understanding the subject and creating the most relevant covers. They scrutinized every image to scout for the most suitable representation of the subject and create an appropriate cover for the book.

The publishing team has been involved in this book since its early stages. They were actively engaged in every process, be it collecting the data, connecting with the contributors or procuring relevant information. The team has been an ardent support to the editorial, designing and production team. Their endless efforts to recruit the best for this project, has resulted in the accomplishment of this book. They are a veteran in the field of academics and their pool of knowledge is as vast as their experience in printing. Their expertise and guidance has proved useful at every step. Their uncompromising quality standards have made this book an exceptional effort. Their encouragement from time to time has been an inspiration for everyone.

The publisher and the editorial board hope that this book will prove to be a valuable piece of knowledge for researchers, students, practitioners and scholars across the globe.

List of Contributors

Milica Manojlović-Stojanoski, Nataša Nestorović and Verica Milošević
University of Belgrade, Institute for Biological Research "Siniša Stanković", Serbia

Emin Turkay Korgun, Asli Ozmen, Gozde Unek and Inanc Mendilcioglu
Akdeniz University, Medical Faculty, Histology and Embryology Department, Antalya, Turkey

Hayley Dickinson, Bree A. O'Connell and David W. Walker
The Ritchie Centre, Monash Institute of Medical Research, Monash University, Clayton, Australia

Karen M. Moritz
The University of Queensland, School of Biomedical Sciences, St Lucia, Australia

Aml Mohammed Erhuma
School of Biomedical Sciences, Nottingham University, Queen`s Medical Centre, Nottingham, UK

Fortunato Vesce, Emilio Giugliano, Elisa Cagnazzo, Stefania Bignardi, Elena Mossuto, Tarcisio Servello and Roberto Marci
Department of Biomedical Sciences and Advanced Therapy, Section of Obstetrics and Gynecology, University of Ferrara, Italy

Abdullah A. Alangari
Department of Pediatrics, College of Medicine, King Saud University, Saudi Arabia

Hiroshi Hashimoto
Professor Emeritus, Aiwakai Medical Corporation, Bajikouen Clinic, Rheumatology, Tokyo, Japan

Fabiana C.P. Valera, Edwin Tamashiro and Wilma T. Anselmo-Lima
Division of Otorhinolaryngology, Departament of Ophthalmology, Otorhinolaryngology, and Head and Neck Surgery, Faculty of Medicine of Ribeirao Preto-University of São Paulo, Ribeirao Preto-SP, Brazil

Amr Amin
Nuclear Medicine, Cairo University, Egypt

Zeinab Nawito
Rheumatology & Rehabilitation, Cairo University, Egypt

Mohammad Zandi
Department of Oral and Maxillofacial Surgery, Hamedan University of Medical Sciences, Hamedan, Iran
Researcher, Dental Research Center, Hamedan University of medical sciences, Hamedan, Iran

Mahboub Bassam and Vats Mayank
Department of Pulmonology and Allergy & Sleep Medicine, Rashid Hospital, Dubai

Pritish Chowdhury and Juri Moni Borah
Natural Products Chemistry Division CSIR- North East Institute of Science & Technology, Jorhat, India

Taner Senyigit and Ozgen Ozer
Ege University, Faculty of Pharmacy, Department of Pharmaceutical Technology, Bornova, Izmir, Turkey

www.ingramcontent.com/pod-product-compliance
Lightning Source LLC
Chambersburg PA
CBHW070718190326
41458CB00004B/1026